Forces of Change

By the same author

Seeds of Change

Forces of Change

An Unorthodox View of History

Henry Hobhouse

Arcade Publishing · New York
Little, Brown and Company

First U.S. Edition 1990

All maps drawn by Neil Hyslop

Library of Congress Cataloging-in-Publication Data

Hobhouse, Henry.
    Forces of change : an unorthodox history / Henry Hobhouse. — 1st
US ed.
        p.   cm.
    ISBN 1-55970-087-4
    1. History, Modern.   2. Population.   3. Food supply.   4. Diseases
and history.   I. Title.
D210.H66   1989
909.82 — dc20   89-18416
                                                                    CIP

Published in the United States by Arcade Publishing, Inc., New York,
a Little, Brown company

10   9   8   7   6   5   4   3   2   1
MV PA
Printed in the United States of America

To my godsons, Andrew Bergen and Jacob Rees-Mogg. Both have helped with this book

Contents

List of Maps

Introduction

All species try to multiply; it is their primitive yet continuous purpose. Mankind is no exception; indeed, *homo sapiens* has become almost unique in an ability to attempt reproduction at any time, any place, anywhere. This awesome capacity has been canalized by custom and history into either marriage or love or both. The urge should not be underrated or its effects discounted. The sublimation of this unique driving force may well have been responsible for much of mankind's artistic and intellectual achievement. Or so we are told.

The subject of this book is more fundamental, and its theme more brutal. Every writer on population has agreed that all species have the capacity to multiply beyond any available food supply. It is mankind's unique quality to be able to increase the supply of food. It was the first great writer on population, Thomas Malthus's lack of faith in that ability (correct at the time) which led him, and many others, to doubt mankind's demographic future. Most of the history of the past five hundred years would be wholly different if this ability had not been developed. Those people who have this ability have an advantage which remains of vital importance, however sophisticated the world may appear to have become. After population growth, the provision of food is the second great force in human history.

The third great force in human affairs has been disease. But disease is helpless in a desert. Any gardener or farmer knows that disease is a function of high populations. The solitary rose does not incur fungoid troubles as easily as the individual plant, one of many; similarly, a sheep's worst enemy is another sheep; humans only begin to suffer significantly from disease when populations reach a certain density. This is why this book starts about five hundred years ago. At that date in, say, 1492, Europe and Asia had only just recovered from the effects of the plague, known in England as the Black Death. That was the last time that the population of the world declined. From a global total of about 360 million in 1340, loss from the plague was immense, 10–15 per cent of the world population. Recovery in numbers did not take place until the middle of the fifteenth century. By 1492, the human population of the earth was just over 400 million. Today, it is between 5 and 6 billion, or 13–15 times as much. The population of Western Europe is only about six times as much; that is half the increase of the world as a whole. But Western Europe, a mere 2 per cent of the world's land area, has been largely responsible for the increase in the rest of the world. There are three reasons why this should be so.

First, most of the useful edible plants in the world are indigenous to Western Europe: so are the animals. Secondly, while ships, guns and navigational instruments were all available to Chinese or Arab precursors, it was Renaissance Europeans who brought them together and made of the opportunity trade and dominion all over both hemispheres. With their agents, plants, animals and diseases, Western Europeans conquered, first the Americas, then Oceania, then most of Africa, half of Asia. This was unprecedented.

It may be coming to an end, since the ascent of the most 'successful' non-European power, Japan, challenges not only Europe, but also the most successful neo-Europe, the United States of America.

Finally, it is Europe and the neo-Europes which have checked diseases, and then 'cured' some of them. One disease has been 'abolished'. Others, less susceptible to human cleverness, have changed their character. Yet others have recently been transferred from animals, or been generated in some way not wholly understood.

So the first theme of this book is that of the Triangle of Forces. This is formed by population growth, food supply and disease. Excessive population growth used to be automatically answered by food shortage, starvation or famine, until mankind found out how to increase food supply. This option is not open to hunter-gatherers, who have no more opportunity to find abundance than predatory lions who follow game, or curious, ingenious monkeys, who seek fruit and nuts, or stately, gracious whales who have to loiter close to their food, ingesting krill. Modern man grows food, trades and exchanges it for other goods and that makes him unique amongst animals. Together with other differences, human attitudes to food make advanced *homo sapiens* wholly distinct.

However sophisticated and remote from fuel food may have become in the Western world, it still represents far the most important human activity. More time and effort are spent on growing, transporting, distributing, marketing, preparing, cooking, serving and eating food than on any three other human activities put together apart from sleeping.

Sleeping, on the other hand, offers few opportunities for entrepreneurial activity, historical imperatives, or world-shaking trends.

Disease, which is the subject of the first chapter, operated for centuries as an automatic system, controlling populations of every species of plant and animal. Humans were no exception. Disease is a much more merciful control system than famine. Death from most diseases is far kinder than starvation. Disease also has three other characteristics. The first is that disease trims, reduces and selects populations. As a population control disease has been far more significant than warfare, even as recently as World War II. Disease is a means of selection; earlier times were those where all adults had to be survivors, not of modern 'childish' diseases such as measles or chicken-pox, but of pandemic killers. Apart from anything else, this favoured people who preferred to be solitary, rather than gregarious. Other characteristics will occur to the reader.

The second point about disease was that it discouraged urban development. Even the best managed ancient and medieval cities consumed people, a very real percentage of the population every year. Until this century, death rate in some cities would be double that of the surrounding countryside, at minimum. In others, the proportion was five times. Birth rates would also be lower. The effects would be that the city was incapable of survival without continuous demographic reinforcement from the hinterland. Cities of any size were therefore rare. When pandemics appeared, populations declined dramatically. Those who were left behind were the least likely to be able to move: the poor, the old, the halt, and the blind. Plagues therefore acted differentially upon urban populations. The mobile, rich, young, fit and fancy-free escaped by leaving the seat of infection. This pattern existed in Roman times and was repeated as recently as the late nineteenth century in places subject to yellow fever for example, a disease not only of cities, but of human density.

Finally, disease was a magnificent agent of Imperialism. This effect started as soon as Columbus arrived in the Caribbean in 1492, and continued until white man's disease had conquered the earth. Smallpox performed wonders for the *conquistadores*. Malaria invaded and weakened resistance throughout the Americas where smallpox had not subdued the population. Measles, influenza, the enteric disorders weakened native peoples with whom white men came into contact. Some diseases were transported across oceans by mankind, almost all since 1492. Columbus took with him malaria, smallpox and measles and brought back syphilis. The slave trade took yellow fever and *Falciparium* malaria from West Africa to the Americas and then to the rest of the world. Every conceivable white man's disease was taken to Australia, a continent far too empty of humans to support much indigenous disease. Both Australia and the

Amazon Basin, an area only slightly smaller, were thinly populated, yet huge populations were killed by white man's diseases, till the native peoples probably fell to one-fifth of what they had been. This kind of loss, of 80 per cent of a population, had never been experienced as a result of war or famine. It is arguable that, without disease in their armoury, Europeans would never have conquered the world.

As a matter of fact it was Europe and the neo-Europes in the Americas and Africa and Oceania that provided the great increase in population during the period 1776–1890. This was for two reasons. One was trade and dominion which lifted many non-European peoples out of subsistence agriculture. Secondly, Europeans took improved methods of food production all over the world, improving European diets dramatically and the diets of non-Europeans by a significant potential. (Not all non-Europeans took advantage of these opportunities, but they still existed.) Finally, Europeans brought into cultivation huge new areas of the world, sometimes for the exclusive benefit of European crops, but necessarily also for the benefit of the natives.

The nineteenth century is, above all, a hundred years of improved food supply, better technology, improved transport of every kind, the application of intellectual effort to what had been traditional processes. This metamorphosis is often called 'scientific'; but it was frequently the case that Europeans missed the essentials of a successful local practice and had to reinvent a native procedure to make the sowing of maize or the culture of bananas or the preparation of rice or cassava possible in a new situation.

The late nineteenth century, when world population reached 1,600 million, was a time of intellectual optimism, with boundless faith in the beneficient possibilities of science. A hundred years ago, there was no doubt that progress was possible, that intellectual effort was continually making life better; there was no danger foreseen in the growth of population. Malthus, so fashionable in the early years of the century, and proved correct at the time of the Irish famine in 1845, was made foolish by the success, for example, of the Irish in the Americas and in Australia, where they were breeding (and surviving) at double the rate of the highest population increase in Europe. This was not in Ireland, which was unique in the Old World, perhaps, in having a population reduced between 1845 and 1890 by nearly half. Europe as a whole was increasing its population by more than 1 per cent a year, and the neo-Europes by twice or three times that figure. This was partly because there was so much less disease than in the home continent. More importantly, there was ample food, for the first time in history, of a high quality. Because of a manpower shortage in the neo-Europes, people were cherished in a way that made children welcome, nurtured and brought up as the finest physical specimens the world had ever seen. Physical fitness is commonplace today. A hundred years ago, it was a revelation to Europeans how much fitter the neo-Europeans were than kin left at home. Neo-Europeans were not only fitter and lived longer, and reared more children, but they also provided Europe with an increasing proportion of its food.

The restraints of disease and starvation have been largely eliminated; conventional warfare is a much overrated means of population control. World Wars I and II were mere blips on the demographer's charts; in both, disease and malnutrition were more significant causes of death than enemy action; in the conventional war between Iraq and Iran in 1980–8, 1 million were killed, but the 2 countries together in the same period have enjoyed a population increase of not less than 5 million, net of war.

Nuclear, chemical and biological warfare is a different matter. In these cases, non-combatant death rates could make serious inroads into populations. But the consequences are so fearful that great powers shy away from using these weapons, and it has been the virtue of the existence of nuclear weapons since 1945 that has prevented great power conflicts of a violent nature. Great powers have nevertheless not often united to prevent lesser powers fighting; indeed, many small wars are between great power proxies.

Great powers have, by definition, retained the initiative as far as weapon technology is concerned, so that the nastier means of killing remain in few hands. There is one present exception to this rule. An estimated 20–30 sovereign nations outside Europe and the neo-Europes are capable of making chemical weapons of a very unpleasant nature. With a world-wide increase in biological engineering, the same sort of dispersal will exist in biological weapons by, say, 2000 or 2010. By that time, a very serious non-nuclear war could be possible, killing huge numbers of people, by genetic means. It will also be possible to engage in what has loosely (and wrongly) been called 'genocide' in the past.

'Genocide' has usually been practised only unconsciously: the guilty parties have not only been political but also disease, starvation, changes in environment. There have been significant losses. Three-quarters of the Amazon tribes have probably been eliminated. So have perhaps half the Aborigine groups in Australia, many discrete tribal peoples in West Africa. Primitive peoples who carved out a survival-niche for themselves as hunter-gatherers or Stone Age survivors, or Iron Age farmers were not capable of resisting whites. But hundreds of individual species of plants and animals have also disappeared. This is an inevitable accompaniment of change; it may be a mistake to blame Europeans wholly for these losses. Perhaps they would have happened in any case, without record, in the absence of human presence.

The third strand in this book, after the Triangle of Forces and the notable success of Western European diseases, plants, animals and men, is the question of challenge and response. Certain peoples have been significantly more successful than others in overcoming disease and the problem of food supplies. Land use has dictated the very nature of nations far more than any other factor. Three specific examples are treated at some length: the United States, Russia and Japan. The argument must be allowed to speak for itself, but without straining the logic, it is clear that the forces of population growth, food supply and disease have operated in quite a different fashion in each country, to produce three very specific cultures.

All through this book, it is assumed that good food produces a long-term advantage for those people who have enjoyed a better diet than others. Primitive men settled often, for other reasons, on the seashore, and on river banks. Unconsciously they found chemicals necessary for the development of the brain, together with high quality proteins and poly-unsaturated fat. Successful peoples have had significantly better diets than unsuccessful peoples ever since. There is a rather strong modern correlation between protein quality – often fish – and group progress, whether expressed in terms of economic growth, science, technology, management skills or whatever.

This point has not been heavily stressed throughout this book, but is assumed; several kind people who have read the draft have suggested that more should be made of this argument. Unfortunately, as with the inefficiencies of food supply in feudal village communities, or the improvement in protein quality in Renaissance Europe, or the serious long-term chronic shortages of food in France of the *ancien régime*, there are no quantities to make the contention numerate. A dozen graduate researchers, working a lifetime each, could not help. People did not, in most of history, record what weight of what edible they ate. Ingestion statistics have only been available in most countries very recently. Even then, no one ever knows what was wasted in cooking, left on the plate, given to pets, or thrown out as swill or rubbish. It is generally true that many other people could survive, if necessary, on what the modern rich throw away; the better the cuisine, the greater the waste; the poorer the society, the lower quality the detritus and (usually) the thinner the rats.

It is the pollution of the modern world which will produce an alternative control to diseases which have been 'cured', and to hunger, starvation, and famines which have been defeated. There are three important problems already threatening mankind, but which have only become obvious in the past decade. They are the greenhouse effect, the destruction of the ozone layer, and acid rain. It is possible that mankind will drown in his own ordure; this will be true if the causes of pollution are not arrested and reversed rather rapidly. There are not only too many people in many parts of the world, but they are consuming too much; less than 20 per cent of the world's population probably live in a way which could be called truly sustainable. Such lives would be regarded by most 'advanced' people as mind-bendingly boring, unacceptable. On the other hand, increases in consumption at the rate of the last hundred years is wholly impossible to imagine for the next twenty years, let alone the next hundred. A century ago, there were just over one-quarter as many people alive as today. Each person in the then world only used one-tenth, on average, of the fuel we use today. So the same earth has to consume and recycle waste products forty times the tonnage of a hundred years ago. There is no chance that eco-systems can deal with the present problems in some parts of the world. It is inconceivable that there should be increases in consumption comparable to the last hundred years; these increases lead directly to pollution in what is perhaps an irreversible way.

This book, like my first book, *Seeds of Change*, is not written to persuade; it is not intended to be didactic; readers are invited to make up their own minds. The evidence is presented, and it would be foolish to ask people to agree with a thesis which would have to be serpentine to cover every aspect of history since 1492. For that reason, each chapter is free-standing, written to be an open window on its time. People can look through the window and appreciate the view – they are not expected to share the perspective.

CHAPTER ONE

Ill Winds
across the Land and Sea

Disease has only been a recognized historical factor in recent years. Links between disease, population growth and food supply have never been made plain: it is the purpose of this book so to do.

This chapter starts with the Black Death, which is considered to be the most important single event between the fall of Rome and the Renaissance. It was not, of course, 'a single event' like a great battle, but both cause and effect rumbled on for a century, having very wide implications for the whole of Western Europe, in particular. The disease was like a pebble, thrown into a pond, the circles of ripples becoming larger and larger before their force faded.

Disease is far more lethal than warfare. For example, if the Spaniards alone had solved the hygiene problem at sea, the outcome of the Armada would have been reversed. Disease has killed many more people, even if only measured during wars, than all the actions of mankind put together.

Disease was the means by which the Europeans conquered the New World. This began with Columbus's arrival in the Caribbean in 1492, and the process continues whenever whites meet a virgin tribe, in the rain forest of the Amazon, or some other 'undiscovered' place today.

Disease 'cured' has upset not only an automatic system which trimmed and selected populations, but also kept in some kind of balance food supply and population growth. Disease cured has thrown great strains upon Third World food supplies.

Finally, there is the remarkable case of the incurable virus, which changes its very character. The common cold and influenza defeat the doctors. A more serious problem is HIV, which gives rise to AIDS. There is a hint of a suggestion that 'new' diseases might take the form of attacking the immune system itself, not the antibodies produced by the immune system. This would be a chilling reminder of the potential impotence of arrogant mankind on an overcrowded earth.

Two men have influenced the thinking about population growth and natural selection, but not disease, for a hundred years or more. Since they will be mentioned throughout this book, it is appropriate to add a note about them here.

Thomas Robert Malthus *was born in Surrey, in 1766. His father was a country gentleman, a 'progressive' of the day, friend (and executor) of Rousseau. Malthus the younger became a Ninth Wrangler at Cambridge, and was elected Fellow of Jesus College in 1793; in 1797, he became curate of Albury, Surrey. The first edition of his* Essay on the Principle of Population *was published in 1798. There were six further editions during his lifetime, each being more restrained than the last. The impulse for the work was his father's absurd optimism about prospects for the human race. Roughly, father Malthus, like many liberals since, believed that human beings could be made happy, useful, and productive by legislation. Malthus presented for the first time the perception that 'progress' was unlikely, because of the inherent limitations of the food supply. The tendency of mankind's progenitive capacity to outrun food supply was the basis of his argument. A kind, rather jolly man, happily married, Malthus would have been horrified if he could have known of the use made of his name in the word 'Malthusian'. But his book on population triggered off the essential clue in Darwin's mind (see below). Malthus, a benevolent and amiable man survived until 1834, as a 'Professor of Political Economy' at Haileybury College, which prepared young men for the service of the East India Company. As far as is known, he never met Darwin.*

Charles Robert Darwin *lived from 1809 to 1882. Both the Darwins, and his mother's family, the Wedgwoods, were intellectuals of power. He read medicine at Edinburgh, then Natural History at Cambridge. On graduation he was appointed naturalist on HMS* Beagle. *The trip took nearly three years, 1831–4, and included Tenerife, Cape Verde, Brazil, Buenos Aires, Monte Video, Tierra del Fuego, Valparaíso, the Galapagos, Tahiti, New Zealand, and Tasmania. In the Keeling Islands, on the way home, Darwin enunciated his famous theory about coral, which contains the germ of natural selection. Married to his cousin, Emma Wedgwood, country gentleman, FRS, practical animal breeder, Darwin did not rush into print. The embryo was formed in 1835–8; the first notes made in 1842–4; the first paper read before the Linnean Society in 1853. The great book* On the Origin of Species by means of Natural Selection *was published in November 1859. Malthus's theory of population led Darwin to believe that 'Natural selection was the inevitable result of the rapid increase of all organic beings.' Thus Malthus inspired Darwin, and they march together through this book.*

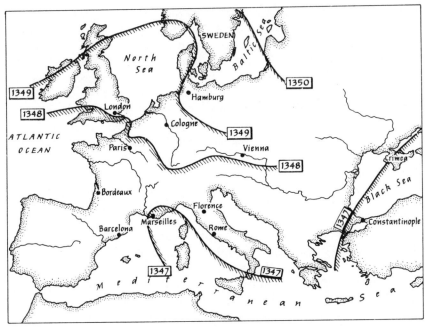

The Black Death: The First European Experience

In about 1300 the population of Western Europe was beginning to reach saturation point. There were local famines in most years between 1290 and 1350. Most of Europe was affected in the years 1314–17. Perhaps the whole of Western Europe was as badly off between 1300–50 as Ireland was between 1800–50. Eastern Europe was less affected, less densely occupied. The limits of technology and husbandry had been reached in the West. There was little hope for the population except for cycles of famine, death, population growth, famine, death and so forth. It was the classic Malthusian situation.

Into this time of great misery came the Black Death, arriving in Kaffa in the Crimea in 1346, and reaching France, Italy, Spain and the rest of the Mediterranean coastline during 1348. Atlantic countries were hit the following year. Finally, the plague reached the north-eastern North Sea and the Baltic in 1349–50. In each country, the plague fanned inward from the ports. It took many months to reach the Volga-Don trade route in Russia. Some parts of Eastern Europe, modern Ukraine for example, escaped the worst effects. In most of Western Europe, the death-rate was of the order of 40 per cent; the more densely populated places suffered the greatest loss. The carrier of the 1346 outbreak was the black rat, *Rattus rattus*. The black rat is not alone in being a plague carrier; there are other potential hosts. In Asia, there are tarbagons, marmots and susliks; in Africa, gerbils and mice; in North America, prairie dogs and ground squirrels. In the early fourteenth century, the reservoir of infection was in the Yunnan area of China; the plague was disturbed and distributed by the Mongols. The Mongols, in turn, found that the host became the black rat, an animal which always lives close to mankind, in the saddle-bags of mounted nomads; in the ships of merchants and warlike sailors; in the cottagers' thatched roof, in bales of merchandise, in ricks of grain.

Pasteurella pestis, the Black Death, bubonic plague, is still with us. It is endemic in certain rodents, harmless to them, like a childhood disease. For mankind, it is a killer. It kills today, as it did in 1346, when it first arrived in Europe. In the most recent outbreaks, in 1947 just before antibiotics, more died, as a percentage of the sick, than did in the original outbreaks in 1346–51.[1]

The Black Death was caused by what would, in about 1900, be recognized as a complicated cycle. The disease does not depend upon the human as part of the cycle. It does depend upon certain sorts of rodent and certain sorts of flea. From the point of view of the disease, the black rat (*Rattus rattus*) and the rat flea (*Xenopsylla cheopsis*) are the ideal methods of propagation. What happens was only really discovered accurately in the period 1900–20.

The preferred flea lives on warm-blooded animals. It is small (about 3 mm long), wingless, can cling on to all types of surface because of hooks on its six limbs, and it feeds only upon its preferred host. Hence, the rat flea prefers rats, the cat flea cats, the dog flea dogs, and in only the most exceptional circumstances is it likely that a particular flea will abandon its host. Fleas, like aphids, are particular parasites. Is it ignorant hysteria for a modern mother to become upset about fleas on the family pet? Or is it some deep-seated tribal feeling about the Black Death?

There have been more than twenty generations since the Black Death. Before the middle of the fourteenth century, there was no flea-borne disease to compare in horror with *Pasteurella pestis*, yet probably 90 per cent of the population carried fleas and other parasites, such as lice. The rat flea, and its habits, would probably change human toleration towards the lice, fleas and nits which humans have carried since time immemorial.

When a plague-infected rat or other rodent dies, the fleas leave the corpse as the body temperature falls. If temperature and humidity are suitable, fleas may remain without a host for at least fifteen days. During that time, they become hungrier and hungrier, and, if they are heavily infected, ravenous.

The peculiar effect on the infected mammal of harbouring the bacillus is to create massive, fulminating, overwhelming septicemia. This is true of an infected human or an infected rat, both of which often die. But the septicemia in the flea does not foreshorten the insect's life. The bacilli multiply in the stomach of the flea, and the stomach gradually becomes blocked. Because the stomach is blocked, it does not nourish the flea. So the insect becomes not only stuffed with a solid mass of bacteria, but also very hungry because it is deriving no nourishment from the blood it is sucking. Ravenous, because the stomach is blocked by the mass of multiplying germs, fleas will jump off the dying host, the rat, on to any convenient warm-blooded animal which happens to be about. Horses, cows, camels, donkeys, dogs, will all attract fleas in this 'blocked' condition. The plague bacillus does no harm to these animals. When the flea chooses a human as an alternative host, matters are very different.

Because the digestive system of the flea is 'blocked' the flea is, as has been explained, very hungry. This makes it an active bloodsucker, taking up to ten times as much blood per day as is normal. None of the blood reaches the flea's stomach, or nourishes it in any way. The sucking of the blood continues until the gullet of the flea is distended and full. Then the flea disgorges the blood back into the wound. This blood is now infected with the bacillus which is blocking the stomach of the flea. Finally, the flea also automatically defecates as it eats the blood; some of the detritus is deposited on the punctured skin of the mammal whose blood is being sucked. There cannot be a more elegant way of spreading a disease. If the bacillus, *Yersinia pestis*, were capable of designing a method of self-propagation, the habits of the flea would come high on the list of available means. Any designer-bacillus would probably decide that no further work could improve on what was already available.

As has been noted, the flea feeding on other mammals apart from man may or may not transmit the bacillus, but the bacillus does little harm to any other animals. It does not even kill as many rodents as it does humans.[2] The bacillus does not seem to benefit from life on all kinds of rodents: rabbits, hares, grey squirrels are not useful hosts.

When a human is infected with plague, the incubation period is from two to eight days. The numbers of the bacilli are initially small, attracted to the lymph glands. The lymph glands are concentrated in the armpit, neck and groin. 'Bubo' is Greek for groin, 'bubonic' meaning 'of the groin'. A groin swelling was commonest in the Middle Ages, perhaps because fleabites were more likely to be on the legs.

The swellings become very large and very painful. If the patient survives, the swellings may discharge like boils, and if the patient survives as long as fourteen days, they may burst. The patient may, of course, suffer from a more rapid build-up of the bacilli. In such cases, massive septicemia sets in, as in the rat, and cases were known of fit men retiring at night and being dead in the morning.

Such a systemic attack by the organism is not unknown in other diseases, but it was the dramatic deaths of so many apparently healthy people which so impressed survivors of the Black Death and all the subsequent attacks of the plague. There is one other curiosity. The flea can take in large numbers of bacilli and transmit the bacteria from man to man. This hardly ever happens. The rat, and specifically the black rat, is an almost essential vector, except when the bubonic plague takes the form of a kind of pneumonia. In such cases, coughs and sneezes spread diseases, notably this one.[3] Ultimately, it was established that the plague takes four forms, all from the same original bacillus.

The first is the establishment of the infestation in the groin and other areas where lymphatic glands are important, round the neck and in the armpits. This manifestation is what gave the Black Death its name: 'bubonic plague'.

Exactly the same bacteria produced a more rapid result and more rapid success (for the disease). This second form took the course of a violent septicemia, which could kill some sufferers in a few hours at worst, and within a few days at best. In this form, the lymphatic glands were overwhelmed without effectively resisting the onset of the infection. Lymph glands characteristically swell when they are in action against some invading organisms, in the same way that the whole body suffers from a rise in temperature when the body is fighting infection. So a disease which overwhelms a patient may do so without any notable swelling of the lymph glands.

The third form takes the course of a violent lung infection. This form, the pneumonic, had symptoms similar to other forms of infection of the lungs. Unlike ordinary pneumonia, pneumonic plague had an expectation of death of 100 per cent, and that within two days. The grim difference between bubonic plague and so-called pneumonic plague is that the disease in the lung produced a far higher death-rate, and the pneumonic form did not require the intervention of fleas or rats. While 10–20 per cent might survive the bubonic form, and the dying would have a period of ten to fourteen days to face the future, they were also not at all infectious during the crisis. Anyone could nurse bubonic plague: it was neither infectious nor contagious.

Pneumonic plague was a death sentence to anyone within range of the patient's coughing or breathing or spitting. No one, originally, knew that the three forms described here were the three manifestations of the same organism at work. There was a fourth form, also thought to be a different disease.

The so-called 'pestis minor' was in fact a simpler matter. This 'disease' occurred when the resistance of the body to the bubonic infection success-fully defeated the bacillus. This happened in a minority of cases, and the proportion did not appear to change much in the six hundred years during which the plague was observed. The Black Death, unlike measles or smallpox, did not become milder during the time it was observed by increasingly skilled and better-equipped doctors, health workers and pathologists. In technical language, the disease did not attenuate.

Between 1347 and the first use of antibiotics against the plague in 1947, there were over one hundred recorded outbreaks known to European history. There may have been several hundred others.

Deaths in the first wave before 1360 varied widely, but if modern experience[4] is anything to go by then the death-rate would not have been less than 30–40 per cent over the whole continent of Europe. This average includes those areas which the plague did not touch.

Massive work on the subject of births and deaths at the time have been done, but most of it has been in England, with a few scholars working in Northern France. In the Mediterranean countries, death-rates could have been much higher than in England, where they were about 35 per cent. In much of Europe east of the Rhine and north of the Alps, no kind of parish records have survived in many areas, and no convincing estimates have been made of either birth- or death-rates. There were recurrences of the plague in every European country. There were everywhere at least four more waves of infection in the century following the first wave of 1346–50.

The Black Death is important for a number of reasons. It is the first plague of which subsequent centuries have any clear idea of cause, effect, and numbers affected. It radically altered the nature of life for the survivors. The creation of a shortage of workers, particularly skilled urban workers, changed the relationship of people to money, gold or land or any other store of value. (The same sort of process had occurred in the third century AD in the Roman Empire, and with much the same effect. We have no data on the cause.)

Before the plague of 1346, the fashionable Christian religion was much in tune with the teachings of St Thomas Aquinas. An easy man to love, Aquinas formed a synthesis of the principle of truth. He held that authority was revealed by the human senses and by experiment, and by experience as well as faith. He died in 1274, and was canonized a few years before the Black Death. How could the optimistic, rational system of Aquinas stand up to the huge death-rate caused by an inexplicable organism which no one could see, or attach in any way to fleas, rats or ships? Fatalism, superstition, fear replaced faith and reason, and the incipient Renaissance was delayed at least a hundred years.

In the absence of any rational explanation for the plague, and the horror of the inexplicable, reason itself went out of fashion. It was not a question of a 'sleep of reason', but of a much more serious flight from the intellect. The inexplicable could only be made acceptable by means of fatalism, the will of God, millennialism, which is that the world is about to end and that the Kingdom of Heaven is at hand.[5]

There was a considerable difference in the death-rate of various classes. The Second Plague of 1362, and the Third Plague of 1369–70 killed more children, more priests, more landed gentry than the First, which was noted for its effect upon the aristocracy. There were, of course, many more outbreaks of the plague. In England, where there is the best opportunity to check the records, there were outbreaks in 1375, 1379, 1381–2, 1383, 1387, 1390 and 1399–1400. In the fifteenth century, there were nearly as many local or regional epidemics. There were nineteen, including the outbreak of 1470–1, which rivalled the second and third plagues. In the south-east, mortality reached 20 per cent.[6]

Superficially, life went on. The Hundred Years War with France (1337–1453) was not significantly interrupted. The Wars of the Roses in England (1455–85) was fought against the plague background. In the Mediterranean, the rivalries between Italian cities, between Latin and Greek, Guelph and Ghibbeline, Muslim and Christian continued. The long-term change was under the surface.

Response to labour shortage was vital. In the West, depopulation of rural areas also depopulated the cities, since it had to be the rural areas which made good the non-plague losses of the cities. Marginal grain areas ceased to be arable, and were often converted to timber, vines and permanent pasture. In England, the area devoted to sheep probably multiplied by three, thus dealing with the shortage of labour as well as the unprofitability of grain-growing on unsuitable land; in sandy Norfolk, new grassland produced a proverb, 'Sheeps' hooves turn sand to gold.'

In Western Europe, the more servile aspects of serfdom came to an end, and the manorial system, already sick, went into a terminal economic decline; rents, taxes and wages all became more important than service to the feudal lord. The modern economic system, based on cash, began to be important in the Western rural economy. Wool provided work which became the northern equivalent to wine as a sophisticated trade.

In the East, the response to labour shortage, the depopulation of rural areas, the 'disenchantment' of German scholars, was quite different. Poland, Prussia, and Hungary became great grain-growing areas, exporting grain to the West via the river systems of the Oder, Vistula and Danube. Serfdom was actually only instituted in parts of Eastern Europe after the Black Death. In some parts of the West, a hundred years of plague led to an increasingly free peasantry, Shakespeare's yeoman of England, for example. In the East, there were places where free peasants became tied to the soil, serfs until the French Revolution and after.[7]

In the South, in the Mediterranean, depopulation was in many ways a beneficial agent of change. Timber recovered, as pressure on marginal land ceased. Specialized, profitable crops developed, yielding a higher return per worker: silk worms, in mulberry trees; stone-fruit trees and olives permitted underplanting of vegetables for adjacent town markets; the area of sugar cane increased in the south of Italy and Spain. Wine improved in quality: trade in food and drink became more important.

Agricultural emphasis for the first time for centuries was upon the output per man rather than output per acre, and this induced an increase in the size of individual holdings. Returns as a multiple of what was sown also increased, as unsuitable land was no longer cultivated for grain. Yields per acre therefore rose for reasons unconnected with the husbandry of the good land: rather the abandonment of the poorer fields.

Technology became important as the means to multiply the effective labour of a smaller population: the capital value of mills, both water and wind-driven, nearly doubled in England in the half-century after 1347. There was a net loss of thousands of skilled masons, a trade requiring a very long apprenticeship, and a conspicuous rise in wages, and a net gain of labour-saving devices: animal-driven devices to multiply the power of diminishing mankind.

There is a point made by William McNeill, in his important book *Plagues and Peoples*.[8] The steppes of the Eurasian landmass became a great reservoir of plague, with the various rodents of the plains as foci of infection. China lost nearly half her population during the fourteenth century. But the plague also disconnected China from the West, by destroying the old Silk Route. The caravan-travellers no longer found it safe to cross the grasslands, since whenever they stopped, they would pick up the bacillus. The steppes themselves became denuded of nomads. The settlers at the edges would, if they survived, become comparatively much stronger. There being no population pressure on the nomads, the invasions from Central Asia came to an end. Whether or not the Black Death was the cause, the Mongols were the last invaders of Europe from the steppes.[9]

Flight from the Intellect after the Black Death was not only due to an excess of death amongst the higher clergy.[10] In 1349, Europe had thirty universities. By 1400, twenty of them had closed. The pursuit of profit in this underpopulated continent became more popular than the pursuit of knowledge; there was a shortage of undergraduates as well as candidates for Holy Orders.

There were other, equally serious, shortages. To keep the universities going, teachers were recruited from primary and secondary schools. So the general level of literacy fell. This had two effects. One was the obvious disconnection between ordinary people and the universities which became an important characteristic after the Renaissance. The other was more intriguing. People started to speak, write and use the vernacular in preference to Latin. English became the official language of all lawcourts in 1363. In the same year, the 'Speech from the Throne' in parliament was given in English, not Latin. Norman French, like Latin, fell into disuse in England. French native languages superseded Latin in France, Teutonic tongues in Germany, Holland, Scandinavia. Nationalism inevitably followed language. Jews were impartially persecuted.

It was not only language that was liable to change. Hanseatic towns lost their supremacy to the Dutch and English. Bruges gave way to Antwerp. Transalpine trade became a preserve of Southern German towns like Augsburg, which developed as a great entrepôt. Only Venice, the richest city in the West, remained at the top, distancing herself in wisdom, wealth and glory from her rivals.

All over Europe the tax base in this new age of money was wholly altered by the Black Death. Land was no longer an absolute source of wealth. In the absence of manpower, land became relatively worthless. More than 10,000 villages disappeared in Western Europe. Some towns had lost half their people, and more than half the houses were unoccupied. New taxes, like the English Poll Tax, in 1381, produced violent, negative reactions. And not only in England, but also in France, Germany and in many Italian cities. The new values placed upon the worth of the individual were to point the way to some sort of consultative, if not representative, government. This was certainly true of taxation in more than one country, and it was because of the substitution of money taxes for feudal dues that this became a truth.

No society accepts readily a change in tax base.[11] The largest change in Western civilization was the substitution of money taxes for feudal service. In achieving this change, rulers of every Western country had to negotiate many kinds of accommodations with their peoples. The horse would have to be consulted by the rider. This anteceded, by several centuries, the idea that the horse should elect the rider. In fact, of course, horses have, throughout history, known which riders were best for them. In time, peoples of almost every Western country would achieve the same result, by a variety of means. It was the Black Death which either accelerated the process, initiated it, or planted the seeds of change amongst both rulers and people.

It would be wrong to think of the Black Death as a discrete event occurring in 1346–50. The plague continued, on and off, for three hundred years and more in Europe. The effects of the Black Death, and its immediate epidemic rather than pandemic successors, in many ways reinforced what was happening in any case: the emergence of the middle class; the end of serfdom in its more rigorous form; the laicization of society; adoption of new methods of raising taxes which were more susceptible to the taxpayer's displeasure.

There were other effects which were unique to depopulation: the survivors less hungry; the search for 'labour-saving' devices; the silting up of rivers; the abandonment of marginal grain-growing land; there was an ecological reversal, the return of wild animals nearer to centres of population, because of diminished densities of people.[12]

The Black Death and its immediate successors were the most important causal agents in European history between the fall of Rome and the discovery of America. But however much influence ascribed to the huge death-toll and its consequence, the alternative must always be considered. And that was famine. The famine necessary to reduce the population to below its Malthusian ceiling of the early fourteenth century was a horror much worse than any disease. Against such a famine, the plague was positively merciful.

After the plague had done its work, population densities were much lower. In terms of then population, Italy was still the most crowded, at only 2.75 hectares (7 acres) per head. France, Germany and the Low Countries were all placed between 5 and 5.5 hectares (12 and 13.5 acres) per head. Iberia, England, Austria and Switzerland were less crowded, at about 6–7 hectares (15 and 17 acres) per head. Southern Scandinavia was emptier still, at about 20 hectares (50 acres) per head.

These densities were much lower than today but they restored populations to a sustainable degree of sustenance, at the kind of output available from feudal husbandry. Grain yields returned to the levels obtaining two hundred years before. The discomfort of excessive density was removed from huge areas. Famine no longer stalked the land one year in three. Hunger was no longer a familiar event every spring. Lent need no longer mean literally a very long fast. The clock, however, was not put back. Post-plague people were entirely different.

One change was in the distribution of the population.[13] The reasons for this were threefold. First, depopulation affected rural areas more drastically than it did the towns. Though the urban death-rate was probably higher than in rural areas, there was always a post-plague surplus of rural adventurers ready to fill the vacancies in town. There was a continual migration into towns; thus fewer post-plague people were involved in living in the country and living directly off the land. Meanwhile, a rising urban standard of life, not necessarily connected with lower populations, led to the demand for more specialized and attractive cash crops – commodities rather than plain bellyfill. There was a move away from subsistence agriculture and a conscious effort to meet the needs of the market, real or imagined. Wine, wool, flax, silk, hemp, sugar, fruit and the vegetable dyes became important objects of trade. In the north, hops and the newer sorts of barley made for the substitution of beer for ale; beer is longer-lived, a better traveller since hops act as a preservative.

Rural depopulation affected both man and the land. The serfs were no longer tied to the land in the way that dense populations had forced upon both people and lords in pre-plague days. A man could command a money wage, and a lord could not hold a man without meeting those wages, whatever the law might say. The medieval laws which sought to tie Western European men to the land were no more successful in the fourteenth and fifteenth centuries than the laws which Diocletian had sought to enforce in the third century, AD.

Large landowners became rentiers, their rents expressed in money terms; thus they left subsistence and feudal dues far behind and counted their wealth in the same coin as the richer merchants. Despite nostalgic efforts to re-establish a bygone age in an excessive display of chivalry, tournaments and the like, aristocrats and gentry adapted quickly to the new conditions; they had to, or they sank, hardly nodding to the yeomen and merchants, who were on their way up. Social conditions amongst the landed classes in post-plague Europe were a great deal more mobile than in pre-plague times, when land, serfs and produce were commoner indicators of wealth than gold or coin. The greatest change in this area was perhaps the most long-term and the least noticed at the time. In 1340, only the privileged eldest sons of the landed class obtained any part of the real property left by a deceased father; by 1500, most sons, and some daughters, would be left a piece of land by inheritance. Thus did the plague work its long-term effects upon land tenure and the landed classes.

Pressure on the land itself had fallen dramatically since the pre-plague population crisis. Marginal areas fell out of cultivation. Mediterranean lands and the Central European Plain had been deforested before 1340, in order to grow subsistence crops. Huge tracts were allowed to fall back into scrub, then forest.[14] Surplus peasants from West Germany and the Netherlands were free to emigrate to Prussia, Poland, and the Baltic provinces. What had been thinly occupied by Teutonic knights warring against

Slav chivalry became prosperous, a productive part of the European trading community. Western Europe was thinned out so much that wolves, which had been driven by heavy rural population density to the northern limits, returned to most of Germany, France and Italy. They were reported in the suburbs of large towns like Paris, equivalent to the modern urban fox who rummages amongst garbage dumps.[15]

The Black Death reversed the kind of population/density/excessive arable syndrome which impoverishes Africa today and used to beggar India before modern methods were adopted in the 1960s.[16] It is the paradoxical effect of a rise in real wages (making for a concentration on output per man) which produces a rise in output per acre. This is because poor land, requiring a disproportionate input of expensive manpower, is abandoned. This raises the yield per acre on what remains, or fresh new land is brought into cultivation.[17]

Above all, the survivors of six generations of plague, taking into account the effect of the selection process of the disease itself, produced in 1500 Europeans who were recognizably very different from those of pre-plague 1340. Novel devices began to be employed to save labour. This means that technology had to make good the losses produced by depopulation. It was largely technology which made people richer, not only the fact that depopulation meant the abandonment of the less profitable processes and means of production. Grinding mills of all kinds became much more valuable. Fish salted at sea by the Dutch after the plague, made for cheaper, better fish, and richer Dutchmen.[18] Increased demand for noble metals and precious gems at a time of declining manpower made technologically assisted mining essential. Pumps, gunpowder and shaft-driving methods were all adopted, often just in time to transfer the techniques to the New World.

Literacy and numeracy became as essential in the business world of Europe in 1500 as is computer use today. The art of printing came in from China; eyeglasses were developed to help the weak of sight to read; arithmetic became a general discipline amongst merchants; the abacus was revived, from its Graeco–Roman, Arabic or Chinese model, and was in general use in counting houses.[19] Paper halved in true cost between 1340 and 1500, and by the latter date had superseded vellum made from calf-bellies, except for the most extravagant use.[20] Printing, paper, eyeglasses, the abacus, numeracy and literacy were all necessary for the modern world. A sense of time became vital. The compass and the compass-rose, the astrolabe were essential; and clocks were still huge.[21]

The Black Death was as important in its effects on the intellect as in the material development of Western European mankind, or in the side-effects in the physical environment, particularly in the Atlantic countries.

First of all, faced with catastrophe, humans reacted in at least two different ways. One was to be stoical, resigned or fatalistic. The other was to take precautions to avoid the worst effects of the plague. Inevitably, these were selfish; the development of a *sauve qui peut* mentality amongst all classes inevitably meant a parallel breakdown of the corporate, co-operative, community feeling of the early Middle Ages. Yet individualism, not always selfish or hedonistic, may also, at its finest, be wholly creative.

In Italy, post-plague individualism became humanism of a very high order, and wholly necessary for the Renaissance. In the Netherlands, Flanders and the Rhineland, personal mysticism and individual piety developed long before the Reformation, and it is arguable that they were necessary for Luther's work to be done. Above all, perhaps, the decay of the old bonds, the weakening of the sense of collective responsibility, the post-plague unreality of Church, State, Lord and People, prepared the medieval world for the modern age. In one sense, successful post-plague Europeans were selfish, pleasure-seeking, infinitely materialistic and pursuers after leisure through personal wealth. On the other hand, they sought to think for themselves, they made curiosity a virtue, they questioned their contemporaries.[22]

What, during this terrible century of recurrent plague, was the Church doing? Was it promoting the freedom of mankind? Was it reacting, in an obscurantist way, to the works of Boccaccio or Chaucer.[23] Did the Church help or hinder the post-plague intellectual movement which became the Renaissance? What was the Church's intellectual contribution to post-plague society?

The earlier plagues of the Antonine era (AD 160–260) materially helped the Christian cause, since Christians were virtually the only people to offer charity and comfort to the sick and the dying. The mature Church in the fourteenth century signally failed to follow the example of the Early Fathers. There was a high death-rate amongst the monks and nuns in enclosed communities, and probably disproportionate casualties amongst the early plague villages, where priests went about their visiting in the traditional way, spreading fleas, microbes and death as they went. In the later outbreaks of that first plague year in the north and east of England, priests and prelates sometimes cut and run; death-rates at York, for example, were less than at Oxford a few months earlier. Many more left town, in favour of the solitary life. Acquired wisdom dictated that being alone might be prudent; whether or not solitude was physically advantageous, it was devastating to the moral cause of the clergy. They had acquired merit from their courage in the Roman plagues. They were rightly thought to be cowards as a result of their prudence in the fourteenth century. Writers from William Langland, to the village poet noticed the unworthiness of the higher clergy.[24]

Then there were the revenues of the Church. Overpopulation had meant famine, starvation, even cannibalism. Deaths around the 1350s led to a desperate hunt for tithes, for any kind of income from a stricken and impoverished population which would soon be visited by further plague epidemics. The Church, having failed its people, now sought to beggar them.

Finally, there was the question of medicine. Then, as now, the lay population was convinced that medical men should 'cure' disease. This quaint notion rebounded upon the Church in a devastating way. Medical men were all licensed and taught by Church authorities by 1300. There was little or no independence outside the creed of the 'humours'.[25] The beliefs were fixed, unquestioned, never subject to experiment. When up to half the population died in great pain and in horrific squalor, and no churchman or doctor of medicine could help, the intellectual reputation of the Church, its claim to omniscience, became risible. Already occasionally found to be without courage or charity, the Church now also lost its claim to wisdom, power or knowledge.

Not every cleric was, of course, a coward, but the terrible inadvertent damage done by the plague to the Church was a necessary prerequisite of the Reformation. Without the disrespect engendered by the post-plague behaviour of the clergy, it is difficult to believe that the heirs of Hus or Wyclif would have proven to be Luther or Calvin.[26]

The bubonic plague, the Black Death, rumbled on and on. The most familiar late outbreak was in the Great Plague year of 1665, when London was struck for the last time. It was not unique in the seventeenth century. There had been plagues in Europe of notable severity in 1603, 1609, 1625, 1636 and 1647. None of them, including the Great Plague of 1665, was as destructive as were the plagues in Lower Egypt in 1603, alleged to have killed a million people; there was an outbreak in Naples in 1656 which killed 300,000; a pandemic in parts of China in 1641 is said to have killed 3 million at the very least. These were more deadly than London's last attack, which only killed about 75,000. The Black Death was a visiting horror which appeared as an epidemic, or as a pandemic. The Red Plague, however, was familiar, and occurred everywhere, all the time, throughout Eurasia. It was so familiar that almost everyone of, say, forty years of age, would have survived at least one attack. In some cities, it was comparable to a childhood disease like chicken-pox, inoculating the survivors. It was the first disease for which Western man found an antidote, called 'vaccination'. It was the first disease which in 1981 the United Nations claimed was 'abolished'. It used to be called 'smallpox'. It has changed history.

Only identified at all by the Arab physician Khazes in the ninth century in Baghdad, smallpox was confused with measles at least as late as the Renaissance. So earlier outbreaks of Red Plague could be smallpox/measles. In fact, of course, measles, which is related to rinderpest in cattle and to canine distemper, was just as lethal as smallpox in the early days, and for the same reason. Smallpox is, in turn, related to cowpox in cattle and several other diseases in other animals. Both measles and smallpox emigrated out of animals into people, as did most of the 'successful' organisms in history.[27]

Smallpox/measles both produce rashes on the skin. Smallpox produces much larger pustules. Temperatures in smallpox cases can be as high as 40–41°C (104–5°F). The pulse is very quick; the fever is accompanied by heavy sweating; there is thirst, constipation and a tendency to rigor. There can be convulsions. The disease is confirmed to be smallpox by the rashes in pocklike form on the face, trunk, and extremities. The pox marks on the face are often hideous and disfiguring. The pustules emit an offensive odour; the voice is hoarse, and there is often a copious and uncontrollable flow of saliva from the mouth. The fever abates when the pox appears, but a few days later it returns in a worse form. There is restlessness, delirium and coma. If the patient survives so far, there are other hazards. Septicemia may set in.

There is another form of the disease which involves septicemia at once, without pustules. It is of little comfort to the sufferer from this form of the pox that the patient usually dies before being disfigured. Most people would prefer to live, even if disfigured for life.

It was the lack of disfigurement enjoyed by dairymaids who had caught cowpox from their charges which first alerted Edward Jenner to the possibilities of vaccination.[28] It was wrongly believed by Jenner that one vaccination would last for life, instead of the six or seven years accepted by about 1900. Compulsory vaccination was adopted by Bavaria, Denmark and Sweden, and Massachusetts, and five other States before the Battle of Waterloo. By 1898, the whole of Europe and the United States was covered by compulsory vaccination orders, though there were provisions for 'conscientious objectors'. In the outbreaks between 1900 and World War I, most of the casualties were amongst those who had conscientious objection to the vaccination process.[29]

Europeans took smallpox with them all over the world. In India and the Far East that made little difference, since there was just as much smallpox in Asia as in Europe. The disease is one, of course, of population density. Virulently infectious as is the disease, breath, saliva, blood, clothing are all charged with the virus. Even the dead body remains infectious for weeks on end. So it is a disease of cities, ships, armies; it was known in Mecca in AD 550, in South Europe by AD 590, throughout Europe by 1250. It is likely, therefore, that it came from the more crowded parts of Asia, probably identified in China in AD 317. The recorded losses at that date from what may well have been smallpox in China amounted to about 30 per cent of the population in thirty years.[30] Similar losses occurred in the first outbreaks in India, Arabia, and the Mediterranean. By 1492, the whole Eurasian landmass can be seen as having an endemic smallpox which was caught and survived by large numbers of children every year. There are certain caveats to be entered.

Dark-skinned people were said to be more susceptible than those who were fair. Once acquired, the disease was said to inoculate for life. Urban losses were far higher in those cities which were untidy, badly drained, and so forth. The rich, of course, by reason of living in a less huddled situation, were less likely to catch the disease. Those who lived in warm countries were more susceptible to infection transmitted in higher ambient temperatures. This was the reverse of the experience with the Black Death, where the inhabitants of Northern Europe were closer to the rats in the winter than in the summer. Smallpox, though, was much less devastating to the nomad than the Black Death which lived in the rodent host. Smallpox, the Red Death, was dependent upon crowded, static mankind for its successful migration from host to host.

Smallpox was at its most effective when the virus was introduced to new, crowded communities, innocent of any previous experience of the disease. The first epidemic in the Americas came in 1518, in Hispaniola, the island which is now divided into Haiti and the Dominican Republic. The inhabitants were said to number one million in 1498, when Columbus made permanent settlements six years after his first voyage. No one, of course, knows who counted the Amerindians, but all the Spaniards agreed that they were feeble and simpleminded. In the absence of the sought-after gold, sugar was introduced in 1506; and one of the first shipments of African slaves in 1512. In 1520, the Spanish historian Bartolomé de Las Casas reported that only 1,000 Indians survived the Red Plague.

If so, then this would have explained to the Spanish how the victory in Mexico was achieved in the next few years. Smallpox landed with the relief expedition which sustained the Spanish *conquistadores* in 1521. Aztecs, bewildered by death as soon as they had contact with the Spaniards, and sharing with the Spaniards the belief that death from disease was an indicator of God's disapproval, surrendered to Hernando Cortés and about 600 Spaniards, plus a small number of Amerindian allies. In the case of Mexico City in the 1520s, it is clear that smallpox had found an ideal home. Mexico City had, perhaps, 60,000 homes in 1520, with a population of 300,000. Within a month of the siege, a third of the population was said to have smallpox, and another third were feeling unwell. In the end, Mexico probably lost 90 per cent of its original population within a decade. Not all of these were victims of the Red Plague; there were losses from malaria, measles, influenza. Yet Spain was teaching in its schools as late as 1980 that they had triumphed because of a superior civilization, the use of horses and gunpowder, and the faith in victory which came from having God on their side. Even so, for 600 men to defeat an army of 100,000, and a nation of, perhaps, 2–3 million, is carrying the superiority of the moral over the material a little far.

Smallpox had reached Guatemala by 1520, and the whole of the Spanish Main by 1526–30. Prepared for defeat by the arrival of Spanish pestilence before the actual invaders themselves, the Inca Empire in Peru was no more of a match for Pizarro than the Aztecs had been in Mexico for Cortés.

The Spanish who arrived in Peru were virtually inoculated against the Red Plague by reason of their previous experience. The Incas reacted to the smallpox plague as did the Aztecs. It was a visitation of God upon a wicked people. Such was the reaction in Europe when a new disease appeared. It was to be a universal reaction of all peoples everywhere to new forms of disease until at least the nineteenth century.

There was a great deal of obscurantism about disease. For example, Napoleon I vaccinated his soldiers against smallpox by using the then new methods of Jenner. His enemies did not. They suffered. The Grande Armée did not. Yet his nephew, Napoleon III, allowed his army *not* to be vaccinated. Twenty thousand French soldiers died in the Franco-Prussian war of 1870. The Prussians lost very few, if any, to smallpox. The French Army, defending France, spread smallpox amongst French civilians. The vaccinated Prussians did not.

In 1904–5, during the Russo-Japanese war, the Japanese army was vaccinated, the Russians were not. The Japanese deaths from smallpox were negligible. The Russians lost five times as many men from disease as they did from battle. They lost more men from smallpox alone than they did from enemy action. But typhus, in 1904–5 and before, was the great wartime killer.

Typhus was a new disease in 1492. It came to Western Europe from the Levant, the first cases appearing in Spain in 1490. It was then taken to Italy by Spanish soldiers. The first mass European outbreak was in 1494. Thereafter, typhus was the most significant disease of armies, of the poor and crowded urban proletariat, of jails. It killed more soldiers between 1500 and 1914 than all military action. In cities, more died from typhus than from street accidents, crime and starvation. In jails, typhus killed far more than ill-treatment, torture or execution: it became known as 'jail fever'. Judges dreaded contact with prisoners, and smelt their posies of herbs and flowers in an effort to ward off the dreadful unknown ailment.[31]

The path and pattern of the disease was not known until just before World War I. In turn, the knowledge of how to prevent typhus led to the infinitely more lethal conditions of the trenches in France in 1914–18, which would have been impossible if clever men had not 'discovered' the typhus cycle. The clever men, of course, were acting from the best principles and the best motives, humanitarians all.

Some diseases are directly contagious or infectious; the pathogens pass from animal to animal by contact or the sharing of breath or by mouth. These are some of the most important human diseases besides smallpox: TB, measles, scarlet fever, chicken-pox, mumps, 'flu, and whooping cough. All have been in turn fatal, then serious, then endemic, then 'childhood' diseases and relatively harmless. Occasionally, a new strain appears, and becomes, successively lethal, then endemic, and so forth. Drugs have been found to deal with some of these diseases, notably TB. There is a vaccine for whooping cough. Most of the rest have become successful as diseases go.[32]

There is another group of diseases, where there are at least two hosts involved. The Black Death, *Pasteurella pestis*, 'bubonic plague' needs fleas and rodents, as has been seen. Sleeping sickness needs the tsetse fly and cattle. Typhus was a third disease which moved between rats and humans and killed differentially. These double-parasite diseases were much more difficult to discover and 'cure' because of the sophistication of the pattern established by the successful organism. In short, all these 'successful' organisms established patterns difficult for humans to detect and interdict. Lateral thinking was required to trace the life of the parasites.

Typhus was no exception. For four hundred years, the problem was thought to be the smell of the great unwashed. Indeed, the poor smelt since they could not afford to be clean. The poor also had typhus; they were probably twenty times as likely to have typhus as the rich. QED.

This kind of proof by association was common enough until this century. Malaria was connected with swamps, not with mosquitoes and plasmodia. The Black Death was connected with crowded cities, not with *Pasteurella pestis* and rats. The Red Plague, smallpox, was connected specifically with dirt, litter and unburnt rubbish as late as 1890–1900, even though vaccination could be proved to prevent it. The secrets of typhus were only unravelled a few years before World War I.

Typhus, according to an up-to-date account before the mystery was solved, had four stages. The first is that of incubation. This lasts from 7–10 days. 'Languor' was said to be the only symptom. As languor could be caused by many other factors, from insufficient nutrition to depression, this clue was not exactly helpful.

Then there are the symptoms of the second stage: rigor, chilliness, prostration, sleeplessness, feverish headache, and a temperature of 39–40°C (103–4°F). The pulse is rapid, the patient is at first excited, and after a week may become as feeble as the pulse. The tongue is at first covered with white fur, then brown and dry; appetite is lost, constipation is characteristic, urine diminished and highly coloured.

The third stage is that of the rash, which is very dark, the spots mulberry-coloured and often accompanied by a subcutaneous haemorrhage. The patient lies with his eyes open, on his back, with a stupid expression on his face, apathetic, but in the worst cases with a wild and maniacal look. The patient may also mutter incomprehensibly.

The fourth stage, at fourteen days, is the crisis. There is an abrupt lowering of temperature, a return of normality to the alimentary system, and a recovery. Alternatively, the patient may die. Death-rates from the disease came down from the high point when the disease was 'new' to an average of about 18–20 per cent which was noted in scores of statistical studies at the turn of the nineteenth century. At this level, typhus would have made World War I impossible.

The discovery of the cycle was rapidly followed by prophylactic measures which were developed during the two Balkan Wars of 1912–13. The cycle involves rats and their fleas, as with the Black Death. But the rat flea and the rat live happily with typhus and recover from any attack. The flea transfers its own parasitic passengers to the human louse, which then sucks human blood and infects one human after another. Certain prerequisites exist.

The virus *Rickettsia prowazeki* kills the human louse, as well as infecting the human being, guinea-pigs and monkeys, which, unlike the rats and the rat flea, are killed. Before death, the human louse not only can infect its own human host, but also move from human to human. Thus, proximity is necessary to the success of the disease. The louse may live happily on an immune native, but jump to a stranger, who is then infected.

Typhus needs cool climates, people in mass, especially strangers, the difficulties of hygiene associated with war and famine, and the retention on the body of foul clothing. Jails were, of course, ideally suited to the spread of the disease. Yet, though the disease was rampant in the eighteenth century, and though ships were often filled with jailbirds, outbreaks on board ship were rarer than in the army. This was presumably because ships were intolerable for the officers, without hygiene. There was also an

ample supply of sterile water for washing. This came, at ambient temperature, from the sea. The lesser mortals in the army, however, had to suffer
and die until the cure was discovered largely by the American Typhus
Commission in the Balkans just before World War I. First, remove
clothing, steam or boil same. Bathe soldier. Spray him with petrol (*sic*).
Examine soldier for lice and nits. Allow him to get dressed in sterile
clothing.

This procedure was standard in the Western armies once the static
warfare of the trenches had become normal. Troops were deloused every
time they left the trenches, and before they returned, say every two to
three weeks. On the Eastern Front, in Serbia, Russia, and in Poland,
typhus raged from the beginning of the breakdown of effective resistance
to the Germans, which was as early as the winter of 1914 in the case of
Serbia. Losses in Eastern Europe due to typhus in the period 1914–21 were
at least double the casualties by direct action. It was only the prophylactic
measures which made possible trench warfare.

Ironically, the good men who solved the problem, those hardworking
doctors, nurses and health workers of the American Typhus Commission
were many of them Quakers. All of them believed in peace rather than
war. Yet, their efforts to prevent typhus enabled trench warfare to be
developed in a way impossible to conceive without delousing stations.
Out of their efforts came the ritualized slaughter of World War I in
France. Perhaps this irony, like so many other ironies, is grossly unfair. If
the Allies had not been given the benison of the work of the Commission,
perhaps the Germans, much more alive to health and hygiene than the
French or Belgians, would have deloused their troops first. In that case, the
Germans would have won the war in the West as they did in the East.

It is entirely possible that if Russian delousing had not broken down,
the Russians would not have lost; in that case, no 1917 Revolution, no
Communism, no Nazism, no World War II, perhaps. These are extreme
hypotheses. There is no doubt, however, that, from 1494 onwards,
typhus was a more important factor for armies than strategy, tactics,
weapons, courage or leadership. Human beings, of course, do not like to
think of such matters. How dull history would be if it were always due to
some causative factor invisible to the naked eye.

Typhus, of course, was not only a disease of armies. It changed history
first in Naples in 1494, where it made the continued siege impossible. The
French king, Charles VIII, discharged his soldiers who survived the
typhus-ridden investiture of the city without the formality of terminal pay
or transport to get home. Not unnaturally, they lived off the country; in
doing so, they spread typhus wherever they went. No one knows how
many reached France, but it is certain that the attempt killed many more

innocent Italian civilians than the actual warfare. It is possible that winter
warfare became even more difficult than it had been before because of
typhus in cold countries. Soldiers, huddled together to keep warm, may
well have produced a death-rate too high to contemplate. Hence the safer
summer 'campaigning season'. Typhus, of course, like other diseases,
became milder. But as a killer, it exceeded all human efforts even in that
most savage of all conflicts, the Thirty Years War. Typhus was particularly lethal in Germany in 1618–48. During that time, Germany suffered
so much as to reverse the advances made during the Renaissance itself, and
to make of parts of Germany a cultural and intellectual desert. Typhus, of
course, killed half Napoleon's army which went to Russia in 1812. Despite
all the great man's efforts at vaccinating his troops against smallpox, no
one could, at that date, have prevented typhus.

The disease was selective, in the Darwinian sense, like all diseases. It
killed more Northerners, more men, more gregarious people rather than
individuals, and above all more poor people. The death-rate in prisons was
such as to make a penal policy hardly necessary.[33] Above all, perhaps,
typhus destroyed the already weak, those who were ill-fed, half-starved,
those on the way to death from famine. In this case, was it more merciful?
Perhaps half or more of those who died in the Irish Famine would have had
the disease as the proximate cause of death.

It followed, therefore, that individualism, cleanliness, sufficient food
and a sharp sense of the disagreeable nature of most other humans were
protective instincts which were selected over the four hundred years
during which typhus occurred in armies, slums and prisons. 'The great
unwashed' became a group to be avoided, potential killers. It would be
interesting to know whether the fever made more obvious class distinction, pity for the victim, or a useful desire to find a cure. Whatever may be
thought by anachronistic moderns, the evidence of the time does not
suggest that typhus sufferers were regarded by the majority as anything
more than people to be avoided. The avoiders of typhus were the selfish,
the rural, the clean, the well-fed, and those who had no desire to commune
too closely with others. The sharp distinction between countries with
and without a long history of typhus will not escape the amateur of
history.[34]

If people could escape typhus by their own prudent behaviour, no such
possibility existed with malaria. This disease like bubonic plague and
typhus, depended upon a parasite invading another host. The host was, of
course, the mosquito. Everyone knows this today, but until 1910, or
thereabouts, few knew anything of the lifestyle of the vector, the mosquito; the internal meanderings of the parasite in the mosquito and in the

human bloodstream were other mysteries. Malaria (bad air) is a disease ascribed in history to swamps, the night air, heat, and in the nineteenth century, to the mosquito. So people sought hilly land, or running water rather than stagnant lakes and ponds, were careful where they slept, went into the hills in the summer and, latterly, used mosquito nets at night. Malaria is a disease which, almost uniquely, was diminished in intensity, if not cured, before anything was known about its progress in the human body. The whole amazing story of quinine has been told. Its influence on history has been profound.

In this book, two particular aspects of the disease are to be unfolded. One is not widely known, the other is original. In 1492, malaria was endemic in the Mediterranean. It was also much commoner in north-west Europe than anyone would imagine today. Holland, Denmark, southern Sweden and Norway were mildly infected all the time; in parts of undrained England, in the Fens in particular, malaria, if not a killer of many, was an annual occurrence. The last person to be found to have died of native 'English' malaria was in Essex in 1924.

Malaria was no respecter of persons. It could not be avoided by repulsing the poor, as with typhus, or avoiding bubonic plague cities, or refusing to get close to someone who might have been in contact with the Red Plague, smallpox. Nor was there any ameliorative agent before quinine, nor was quinine freely available to any but the rich before about 1860. So thousands of travellers, merchants, people from low-lying areas all over Europe were sufferers and losers. The disease of malaria was, like typhus, highly selective, but in quite different ways. It operated against landlubbers, since North European mosquitoes could not survive at sea, against summer travellers, against rural dwellers in low-lying locations. The disease, of course, is recurring, so that people would be made lethargic and insipid and ineffective long before death appeared over the horizon. It was taken by Western Europeans all over the world, like every other white man's disease.

How much of a killer was malaria in the Americas? While the mosquito could not fly far overseas, the insect could recycle in the ship's bilges in a warm enough climate. The southern route taken by Columbus in the summer of 1492, via the Canaries, could well have brought the disease to the Caribbean in that year. In contrast, John Cabot's voyage to the St Lawrence in 1496 would not have made possible a continuous breeding programme for the marine mosquito. Nor was the European mosquito necessary to the success of the disease in the Americas. Enough sailors carrying endemic malaria could have arrived in the Caribbean or in Canada and been bitten by native mosquitoes to have started the cycle going even if the ship had been clear of any European insects. There are four hundred sorts of mosquitoes. Sixty are vectors of malaria. Of the sixty, thirteen are native to the Americas.

So, one way or another, malaria was one of the gifts the Europeans gave to the Americas besides smallpox and measles. While smallpox and measles killed, and killed swiftly and with indiscriminate success, malaria of the European type of 1492 was spread throughout the Americas. The survivors of smallpox and measles were profoundly affected by malaria. The survivor of malaria was like all other survivors before quinine; they were listless, anaemic, and with a badly damaged liver, had probable cancer of that organ, and a shortened lifespan. The Europeans (descendants of perhaps fifty generations of malaria) survived rather better, even without quinine. Malaria, unlike smallpox and measles, was not a quick ally for the European, but a long-term one. Taking malaria with them throughout the double continent, the disease had a long-term effect. Resistance was lowered, slowly. It produced the death of cultures, rather than people. Vigour disappeared, passivity and debility became the order of the day; optimism fled. It is almost impossible for a malaria victim to be anything but fatalistic, a chattering weakling during the recurrent attacks, listless and fearing the next when apparently 'normal'.

How could a native civilization survive such an attack, even if smallpox and measles had selected the survivors? Malaria was a more insidious foe. The real irony, of course, was that the (South American) cure was generally only available to the whites, who doled it out in every country to their slaves, serfs and workers. It was a form of Imperialism which a mad biotechnologist might have invented. An incurable disease is introduced. The ameliorative agent is 'discovered'. The control of the agent remains in the hands of the Imperial power. Why did Marx not include the malaria/ quinine story in his catalogue of European capitalist crimes? Simply because Marx, who died in 1883, never knew about malaria, its cycle, its parasites, its 'cure'. More importantly, Marx, like lesser men, ascribed all human misfortunes to other human actions. What price willpower in the victims of malaria?

The other point of the malaria story has never been properly considered. It is known that the much more lethal form of malaria, *falciparium*, was unique to West Africa and taken to the Caribbean. It is also known that native West Africans are partially immune to *falciparium* malaria because of the recessive in their genes. It was for this reason that Negroes[35] became the ideal workforce in the Caribbean into which the non-immune whites had introduced West African malaria in company with the slaves they had brought over by ship. *Falciparium* is a much more lethal strain than the ordinary, European type called, today, *Vivax*. This malaria was endemic throughout the Old World, an acknowledged minor drag upon enterprise and effort throughout written history, 'swamp fever', 'marsh miasma', or 'palundine poison'. Malaria was recognized long before the name was invented as a problem in many areas. But Eurasians from China to Portugal learned to live with the debilitating effects. The whole of the African shore of the Mediterranean and the Indian Ocean also contained millions of people who had experienced and survived the disease. It was a nagging familiar. As with other endemic conditions, it produced a population largely resistant to the worst effects. In a competitive world, those who did not overcome the depressing effects did not thrive.

Plasmodia falciparium was quite another matter. It was confined, before the Portuguese voyages, to the West African lowlands, where the native Negro population had developed an in-built genetic resistance. The invading Arabs and other Muslims stayed in the highlands, and did not survive the penetration of the rain forests, swamps and deep river basins. Nor did the medieval Arab trade routes across the Sahara permit of any recycling of the mosquito. Few mosquitoes would survive for more than a day in the desert. Few men with *falciparium* malaria would survive much longer, walking north from Timbuktu.[36]

So Negro slaves, perhaps 1,000 a year, brought north from West Africa by Arab slave-dealers before 1400, did not bring with them *falciparium* malaria. After 1440, the story was different. At least 500,000 West African blacks were brought in to Portugal in the 150 years after 1440. They were set to work in the south of the country, and made possible agriculture in what had been the empty Alemtejo, once the granary of Portugal, but barren since the Moors had left. *Falciparium* malaria needs a mosquito, like other malaria, in which to develop. *Plasmodia falciparium* needs a temperature of at least 20°C (68°F) to spread. At that constant, it needs twenty-one days to evolve in the mosquito. At 25°C (77°F) the time is cut to seven days or less. Southern Portugal in the summer became a killing ground. The survival of the immune Africans made Portugal south of Lisbon a black colony. Did *falciparium* also spread to southern Spain? Can it explain much of the decay in the Iberian spirit in the first century after 1492?

The effects of *falciparium* malaria in the Americas were lethal to the whites, as the *Plasmodia vivax* was destructive of the Red Amerindian. The whites brought malaria from Europe in all of Columbus's voyages, and it spread all over the Caribbean. Every Spanish *conquistador*, every Portuguese settler, every French, British or Dutch buccaneer brought malaria of the *vivax* type from Europe along with the measles, smallpox and influenza to every part of North and South America. This is documented from Quebec to the River Plate. The Europeans, after 1517, brought Negro slaves from Spain and Portugal to the Americas. After

1530, there was a direct trade from West Africa, which went on for three hundred years. During that time, millions of slaves, and billions of mosquitoes carrying *Plasmodia falciparium* were brought over. European death-rates in the West Indies were sometimes twenty times as great as at home. Some were victims of *falciparium* malaria, others of yellow fever.

Yellow fever is carried by the same sort of mosquito and it was brought by ship from West Africa. The insect can only survive in a much narrower temperature range than the *falciparium* mosquito; the fever is an elegant illustration of how Europeans have made disease international.

Yellow fever did not appear as early as malaria. If so, there would be evidence since the 'yellows' were regarded with an even greater and more justifiable horror than the *falciparium* malaria. But yellow fever depends upon a mosquito even more particular in its requirements than the type responsible for *falciparium* malaria. The unique mosquito is called *Aedes aegypti*. It loves mankind, in its original home Egypt, a minor irritant. It is a parasite of man. It cannot breed in 'natural' water which is above mud or earth or sand. Nor can it breed in running water. So it must find a man-made object, or a fallen tree or a rock enclosing a quantity of stagnant water in order to perpetuate its species. The stagnant water in bilges or barrels in ships are ideal. So *Aedes aegypti* became a great traveller, but on certain conditions. The mosquitoes also have a very narrow range of temperature. This must always stay above 24°C. Unlike some mosquitoes, *Aedes aegypti* cannot survive even one night at a lower temperature. Death intervenes at a drop of only 1° below 24°C (75°F). This gives a new meaning to the phrase 'one degree under'. For this insect *Aedes aegypti* one degree under means death.

So this mosquito thrives only in the tropics. A ship carrying the insects and the eggs would not normally bring the yellow fever north to Europe, or south to South Africa, or east to India or China. Yellow fever, unlike *falciparium* malaria, was uniquely brought across the Atlantic, always within the temperature zone above 24°C (75°F). Blown north on a voyage to the Caribbean, or south on a voyage to Brazil, the mosquito usually died. The fever was first noted in Bridgetown, Barbados, in 1647, and in Havana the next year.

'Yellow Jack' as sailors knew it, killed all the time while the ship was in the tropics. Sometimes, slavers were left with only a few white survivors, occasionally with none. The immune black slaves then starved to death. Ashore, in tropical America, it was the greatest killer known to the eighteenth century. Sometimes whole regiments of soldiers were wiped out. A ship on a trip in the Triangle England–West Africa–West Indies–England might lose half its crew from yellow fever trading round the islands of the Caribbean, even if the mosquito had not been picked up in West Africa. In hot weather, the fever went north as far as New Orleans, Florida and Texas, and was so feared as to empty the towns along the Gulf Coast in a hot, bad year. It also went as far south as Rio de Janiero, in the southern summer.

Exceptionally, yellow fever moved as far as 40°N in both hemispheres during the period 1793–1821. Did the nature of the mosquito change? Or were the then northern summers exceptionally hot? The disease appeared in Philadelphia and in Cadiz, Lisbon, Malaga and Barcelona. There was a single outbreak in Lisbon in 1857, killing 6,000 in six weeks. There have been no recorded cases in the Eastern Mediterranean. Death-rates have been greater than with any type of malaria, and the disease was quite early connected with mosquitoes, if the wrong ones, with high temperatures, with stagnant water and with dirt.[37]

The final blow to the white man's pride was the Panama Canal, which virtually had to be abandoned because yellow fever defeated the contractors. The death-rate between 1890 and the end of the old company in 1901 was of the order of 50 per cent of those involved. 'Sanitation' became an essential prerequisite of the new company. The mosquito was defeated by drastic measures, and the Canal was built. Yellow fever is not only defeated by dealing with the mosquito. There is an inoculation, which confers upon other races the immunity which made the black West African the essential labouring race of the West Indies. Ironically, if the whites had never traded slaves in West Africa, then yellow fever would never have left the Bight of Benin. The disease was brought to the Americas by slavers: it was the disease which later made black slavery essential.

Mosquitoes were defeated by the United States doctors and engineers and sanitary workers by drastic use of petroleum products. Bilges, stagnant water ashore, lakes and ponds were all sprayed with kerosene. Before DDT, this was a standard procedure all over the Caribbean, and much of the rest of the Americas. Wooden ships harboured the mosquito much more easily than modern steel vessels. New building construction did not permit nooks and crannies which allowed insects to cycle and recycle. Commercial management of land did not allow stagnant pools of water. But it was the Sanitary Commissions of various kinds which, in the days before DDT, made yellow fever and malaria much less of a problem. DDT itself transformed the situation.

The liberal use of DDT at the end of World War II destroyed the home life of the mosquito. DDT also destroyed many other insects, including the enemies of mosquitoes. Its lavish use has had two uncovenanted consequences. The first result was relief. Thereafter, population growth took over, and relief sometimes disappears. Greece was relieved of malaria for the first time in history: only then could Greece become a tourist paradise. In Bangladesh, one of the poorest countries in the world, tourism is unlikely. Population increases at a rate which doubles every twenty-five years, far beyond the possibility of enough food. The density of population in Bangladesh is over 6 people per hectare (14 people per acre) compared with 4 (10) people in the Netherlands or southern England, or 1.5 (4) in New York State as a whole. By 2000 it is likely that Bangladesh's population will be 10 people per hectare, an ecological disaster. This has been the effect of defeating disease in many parts of the world, and will be noted in due course.

The other problem, revealed by the success of DDT, is the polluting effect of wonder cures. DDT was found all over the world by 1955. Like strychnine, DDT can never be denatured; it cycles and recycles, poisoning the environment. It is found in the bloodstreams of Antarctic penguins, and in fish which are eaten by mankind, whose detritus returns to the sea to pollute other fish or the very rain which falls on the other side of the world. Pollution by substances which can never be broken down is creating anomalies. Some chemicals, unwanted any longer for their original purpose, cannot be denatured or broken down, so they spend from now until eternity, doomed travellers like Coleridge's Ancient Mariner.

It creates a very real problem if complicated, beneficient substances have side-effects which cannot be assessed before those substances are used over a number of years. To this logical conundrum there appears to be no answer. Not to have used insecticides would have meant that malaria and yellow fever would have remained chronic, mosquito-borne diseases. To use an effective insecticide may condemn the world to pollution at rates which could become irreversible. Fortunately this paradox applies only to insect-borne diseases.

Three diseases which, like malaria and yellow fever, had to wait for the end of the nineteenth century for their suppression, were the alimentary troubles. Of these, dysentery and typhoid fever probably date from the early years of the Christian era. Cholera burst out of India in the early 1820s and is, *par excellence*, an urban disease of the nineteenth century. All three diseases cycle from human to human, via the drinking water and sewage systems or, more intimately, from unwashed hand to food to mouth. Typhoid and dysentery have different symptoms, yet historically, it is difficult to distinguish between the two. Typhoid results in diarrhoea, and fever, and general debility. But the organism affects all the organs, and may live on for years, especially in women.[38] Typhoid fever organisms survive in water, but do not multiply therein. They live in warm air long enough to infect people downwind of the excreta of the diseased. The organism prefers acid conditions, of the pH of a normal stomach. So alkaline soils, water and cold conditions deter mass infection. Typhoid was always known as a warm weather disease, or of the tropics. It took a long time for people to realize that the active organism was inhibited by cold, but multiplied in balmy weather. Typhoid was a great killer of people in cities and in armies. As late as the Boer War (1899–1902) the British lost twice as many men from typhoid as from all battle casualties, and ten times as many as were killed outright by the enemy. It was this kind of loss of life which made warfare so expensive in manpower.

Dysentery was also a great killer. In the Crimean War (1854–7) British deaths from dysentery were ten times those from all killed in enemy action. But dysentery, unlike typhoid, is not carried especially by women.[39] It was originally known in England as 'the bloody flux' since the stomach evacuates everything, then starts to discharge skin, flesh, and blood. Ultimately the unlucky patient dies, as often as not in great pain, of internal haemorrhage, passing stinking matter of a peculiarly nauseous and unique nature. Old-time doctors could smell the difference between typhoid and dysentery a hundred yards away from a sufferer.

Typhoid was prevented by the injection of dead organisms in a vaccine, the process being regularized in most armies before 1939.[40] Dysentery another matter, needing constant care and hygiene to prevent the problem. The prevention is still the same sort of hygiene and sanitation that wise people have practised for centuries. Dysentery is spread by flies, contact with infected people or faeces, and by birds and other animals. Of the two causative factors, the bacillus which causes one sort of dysentery can be killed by the sulfa drugs. Amoebic dysentery, on the other hand, is a subacute, chronic, recurring form of the disease and may persist for years, like malaria; the parasite can cause serious liver problems if untreated. For years, the solution was a derivative of the Brazilian plant ipecacuahana. This contains the alkaloid emetine which, combined with opium, was made up as Dover's Powder, without which no Victorian traveller was properly prepared for the rigours of 'abroad'. It is specific against amoebic dysentery, but it was more widely used. This convenient drug was used for every kind of upset, from diarrhoea, however caused, through Gippy tummy to Montezuma's revenge. Probably the mild dose of narcotic did as much to comfort the voyager as did ignorance of the true nature of the trouble.

Cholera was another matter, because it was a 'new' disease for the European. Like typhoid and some sorts of dysentery, cholera gives rise to fever. Unlike any previous 'civilized' disease, it sprang upon the world at a time when its symptoms were fully noted. It has had a short career in the Western World, as diseases go. Cholera, or some other fever answering the description given by later writers, had been cycling and recycling in the Far East for centuries. A particularly bad outbreak occurred in Bengal, India, in 1816–17. Cholera, unlike dysentery and typhoid, is very rapid. Very often the disease reached the acute stage within twenty-four hours, and has been known to kill within another day.

Unlike typhoid, cholera prefers alkaline conditions, so a stomach of normal acidity can easily destroy the cholera bacillus. The use of purgative medicines, the eating of unripe fruit, or alcoholism may all predispose the stomach to accept rather than reject the organism. In a dramatic demonstration given in the 1880s, the great German pathologist Robert Koch consumed in front of his students a capsule of infected matter from a cholera victim. He made quite certain that the pH of his stomach was below the normal value before he risked his life. Cholera bacillus is also killed by a temperature of more than 60°C (140°F), so tea and coffee are always safe. The reservoir of infection is often drinking water, in rivers or in reservoirs. The bacillus is not killed by adding whisky to water, contrary to what old Indian hands may have told their children.[41]

There were six great global outbreaks in the nineteenth century. The first, in the years after 1817, reached China and Japan in the east, Astrakhan in the north. The next epidemic started in 1826, reached Astrakhan in 1830, Moscow and Berlin in the following year, Paris and London in 1832. Carried to Canada by emigrants the same year, it reached all the North American cities by 1838. The next outbreak reached Europe in 1847 and lasted until 1855. The next two outbreaks, in 1865–9 and 1884–8 were taken from India to Mecca by Muslim pilgrims, and from Mecca all over the Muslim world, and by contact, all over southern and then northern Europe.[42]

The final cholera outbreak was so widespread as to be almost a pandemic rather than an epidemic. From 1892–5, the disease raged all over the world. In Hamburg, in 1892, 50 per cent of those infected died, nearly 9,000 of them. The same sort of story came out of France, England and most of Western Europe. The next year, it was prevalent in the Americas. By 1895, it covered Asia. The situation was so serious that stern efforts were made to 'cure' the problem. These were much inhibited by the received wisdom of the day, which rejected the theory of germs causing disease. Pasteur had discovered the first bacillus (of anthrax) in 1876; Robert Koch found the tubercle bacillus in 1879, and the cholera bacillus in 1883. Yet the Establishment still claimed, as did the great Greek physician, Hippocrates, that sudden epidemics appeared out of the soil, the miasma left there by dead bodies.

This was the perceived truth in medical schools in the 1880s and 1890s, despite the efforts of the followers of the Renaissance germ theory of the Italian Girolamo Fracastoro (1483–1553). Had it been theories of contagion which had instituted the practice of quarantine? Or was it observation? In Venice, quarantine was instituted before 1450, a century before Fracastoro. It became common in every port by 1800. Unbelievably, quarantine was repealed as a compulsory precaution in England, the world's then greatest trading nation in 1896. This was coincidental with early pathological work by Sir Almroth Wright, whose pupils later included the inventor of penicillin, Sir Alexander Fleming. It would not be the last time in the world when an obstinate, almost invincible ignorance coincided with the beginning of enlightenment.[43]

Until the true nature of diseases was revealed by observation, microscope, logic, experiment, thesis, antithesis and synthesis, the Establishment held sway in a bluff, no-nonsense kind of way. Unfortunately, however, there was plenty of nonsense.

As late as 1895, after the work of the French physician Alphonse Laveran in 1881, malaria was still said to be often due to the upturning of virgin soil. This released the miasma. Dysentery, typhoid and cholera organisms were present in the localities where the outbreaks occurred. Against all the evidence, smallpox, bubonic plague and typhus were due to the 'floating atmosphere' of the place, ship or city. Smallpox could be vaccinated against. Plague could be avoided. It was, however, recognized that the building of new jails and poorhouses reduced the incidence of typhus. This is now known to be because rats and fleas live with greater ease in old buildings rather than new, old ships rather than new, old cities rather than new.

Nevertheless, most physicians of the last quarter of the nineteenth century refused to accept more than a generalized explanation for the prevalence of serious epidemics and pandemics. It was back to the times of Hippocrates who had died in 359 BC, or thereabouts. Charles Creighton, a leading medical man of his time, actually wrote a huge, tendentious study, *History of Epidemics in Britain*, in order to disprove the new germ theories of the modern pathologists. This came out in 1891 and 1894, nearly 2,000 pages in each volume. The book was highly recommended by the obscurantists of the day, and the Establishment.

It did not last long at the top. Within twenty years, the theories of Pasteur, Lister, Koch and Ehrlich were as widely accepted as the old 'truth' of Hippocrates was discredited.

Within a generation, every serious infection was at least traced in its course, and avoidance or prevention became routine. It would not be until the advent of the sulfa drugs and the antibiotics that true 'cures' became possible.[44]

One disease, wholly connected with sexual intercourse has always been considered to be avoidable. It is, of course, venereal, and it is called syphilis.

Syphilis is likely to have been brought back from the Caribbean by Columbus's sailors on the first voyage. There is another, non-Columbian history of the disease, which has always been unconvincing, and the evidence accumulates in favour of the traditional explanation. The disease first appeared in Europe in 1493 at Cadiz.[45]

Europeans took with them across the world more than a score of diseases, all of which were fatal in the first instance to the native populations whose bodies were invaded by invisible European allies. Syphilis is the only American disease which has had any success, from the point of view of the disease, in the Old World. After 1493, Europeans took the new import with them all over the world.[46]

Syphilis is spread by contact between people engaged in sexual activity. It is difficult to catch by other forms of contact, except in the tropics, where the ambient temperature may well permit the spirochetes to survive for long enough for non-venereal transmission. The disease appears to have been widespread in the Caribbean and it is known to be passed on in the milk of infected women. Children borne or suckled by infected women are inoculated against more severe forms of the disease; in generations, a whole population could well have grown up with a mild, secondary form of syphilis. This would have been acquired in the womb or in the first few months of birth. At the same time, such a population would never be able to increase its numbers so as to produce market agriculture, villages, towns, and so forth. Can it therefore be concluded that syphilis was present in those Caribbean islands with low, pre-Columbian, populations? It must have been absent in those, like San Domingo, which allegedly had a native population of a million when Columbus arrived. More convincingly, syphilis cannot have been present, except in a very attenuated form, in Mexico or Peru, which had substantial populations, with considerable surpluses which could be used by high priests for human sacrifice.

Such a pattern does not fit what is known of populations which have had syphilis for many generations. Needless to add that no experiment has been conducted, since the true nature of syphilis has only been known since 1900 or thereabouts, since when it has been 'cured'. The timescale necessary to prove the mild, attenuated form of pre-Columbian Amer-indian syphilis must be of the order of at least ten generations. There is nowhere in the world today an isolated community which has congenital syphilis, and which can be guaranteed not to have been reinfected for ten generations. Sailors of every nationality, of course, have spread syphilis for nearly five hundred years.[47]

But sailors were only the first wave of white invaders. They acquired the disease from Caribbean women in 1492, and infected whores or wives throughout Spain on their return next year. Some of them returned with Columbus on the second voyage. These then infected other Caribbean women. By the time that serious Iberian conquest was involved in the early 1520s, Spanish and Portuguese sailors had probably infected women all over the shoreline of the Americas. There was enough infection to ensure disease in those populations which had previously been free from syphilis: Aztecs, Mayas, Incas, certain populated islands in the Caribbean. These would all have been infected by Europeans.

To 'clean' Amerindian populations, the effects of syphilis must have been as serious as the same effects on virgin European populations. Density of people catastrophically declined. The first instance would be an alarming rise in miscarriages. The next a huge increase in babies dying in the first six months of life, shrivelled and wan. Perinatal syphilis has been studied in statistical terms; healthy infants reared to three years number only about one-tenth the number of infants borne by healthy women. Syphilis produces a demographic disaster.

This point, about differential incidence of the disease in the Americas in 1492, has never been examined. It is impossible to prove either way. But syphilis would be a satisfactory explanation of why Amerindian populations were so small in certain areas, and so dense in others. There were no other comparable Amerindian diseases. It is also possible that syphilitic syndromes which Europeans would now experience, after the summer of 1493, had all been part of the Amerindian folk-memory in some areas.

It is important to remember that, before syphilis, attitudes to sex were very different. It is true that promiscuity was the luxury of the rich. But certain populations in Europe still offered sexual hospitality to the peaceful stranger, as did almost every 'primitive' people, and as do some Africans and many Eskimos, to this day.[48]

Pre-marital intercourse was no more prohibited in some European societies than it was in the Pacific. It is true that Europe certainly had other sexually transmitted diseases, gonorrhoea in particular. But these problems never had the impact of syphilis in the public psyche. After syphilis appeared, sexual manners and morals were altered permanently. Or at least until modern man thought he had 'cured' the disease.

First, there was a profound decline in the ability of royal and noble families to breed. Henry VIII of England, the Valois of France, the Ottoman Sultans of Turkey, all had difficulties which were unprecedented. So did dozens of aristocratic families. Did the decline of aristocratic vigour precede the demand of the plebs for public power, or did it follow?[49]

Secondly, the kind of sexual ebullience which characterized the lifestyle of every Italian family of the day, Medici, Borgia, Sforza, came to a sober end. The first priest died of syphilitic symptoms in 1496, the first bishop in 1506, and the first Pope in 1516. The career of Lucrezia Borgia, overstated as it has been in fiction, could never, for example, have existed after syphilis.[50]

Thirdly, and as a consequence of the experience of the thirty years 1493–1523, both northern 'Protestants' and the southern Counter-Reformation Catholics became 'puritan'. The kill-joy streak in humans, never far below the surface, became an absolute necessity to preserve the family, the tribe, the race. In this connection, it is arguable that papal folly and excesses in the period 1460 to 1520, which were such a causative factor in the Reformation, would have been impossible in the Age of Syphilis. It is impossible to imagine Renaissance papal behaviour if Columbus had sailed a hundred years previously.

Fourthly, women had another reason to fear men besides the loss of virginity. Syphilis ruined lives. Certain classes of men were more suspect than others. Aristocrats acquired a reputation for raffishness, sexual irresponsibility, an inability to reproduce which may well have helped the development of the modern world. The effective aristocracies, which survived in some European countries in all their vigour, were renewed all the time by new blood. The middle classes, meanwhile, developed a strong sense of sexual ethic which would one day be called 'Victorian', sometimes an adjective of contempt. (This contempt could only be expressed by those who ignored the fact that syphilis raged throughout Victorian England, except amongst those who were prissily careful.) Sailors ever since Columbus have had an especial reputation, not always good.

Finally, there is a point never before made about this revolutionary disease. Syphilis was the first disease in human consciousness that was obviously the direct result of human action. In an era innocent of any knowledge of germ, bacterium, virus, or causative agent of any kind, syphilis taught every European a lesson within a century. Cause and effect. Leave the unclean alone. Do not engage in pre-marital intercourse, or promiscuity. Plan marriages with children in mind. What would be called the bourgeois virtues combined with the sixth Commandment. Indulgences, even Papal Indulgences, could not cure syphilis.[51]

For four centuries, nothing cured syphilis. Then in the late nineteenth century, a long and painful course of mercury effected a cure. But the cure was often worse than the disease and gave rise to the sailors' saying: 'Better

the disease than the cure.' Ehrlich invented two complex combinations of
arsenic in the period 1910 to 1914 which were widely used to limit the
damage from syphilis during World War I. But the real 'cure' came from
antibiotics. This occurred in the late 1940s.

Antibiotics promised to 'wipe out' syphilis. So said optimistic pathologists and the people believed them, as people do, when they want to
believe. The combination of a 'cure' for venereal disease and a birth-
control pill which was nearly 99 per cent effective led to the sexual
revolution of the 1960s. This in turn lasted until AIDS (Acquired Immune Deficiency Syndrome) came along.

AIDS has in some places already begun to produce social results similar
to those following the arrival of syphilis five hundred years ago. But because of the precautions immediately made obvious and necessary in the
First World, AIDS has a less chilling effect now than when it first arrived.

Public attitudes to AIDS differ greatly. In some areas of the United
States it is seen as a needle disease, in others, not. In Europe, it is more
associated with "unsafe" (unprotected) sex. In the USSR, it was originally seen as an import and a sexually-transmitted disease; today, with
glasnost, the shortage of needles in Soviet hospitals and their repeated
reuse, sometimes with insufficient sterilisation, are common knowledge.
In China there is more homosexuality than drug abuse. In Japan, AIDS
is not seen as a local problem. In Africa, it is a major killer.[52]

AIDS was the first disease to challenge Western medical triumphalism.
It is different, perhaps unique, in attacking the immune system, rather
than antibodies. As it is not susceptible to injection of either the live or
dead virus, there is no traditional protection or mitigation. The search for
drugs to combat the disease has tended to follow two lines of development: the first, for an inhibition to prevent HIV becoming AIDS; the
second, to delay or prevent the inevitable end. Neither drug has yet
proved possible, despite certain optimistic signs. There is no doubt in
some quarters that the enormous resources now deployed will one day
prove successful.[53]

At one time, it seemed likely that survival of the bourgeois virtues, the
family, the framework of gentle society would depend upon the reasser-
tion of values existing before the subculture of the 1960s marginalised received behaviour. This has not proved to be the case. Freedom of sexual
association has once again become the norm in some places in the Western
World, while permanent partnerships are the ideal elsewhere. Personal responsibility in many ways is very much back in fashion. It is difficult to
know how much of that difference compared with twenty years ago can
be credited to a change in sexual mores, in turn due to AIDS.

The tragedy with AIDS, which will make the impact far worse than appears at the time of writing, is the long, long incubation period. This makes the situation far graver than anyone is now (1989) prepared to admit in public. AIDS could, for example, destroy one-third of the population of tropical Africa. As in the case of the bubonic plague in Europe six hundred years ago, this would have profound consequences. Because it is currently incurable, AIDS is the first disease since 1347 which is likely to have similar consequences to the Black Death.

Apart from the special consequences of the diseases described, there are four general effects of disease in history.

First, there was nothing that the individual could do about most diseases before about 1800, when smallpox inoculation became available. Then there was an interval. All the great advances in bacteriology and medicine have virtually been in the last century. The major diseases already described had general and important effects, of which the individual certainly was not aware at the time. Usually the nature of the disease was not known to contemporaries.

Disease trimmed and reduced populations. Chronic diseases were present in Eurasian populations most of the time. The more obvious were malaria and smallpox, which many survivors suffered more than once. But it is likely that more people died from alimentary disorders than from all other causes put together. These ranged from typhoid to dysentery to various local enteric fevers to salmonella. Stomach diseases do not need mosquitoes, or rats, or lice. Enteric disorders cycle and recycle, between the human, his sewage and his water supply. Local populations can become tolerant of a local set of organisms which will kill the visitor. In the days before piped water supplies travellers were often in grave danger. Safe sewage and water systems were not in place in most of Western Europe much before 1900. Sometimes the water improvements cleared up the local trouble before the medical men had properly diagnosed the nature of the problem.

The second effect of disease followed from the first. Dense communities were not really self-supporting in statistical terms until recently. Large towns encouraged all sorts of infections, and often required five to ten times as many immigrants to supplement those who survived perinatal death. In London, before 1750, death-rates would range from 5–10 per cent of a population then above half a million. This figure would include all deaths, including those from diseases not noticed here, TB, cancer and influenza. Children of every age would be included. The crude death-rate of adults was double the number of baptisms, and probably three to four times the number of conceptions.

Between 15,000 and 20,000 immigrants a year (or more than 3 per cent) were needed just to maintain numbers. Later, immigrants increased the total population. Other cities were in the same position. It is almost certain that great centres in the Third World are in the same position today, but no reliable statistics exist. Calcutta, for example, must bear much resemblance to eighteenth-century London or Paris.

The third effect was when Europeans followed Columbus all over the world. They took with them a massive armoury of disease. This killed the natives at the point of contact, as described with Cortés and the Aztecs. This condition was repeated all over the world. Disease landed in the Americas, and spread ahead of the Europeans; disease landed in New Zealand and Australia with the first Europeans. By the time that later Europeans 'discovered' the Maoris of the centre of the North Island in New Zealand, or the Aborigines of the area north of what is now Adelaide, Australia, the natives were already suffering from syphilis, smallpox, influenza, measles and so forth. The same process fanned ahead of the Russians in Siberia and Central Asia, an Asian empire nearly twice the size of the United States.

Every area of the world has been transformed by the ecology of European disease. In the tropics, the local populations have been wholly rearranged, usually for reasons not unconnected with disease. Blacks were imported into the Americas; Indians replaced the natives in East Africa, Fiji or Malaya; Chinese coolies were taken all over the Pacific. Only in West Africa were the residual natives left alone after the slave trade was abolished. In temperate countries, native populations were largely destroyed and replaced by Europeans; the countries became neo-Europes. This process would have been impossible, if the native populations had been resistant to European diseases. As it was, the European victory was won by invisible allies who were never given the credit they deserved. In fact, it was often the microbes who deserved the medals, not the heroic men.

Finally, there has been the dramatic effect of curing disease. Apart from hygiene and sanitation which took place largely before 1914, advances in pathology have been most dramatic since 1945. Since that date, world population has increased by a rate much greater than in the previous forty years. Between 1905 and 1945, world population increased by less than 50 per cent. Between 1945 and 1985, it has just about doubled.

The great increase is due to an improvement in two areas, food supply and disease control. The dramatic increase in control over most of the diseases which have checked and trimmed populations since time began is the more obvious. Which is more important may appear to be evident later on in this book. The combination has sometimes been ecologically lethal.

There is one other possibility in the realm of disease about which there can be no kind of proof. It is possible that disease, which has for century after century been fighting a war with man's ability to resist pathogens, has now changed its very nature. It is possible that, instead of attacking anti-bodies directly, and provoking a form of warfare in which millions of active pathogens are defeated by millions of active defenders in the animal or human body, diseases may have changed into organisms which attack the immune system itself. There are three human diseases; two in cattle; one in sheep; one in cats; they were unknown a generation ago, and now threaten each species rather seriously. This is very important for mankind, if correct. Some of the animal diseases could well transfer to humans. Humans, in turn, could not defeat these diseases *en masse*. It is possible that by the end of the century, pathologists and biotechnologists may have defeated AIDS's ability to destroy the immune system. But how could humans defeat twenty different diseases, each of them behaving like AIDS, none of them transferred sexually? Such a course would restore disease to its traditional role as one of the Forces of Change. Such a future might quite easily terrify the optimists. On the other hand, it would be a rather *elegant* cure for the population/pollution problems which now exist. These are rendered all the more powerful because of the defeat of the conventional diseases which attack human anti-bodies.[54]

Notes

1   It is almost certain that a woman in New Mexico died of undiagnosed bubonic plague in 1987. A new theory about mutation in the basic bacterium *Yersinia pestis* was developed at the University of Umea, Sweden in 1987–8. This was disputed by Professor Gillett of the London School of Hygiene and Tropical Medicine in August 1988.
2   If a disease killed more of the animal host than it did of humans, it would very quickly reduce itself, the disease, to impotence. Or, more properly, the disease would never have become a threat of any kind, let alone a pandemic or epidemic.
3   The nursery rhyme 'Ring-a-ring-a-roses' refers to the string of lesions round the waist, found in people with bubonic-type plague. 'Atish-oo, atish-oo, we all fall down', relates to the pneumonic method of spreading the disease by droplet exchange.
4   India, 1907–25; Manchuria, 1920; Egypt and East Africa, 1930s; China, 1945.
5   Millennialism named after hysterical feelings current in AD 1000 that Christ would return to earth 1,000 years after his birth. This apocalyptic faith is commoner in the Jewish and some other Eastern faiths. But it was the anti-papal party in the Middle Ages, and the German and Swiss reformers who later encouraged a belief that the end of the world was nigh. It was not difficult to find converts at the time of the Black Death. Superstition overcame belief: scepticism replaced curiosity; some people refused to think or feel at all about the future, living only for the present. Amongst others, the same choice as was presented in time of trouble in Rome: drink deep, be merry, for tomorrow, we die. Or become a stoic, albeit perhaps a Christian stoic, and survive.

6   The Paston Letters present a picture of life in Norfolk in the years 1422–1509. The Paston family rose socially from being prosperous peasants, cultivating about 40 hectares (99 acres), ('kulaks' in Stalinist terminology) to the Earldom of Yarmouth. They rose by marriage, education, the Law, fast footwork during the Wars of the Roses, from 1455–85, and sheer ability during several generations. The important point here is the effect of the plague upon their lives, even as late as the late fifteenth century.

7   France, 1789; most of Germany, 1808; Austria, 1811; Hungary, 1813; Russia, 1861.

8   William H. McNeill, who first popularized the effects of disease in history, with his brilliant book, *Plagues and Peoples* (1977), also attaches great importance to the factors which, by their epidemiological effects, have an important new causative significance when the factor is abandoned. McNeill has drawn attention (amongst others) to the problems arising from the absence of dirt, also known as cleanliness (poliomyelitis); the use of fast steamships instead of slower sailing vessels, which gave too little time for the incubation of certain diseases; and cultivation of waste ground as populations increased which destroyed the habitat, not only of rodent hosts of bubonic plague, but also of malarial mosquito. McNeill's book in no way suggests the idea of any control system operating as between disease, food supply and population growth. With the prudence of a professional historian, he does not extend his arguments further than colleagues can be carried. There is also a vast literature of a usually anthropological nature about the link between demography and disease. Numbers are often lacking in these papers. McNeill's illustrations of the disease-factor and of weaponry (*The Pursuit of Power*) were, he said, to make good deficiencies in his *magnum opus, The Rise of the West*. If so, he is one of the few historians who has written a great work and then two more, as 'footnotes' in his own phrase. These acts of amplification to an already major effort must place him on the shortest of short lists of contemporary historians.

9   It is worth noting that Mamelukes recruited their successors each year from the steppes. The Mamelukes, most of them being castrated, reproduced by buying blue-eyed blond boys from Circassia. This lasted from 1382 until Napoleon brought the system to an end in 1798. The plague effect was that Egypt became the worst affected place in the Mediterranean after the key date, 1382. The side-effect was that Egyptian decadence, assisted by the lack of Mameluke commitment to the future, rendered Egypt a soft target. The true rulers of Egypt remained what they had always been, even after the Turkish triumph in 1517: the ratio between population growth, a nearly fixed food supply provided by the Nile flood, and the plague which modified the ratio. It was plague which kept the Egyptian population from exceeding the ancient total of 3–5 million before 1800. This ancient total was always within the ability of the marvellous Nile to afford a decent standard of life and, in Roman times, for example, to produce rations for another one million or two.

After Napoleon (and Nelson) cut the umbilical and plague-producing cord between Circassia and Cairo in 1798, matters changed. Plague modified itself in Egypt, ceasing to be chronic; the next serious outbreak was in 1844, by which time population had increased from 3.5 million to 5 million. By 1900, it was 10 million, by 1950, 20 million, and today it is well over 50 million. By 2000 it could be 65 million. Cairo, capital of this unbridled country heading for population-induced poverty, has a population of about 20 million. Most of them are very poor, living in shantytowns, alive only because of the healthy climate, which makes many diseases 'unsuccessful'.

10 More than a third of all cardinals, bishops and archdeacons died between May 1348 and March 1350 in Western Europe.

11 In 1988–90 the English suffered the same phenomenon. There was the substitution of the community charge for the rates (a property tax). There were cries of 'Poll Tax' and shades of 1381, when Wat Tyler's march on London led to a general rising against lawyers, serfdom, and the right to rent land for low cash payment, not for services rendered. In fact, the grievances of the peasantry were general; it was the occasion of the change in tax base which triggered the revolt. The same phenomenon has occurred in France, Germany and other countries. It probably happens because the tax-paying classes are temporarily united with the poor in resisting a change for the worse in their circumstances.

12 Wolves became bolder, taking animals and young children in daylight; the habit of huddling in villages, abandoning isolated houses, became *de rigueur* in many Continental countries.

13 In 1340, most of the population was directly engaged in agriculture. If, in 1340, 90 per cent of the population in any area lived in villages of less than, say, 250 people, then in 1400, that proportion would have been reduced to about 75 per cent. See footnote 22, this chapter.

14 Most European forests thus date from 1350 or later.

15 Huge numbers of foxes reverse-commute today into towns, at night, to feed. Others live in waste areas and in parks in towns. Perhaps 50 per cent of the fox-population in modern England is urban, but not for the same reason as in the fifteenth century.

16 Post-plague returns for seed sown/seed harvested rose in Western Europe as follows: wheat, from 4.1 to 5.5; barley, 3.7 to 4.8; oats, 2.5 to nearly 4. In some marginal areas, pre-plague ratios were below 2–1. After the plague, marginal areas were not cultivated.

17 East Germany and parts of Poland became comparable to the MidWest of the United States in the late nineteenth century: a granary for Western Europe.

18 It was herring which gave the Dutch a first chance to lift themselves. Herrings were an analogue to wool in England, and of the same kind of relative value to a country of one-third the English population.

19 People can use an abacus even if they can't count properly; the modern comparison is with check-out devices for the innumerate.

20 No idea of the volume of paper production is generally known, but other evidence suggests that by the time that printing came along, paper was available and plentiful in almost any market town. Certainly this was true in England when Caxton set up his press in Tothill Street, Westminster in 1477. Printing could never have occurred without the previous development of paper.

21 Clocks at Wells or Salisbury had not been reduced in any way to make them portable. Early mariners still used a sand-glass, marking off 30 minutes. Water-glasses were also available, more accurate since water is more fluid than sand, less accurate if not temperature compensated. 30-minute glasses were calibrated against known accurate clocks. Columbus set his by the cathedral clock at Cadiz, before crossing the Atlantic. Someone then turned it over every half-hour till he returned the next year. That was the theory. Medieval clocks were authentic and long-lived; that of Dover Castle, made in the plague year of 1348, was exhibited in accurate action at a Scientific Exhibition in 1876.

22 The village ethos in the pre-plague Middle Ages can be savoured today in a third world country. The collective decision is all important; consensus is promoted without the rigour of debate of an intellectual nature; there is normally only one answer to most questions. Present-day Europe has, in the end, the plague to thank for its freedom of choice.

23 Geoffrey Chaucer, 1345–1400, son of a tavern-keeper and wine-merchant of the City of London. Page in the service of the Duke of Clarence, 1357 or 1358. In the King's service in France, 1359. King granted him a pension in 1367, and he was on the royal service abroad in 1370, 1372–3, 1376, 1377, 1378. Much of his subject matter was derived from Boccaccio, see below, but Chaucer's output, in English, was probably greater. The first great English poet, Chaucer left his most important work till the prime of life, starting it in 1387, when 42. *The Canterbury Tales* was never finished, but remains the greatest work of the greatest English poet before Shakespeare two centuries later.

Giovanni Boccaccio, 1313–75. Unlike Chaucer, Boccaccio was an adult throughout the Plague. Until 1350, he was a successful courtier, story-teller, scholar, the romantic lover of the lady Fiammetta. After 1350, he became a diplomat, and an early Renaissance scholar. This worthy existence did not prevent him writing his most famous work, *The Decameron*. In this (not always bawdy) compilation, ten days are spent in escaping the Plague. Ten people (hence Decameron) seven women, three men, tell ten tales each, one hundred in all. The effect of this great collection of romantic and classical folk-tales which had wandered round Mediterranean civilizations for five hundred years was considerable. Amongst the English, Shakespeare, Sidney, Marston and Fletcher as well as Chaucer borrowed from the Decameron. So did French, Italian, Dutch, Spanish and German writers. So did Dryden, Keats, Tennyson, Longfellow, Swinburn and George Eliot. The Decameron is still being used as a source book, on television, almost daily. There is never any acknowledgement, of course.

24 William Langland, 1322–1400, author of *Piers Plowman*, wrote: 'So we need an antidote strong enough to reform these prelates who should pray for peace but are hindered by their possessions. Then take their land from them, you nobles, and let them live on their tithes. For surely, if property is a deadly poison that corrupts them, it would be good for Holy Church's sake to relieve them of it and purge them of this poison before it grows more dangerous . . .' Penguin ed., pp. 194–5.

25 The dominating theory of disease was the humoral, which has always subconsciously influenced thinkers on the subject. In this doctrine, the body contains four humours: blood, phlegm, yellow bile and black bile. Health is dependent upon the correct proportion and mixture. This passed into the psyche of ordinary, non-medical people ever since Hippocrates (?460–377 or 359 BC). More lasting was the Hippocratic oath, which was that service to the patient was of the highest importance; and the importance of the healing power of nature. It is vital to remember that in the Middle Ages there were few doctors of medicine in Western Europe, fewer still after the plague.

26 John Wyclif, 1329–84. Scholar and teacher at Oxford University, and Master of Balliol in 1360. In 1374 became Rector of Lutterworth, Leicestershire, and in the same year sent by the government on a mission to Bruges about Papal abuses. Wyclif believed that the temporal power should be paramount, that the secular power should control the clergy. The Pope became an enemy, who addressed bulls to the King, the Bishops and the University of Oxford. His allies were the common clergy, the merchants and some of the nobility. Wyclif started to

translate the Bible, denied priestly absolution, confessions, penances, and anticipated many of the Protestant objections to papal misuse of power which Luther
identified in 1517–22. Like Luther, Wyclif died in bed, but his bones were dug up
in 1428, burnt and cast into the river. His followers, the Lollards, survived till the
Reformation and his works influenced others such as Hus, see below.

John Hus, 1369–1415, son of a peasant in Bohemia. Educated Prague University; became Rector, 1402. Highly critical of senior clergy, followed Wyclif's
Lollard views, partly religious, partly social. From 1410, Hus preached
courageously against his spiritual enemies, and worked and wrote energetically
until driven from Prague by the Church Establishment. Even King Wenceslaus
could not save him. Seized, thrown into prison, tried at Constance in May 1415.
Burnt at the stake, 8 July 1415. His death was followed by an uprising of the
enraged Czechs against the Holy Roman Emperor, Sigismund, in the so-called
'Hussite Wars'.

27 The logic runs as follows. A parasite, to be successful, must multiply, like any
other species. It must not be so successful that it destroys its own host. (See
footnote 2, this chapter.) It is therefore essential that the host of the parasite should
survive, or that some hosts should survive. An ideal proportion has to be more
than half – this is in the verdant country which harbours both logic and pure
mathematics.

Both smallpox and measles could well have leapt out of animals, in which they
had proved to be less than successful. This was true of the transfer of myxomatosis
(a relative of smallpox) from the guinea-pigs of South America. Myxomatosis
passed through the Brazilian rabbit (which is not really a rabbit) into the European
rabbit in the neo-European country of Australia. Both transfers were effected by
men moving infected animals. This transfer has happened under the eyes of
pathologists from every kind of country. Amongst guinea-pigs, the disease was
relatively harmless, as it was in the other Latin American rodent, the Brazilian
rabbit. In the European rabbit, on the other hand, the death-rate was at least 98 per
cent at first, and over 95 per cent in every succeeding pandemic. The breeding
abilities of rabbits, however, are great enough to combat these huge losses; there
have been over 200 generations since the first introduction of myxomatosis into
Europe in the summer of 1952, and there are still many rabbits about. The rabbits,
however, have changed their habits. Survivors largely live above ground, perhaps
because folk memory suggests that a flea-spread disease is best avoided by
abandoning underground homes. The nature of European rabbits since 1953, their
habits, their social organization, all these have changed just as disease changes the
lifestyle of humans. Social scientists should be busy amongst the bunnies.

28 The first person in the world to be injected with live cowpox 'matter' was
eight-year-old James Phipps. That was in 1796 in the village of Berkeley in
Gloucestershire.

29 The Chinese, as always, had previously had a different method, which was for
the patient to breathe in live smallpox 'matter' into his nostrils through a straw.
This procedure had a death-rate of about one-fifth. It was fashionable amongst the
richer, most sophisticated Europeans before Jenner, and amongst Moslems. Lady
Mary Wortley Montague (1689–1762) wife of the then British ambassador to the
Porte in Constantinople in 1716, had brought this method back to England in
1721. It became general in Russia in the 1770s, and in France, because of Louis
XV's death from smallpox (1774). Frederick the Great of Germany introduced
inoculation into the court at Potsdam in the 1770s, and George Washington

inoculated a large proportion of the Revolutionary Army after Bunker Hill in 1776. It was notable that the conscientious objectors did not long survive.

30 These figures come from the *Imperial Encyclopaedia*, compiled in 1726 which repeats a great deal of the work of the scholar Ssu-ma Kuang, of the Sung Dynasty (960–1279). See William H. McNeill: *Plagues and Peoples.*

31 English judges still carry these posies in official processions, though prisoners are no longer lousy.

32 There is, of course, always a danger that a new strain of disease will prove lethal, or will emulate chicken-pox and encourage a relative into the human body. Chicken-pox, now relatively harmless, permits the ingress of the parasite which causes shingles many years later. Shingles is painful, quite unlike chicken-pox.

33 Death from disease was often considered a kinder fate than public execution.

34 Japan only became obviously lousy and carrying any kind of typhus in the summer of 1945; it is possible that the pathogen was brought over from Korea or China, and that the national breakdown at the end of World War II made it too difficult to contain the disease by hygiene.

35 All negroes are black. All blacks are not necessarily negroes. In this book, a negro is one who has sickle-cell anemia, and therefore an antidote to malaria in the blood-genes. The importance of this recessive factor is explained at length in the Quinine chapter of *Seeds of Change* by Henry Hobhouse, Sidgwick & Jackson, London, 1985.

36 The four pre-Renaissance slave-routes were from Timbuktu to what is now modern Algeria; from Lake Chad to what is modern Tripoli; from East Africa down the Nile; from Ethiopia and East Africa to Oman. Only the slaves gathered to walk north via Timbuktu would have come from a place where *falciparium* malaria was endemic.

37 The connection between stagnant, dirty water and the yellow fever mosquito raises the question of how the disease ever started in a world in which humans were not densely packed enough to produce dirt, and stagnant water. There has to be a satisfactory philosophic explanation.

38 There are numerous cases of female cooks, bakers, dairymaids, acting as carriers over many years. The longest known case was for fifty-two years, during which the woman showed no signs of the disease. How many men did she infect?

39 Unlike typhoid dysentery was in no way affected by the introduction of Florence Nightingale and her nurses in 1855.

40 In some armies, anti-typhoid vaccines were in use as early as World War I.

41 The antiseptic virtues of alcohol provided a fashionable excuse for the ingestion of hard liquor. Earlier, it was the reason for the use of wine and water mixtures, and of 'small beer', a very weak brew which, however, was safe to drink. Hot drinks were also safer than water.

42 Pilgrimages have always been great disease distributors. In India, it was the confluence of Hindus at the holy city of Benares that spread cholera throughout Hindustan; in Europe, it was returning pilgrims from Jerusalem who were responsible for bringing back one kind of tuberculosis. Pilgrims to Mecca exchanged and encouraged smallpox. Pilgrims to Canterbury or Rome spread disease on both outward and return trips. The Pilgrim Fathers, to make a point, brought smallpox, measles, and influenza to the Amerindians of Massachusetts, even though it is known that some sort of killer-disease had already spread from the French in Nova Scotia in 1616–18. The point is made. Pilgrims who, in the

Middle Ages, may have out-travelled soldiers or sailors, spread disease wherever they went, as did every other traveller.

43   Sir Almroth Wright, 1861–1947, was responsible for training innumerable fellow doctors in the pathology of parasites. In World War I, he successfully introduced antityphoid inoculation into the British Army. He was present, as a young student, at the early lectures by people like Robert Koch, whose work on septicemia (1880) led to his identification of the TB bacillus in 1882, and of cholera in 1883. Wright, in turn, gave Alexander Fleming (1881–1955) the impulse to develop penicillin with Howard Florey (1898–1965) and Ernest Chain (1906–79). Since Robert Koch had sat at the feet of both Lister (1827–1912) and Pasteur (1822–95), there is a fine, almost apostolic succession through the work of Almroth Wright.

44   By the 1960s, it was predicted that 'most' disease would be eliminated. One has been officially 'abolished' – smallpox. If it ever returned, the carnage would be at a level comparable to the Black Death, since inoculation was also 'abolished'. Measles, chicken-pox, German measles, whooping cough and some other childish diseases have been controlled by prophylactic inoculation or vaccination. Malaria, once optimistically put into the 'to be abolished' column, has, in fact, become much more serious, perhaps now affecting 10 per cent of the human race.

45   The non-Columbian explanation involves yaws, a spirochetes-infective disease which resembles leprosy in its worst effects; it shares with syphilis only its transmission by spirochetes. Syphilis is venereally transferred. Yaws is spread by a spirochete, indistinguishable from that of syphilis, but entering the body through non-venereal contact. Yaws was probably classed as 'leprosy' in the Middle Ages, if it had not then died out. After Columbus, syphilis broke out virulently in Europe, travelling everywhere by venereal means. Yet the yaws' spirochete and that of syphilis are hard to tell apart. The only explanation, if the non-Columbian history be correct, is that the spirochete abandoned one method of transferring itself from host to host, and changed the paths of infection which would be essential in view of the different methods of entry into the human system. This is not impossible, but as has already been said in the text, unconvincing.

46   Apart from syphilis, the only other notable Amerindian diseases were Carrion's disease and Chaga's. Neither of them survives a journey across the Atlantic. See Manson's *Tropical Diseases*, Baltimore, Williams and Wilkins, 1972.

47   Such a community might have been the descendants of those survivors from the mutineers in HMS *Bounty*. But by now, the inhabitants of Pitcairn Island have been disturbed too much to be a suitable case for investigation. By 1858, only a few families were willing to remain on the island. By 1900, the survivors were showing 'a deterioration of morals, intellect and energy'. Are these not the symptoms also shown by some Amerindians, but not others?

48   In societies in danger of collapse through inbreeding, this hospitality may have offered the tribe a genetic pathway to survival. In other words, it could have been a strong instinct.

49   Historically, plebs have always sought to acquire more power, or equality, or social justice. Patrician resistance to this process required overt acts of wisely deployed strength. A minor weakening of the patrician resolve would result in loss of power.

50   The BBC produced an extraordinary mini-series on TV about the Borgias. Replete with Renaissance cruelty and lust, and wonderfully caparisoned, it provoked one critic to complain that there was too much sex, a lot of it incestuous.

The tone of the series was explained, said the TV critic of the *Financial Times*, if you realized that the following exchange took place: Cesare Borgia, to his sister, Lucrezia: 'You're better in bed than Mum.' To which Lucrezia replied: 'That's what Dad says.'

51 In 1319, one fine at Avignon for Indulgences was as follows: 'A nun who has abandoned herself to several men in succession, either in or outside her convent, and wants to rise to the rank of abbess, should pay 131 pounds.' This was quite a lot of money, about £500,000 in today's coin. But it would not have saved anyone from the scourge of syphilis.

52 Both China and the USSR, as well as other countries, are using blood-tests to control the entry of long-term visitors suspected of carrying either HIV (Human Immunodeficiency Virus) or subsequent AIDS. It appears positive that HIV must precede AIDS by a gap of at least 6 months and not more than 6 years. HIV has been traced in tears, saliva, and urine, but it is still believed (in the United States) that no evidence exists for believing that HIV may be transmitted through an exchange of these fluids. People in Africa are not so sure. A new cause of death has crept into the literature, AIDS-related complex, or ARC. It appears likely that infected people can proceed from HIV to ARC without AIDS itself being diagnosed. It should be stated at this point, perhaps, that the effect of HIV, AIDS or ARC on human conduct is multiplied many times by the horror of the form of death and the prominence of homosexual or promiscuous media people who figure as victims. If a million people actually die of the syndrome, it is a fair calculation that ten or twenty times as many will avoid the disease by modifying lifestyles. This happened with syphilis since many early victims were aristocrats whose example was in those days followed.

53 The task is made more difficult by the very nature of the disease's attack upon the immune system. Every other successful 'cure' has reinforced the anti-bodies or stimulated their production. This is not possible in the case of drugs designed to combat AIDS.

54 The word *elegant* in this connection is wholly scientific, as is its use on page 69.

CHAPTER TWO

Bread to
Make the Old World Strong

The steady rise in world population since the fifteenth century has only been made possible by increased food supply. In 1492, in Western Europe, there was more food available per head than ever before, and the techniques to increase this potential still further were known. No one knew it at the time, but only in Western Europe were there means of feeding the whole world five hundred years later. It would be technology worked out by unscientific men which would produce the first increases; much of the daily practice on farms in the Renaissance was similar to what had been good husbandry in the days of Virgil. The way to achieve it was different: animals instead of men; mills, driven by wind and water; much more flesh eaten than in Roman days. These improvements to classical methods were sufficient until the ratio of humans to land changed as much as it did during the fourteenth century. First, the enormous increase in population in the century before the Black Death; then the loss of more than a third of the people in most areas. This tended to break up the feudal system in proportion to the increase in population from a base sometime about AD 800.

The second great challenge to the methods of the time was in the period before and during the Industrial Revolution. In the second half of the eighteenth century, the English population had increased by more than half; in the next fifty years, it more than doubled. In the hundred years 1750–1850, the population increased by three times, from 5.5 million to 16.5 million, and 2 million people emigrated. Nearly all this increase was produced by English food and, allowing for horses and other animals not normally eaten, such as dogs, every English human was being fed by English soil even in 1850. This was a massive achievement.

There was some hunger, some starvation even, but in an age in which there was little surplus in the Northern Hemisphere, and none at all in the Southern, the English were the first people to have fed themselves from their own soil, yet support such an increase in population. They improved their agriculture in a way which made the Industrial Revolution possible. This was by increasing output per acre. The problem of usefully using every possible acre was answered by the rough and

*ready method of enclosure. This was again a cruel policy at the margin: the many
benefited but a few suffered. But it was a uniquely successful solution to a problem
which was peculiar to Europe, and thus at that time in the world.*

*This chapter is not in any way wholly about England or English husbandry; but
Europe and England taught the world. It was population pressure which made the
English success essential: failure would have resulted in a very different story,
without an Industrial Revolution, without the defeat of Napoleon, and without the
survival of an unprecedented (and unrepeated) increase of population in an already
densely populated land. Unlike every other European country, England avoided
revolution: for that too, agricultural husbandry has largely to be thanked.*

Western Europeans had acquired from the East by 1492 most of the techniques from which they were likely to benefit. After this date, technological leadership, then scientific research and application, passed to the West.
Some of the *technological drift* from China was, in 1492, of recent origin.
Some was yet to come. There were advances which applied to food
production. Cast iron as a technique only occurred in the West in about
1250, so ploughs were made of wood. The concave mouldboard, used in
China in the ninth century BC, took twenty-five centuries to arrive in the
West. The first formulae for the correct dynamic angles for a turnover
plough were not worked out until Thomas Jefferson performed the
mathematics in the 1790s. He was unaware of Chinese scripts only
uncovered by Western scholars more than a century later.

Though the humble wheelbarrow was invented in China and transferred to the West as late as about AD 1200, the most important improvement
to help husbandry was animal harness which the Chinese had invented
nearly ten centuries before. The breast strap was not widely used in
Western Europe before the twelfth century, and the more efficient breast
collar, which did not cut the horse's windpipe, until later. Both were an
improvement on the Roman sling, which was a rope round the neck
passing between the legs, under the belly, to the implement being pulled.

In some countries, notably Ireland, and some of the Baltic provinces,
horses were hitched to the plough by the tail, a practice which limited the
draught to less than a tenth of that available from the same horse using a
modern harness. Partly for the harness reason, partly because horses were
more expensive and more uncommon and partly because of disease, oxen
were preferred as draught animals before 1492. Teams of two were
normal, three were used; a four in hand was a sign of heavy soil, or
affluence. Regardless of number, oxen, which also had the advantage of
working without shoes, walked at half the speed of horses. They also had a
longer working life, were not subject to as many health problems, and
were less attractive as loot. They also provided more and better meat when

slaughtered at the end of their lives. Before 1492, they were yoked or the draught-trace was fixed to their horns. Either way, efficiency was low.

In 1492, 'Agriculture' within the European experience was limited to three areas. There was, in Egypt, a perfect system, more than 4,000 years old, which used the Nile flood and the water and alluvial mud from the Central African highlands. The flood was in August each year. It produced enough plant food to grow a good crop of wheat or barley. The water not only provided enough moisture to grow the crop but, before planting, it killed all the living weeds on the stubble of last year's corn. The crop was planted in the late autumn, when the flood subsided, and harvested in the late spring, after say, 180 days of growth. The stubble burnt in the summer sun, destroying micro-organisms which in other climates would have prejudiced continuous corn production. Then the reliable flood came again, and the process was repeated.

The Egyptian system was a perfect example of a sustainable man-made pattern which cropped nature, and did not exploit or threaten the balance. The ecosystem was not dependent upon science, industrial tools, or added power. As it had existed since 2500 BC, it was capable of feeding up to 10 million Egyptians. More normally, as in Roman times, the Nile fed, say, 4 million at home, and enough was exported to feed the same number again abroad.

In 1492, the population of Egypt was much as it had been in Roman times, 4 million. It was held in check by a whole catalogue of diseases. There were alluvial, flood-irrigated, river-basin cultures operating in China, India, Burma, Siam and so forth, about which Europeans knew little. There were also, in what is now modern Iraq, the Tigris-Euphrates basin, and single river cultures in Greece, Italy and Spain, and in many areas of the Maghreb. There were also, unknown to Europeans, systems at work in the Americas. There was a quite different system at work in Holland, the Po Valley and parts of England. For obvious reasons, irrigation was not an option to those times for a massive increase in food supply. Drainage, with windmills, used after 1350, had reached a plateau before steam came to the rescue. Modern techniques, which make water-use far more efficient, depend upon power to dig channels and build dams, pipes to prevent evaporation loss, and power to pump and distribute water, often by overhead irrigation. In 1492, it is entirely possible that irrigation had reached a limit dictated by the state of the art rather than by economics. There were two other systems with which the Western Europeans were familiar.

The first was the hot climate, Mediterranean, dry-farming technique. The purpose of cultivation in these areas was to conserve moisture, kill weeds, and to grow the best possible crop every second year, or two years out of three.

The techniques of Mediterranean farming had reached a plateau in the first century BC, and were described by Virgil in a passage from the *First Georgic* which could not be improved upon at any time before 1492.

First, learn the peculiarities of your soil and climate. Plough the fallow in the early spring; plough frequently, twice in winter, and twice in summer unless your land is poor, in which case a light ploughing in September will suffice.

Either let the land lie fallow every other year, or else let spelt [wheat] follow pulse, vetches or lupins.

Repetition of one crop exhausts the ground; rotation will lighten the strain; exhausted crops must be well-dressed with manure or ashes. It often does good to burn stubble.

Irrigation benefits a sandy soil; draining a marsh.

Geese and crane and other birds; mildew and weeds are all enemies of the crop.

Careful annual selection of the seed by hand must be the only way to prevent degeneration.

Virgil wrote these lines about 35 BC, and read them to the Emperor Augustus five years later. Like the advice given by Pliny, Varro and all the other writers on agriculture, 'Geoponici', the *Georgics* were in verse, intended for a verbal society, which did not know anything about printing or much about reading.[1]

In North-West Europe, the food production problem was quite different. There was a much older tradition of flesh-eating. As population density rose, the hunter had to become a herdsman. Originally, there cannot have been much difference.[2]

By the time of the stable Roman Empire, with its boundaries on the Rhine and the Danube, Germans in clearings in their gloomy forests were using ploughs as well as living off herds of cattle. The ploughs they later used were claimed to be unique, different to the Mediterranean implements, an answer to the problem of cultivation in heavy soils. Modern research suggests that such claims as those that say that Germans or Slavs gave Europe the true heavy plough in about AD 600 are romantics. The logic is not easily answered.

A plough differs from any handheld digging implement in that the traction of the plough through the soil does the work, and does it continuously. Traction from the draught team is transmitted through the beam and pole and to the stock; this has a leading point which lays nearly horizontal and does the actual job. The stock might well be formed of a tree branch and in the simplest ploughs, the stock and pole might be formed in one piece. The handle which on Greek or Roman ploughs was single, would be attached to the tree-branch of another wood, usually oak. These were the ploughs which evolved all over the Western world before Christ. In some, favoured places, iron was cheap enough to clothe the wearing point of the plough; in others, flints or other hard pebbles were inserted in holes in the wood. The iron 'shoe' would, of course, be used again and again, the wooden parts of the plough having a much shorter life.

Ploughing has always involved huge inputs of power. A hectare of land ploughed to a depth of 10 cm (4 in) involves shifting 1,000 tons of dirt; a depth of 15 cm (6 in) 1,500 tons; a depth of 20 cm (8 in) 2,000 tons. Today, this takes a man and a pair of carefully bred horses, working effectively at about 2 kph (1 mph), about 20 hours. No pair of horses could do more than 8 hours a day at this work, so that 2 hectares, or about 5 acres, was work for 5 days; one day's light work, and one rest day made up the week.[3]

There was at one time a great school of Anglo-Saxon revisionists who produced a golden pre-Norman past which included a heavy wheeled plough, drawn by eight oxen. This was said to have been brought by Teutonic invaders soon after the Roman withdrawal. These early Anglo-Saxons changed the landscape, the myth continues, by bringing into cultivation the heavy clay lands of the Midlands. Yet these stories from some golden past no more stand up to analysis than does King Arthur. In fact, Camelot is probably easier to 'prove'.[4]

The habit which the Saxons *did* bring to England was that of flesh-eating. In the post-Roman centuries, with the density of population probably existing in the Midlands, much more food would have been produced per acre by grazing cattle or sheep than by trying to grow wheat instead of grass. On a Midland pasture, of a low botanical composition (largely agrostis, not much clover) and without any input of fertilizer, the annual yield could be of the order of at least 50 kg of beef per hectare (45 lb per acre), twice as much as lamb. This far exceeds the net yield of grain at the same date, with the technology then available. It was only the density of human population, demanding high grain output per acre which dictated the ploughing of clay lands. It is unlikely that this took place much before the time of King Alfred (849–900). The population of England after the retirement of the Romans in the fifth century is unlikely to have exceeded 600,000. Population did not reach the high Roman figure of 800,000 before Alfred's reign. At the time of the Domesday survey (1086), it was about twice that of Alfred's time. Despite Danish invasion, or because of Viking vigour, the population doubled in less than two centuries, a high rate of increase at the time. If the clay lands had to be cultivated, it would not have been until the High Saxon Age during and after Alfred the Great.[5]

Having been ploughed, the soil has to be harrowed in order to break down the clods or to make a tilth for the seeds to be able to germinate. The rule is simple. The bigger the seed, the coarser the tilth; winter-sown grain requires a cloddier tilth than grain sown in the spring, so as to protect seedlings from the winter weather; in some soils, too fine a tilth produces too many weeds. Grain is at one end of the condition required; onion seed is at the other. Both were widely grown from 2000 BC all over the Mediterranean. Harrows of all types are used to prepare the ground and cover the seed. They have probably been used longer than ploughs. In suitable wooded country, they can be made in an hour by cutting thorns from bushes. But man-made harrows, wood frames into which were fitted iron spikes, were used from Roman times. So were roller harrows, made of tree-trunks spiked with large iron nails. Horse draught came in for breaking down clods, or covering the soil, on account of the speed of the horse and its ability to beat the changeable weather of the Atlantic countries. The square or triangular wooden or steel frame with spikes is still widely used. But there are other modern harrows, based on steel technology, and using discs, or chains, or springs. These were all developed in the nineteenth century. More recently, the power take-off available on oil-driven tractors has given birth to power-driven harrows which can produce the correct tilth at one 'pass' of the tractor; these can change the nature of tilth during work to suit difficult fields with several soil types. As with modern ploughs, these implements move tons of earth in each hour of work.

Sowing seed is still most efficiently performed by hand. No implement can beat a good man walking at 5 kph (3 mph), with the seed in a sheet suspended from his shoulder. It is the cultural necessity to place fertilizer in close proximity to seed which justifies the expensive and complicated seed-drills now in use. Nor can men be found to walk the distances required to do a day's work as a biblical sower. Such a task for a day would involve 40 km (25 miles) in 9 hours of sowing, planting in all, 20 hectares (50 acres). Such a machine-beating output can be achieved only in a few industries, and in very few operations. But men do not like such effort, today, even in agriculture.

Harvesting is another matter altogether. The scythe man, served by two or more men or women tying up the sheaves, was known in the Middle Ages, even in Roman times. Sickles of every shape and size were developed in the Middle Ages. But it was commoner to harvest in earlier times by merely cutting off the heads of grain. Carts were used for this purpose by pre-Roman British Celts, and very efficient they were, capable of harvesting 10 hectares (25 acres) a day, with one or two men pushing the cart, and another two emptying it at the end of a 'bout'. A gleaner was, of course, also needed, to pick up short-strawed grain missed by the cart, which had fixed in front a device described by Pliny as a harvesting comb. These carts were pushed, in the Mediterranean, by slaves, mules or oxen, in Britain by one or two men, never by horses. Grain was threshed by hand in a basket, or by a winnowing fan, hand-held and operated, or by the wind, which is free. Not until the seventeenth century did the winnowing machine reach Western Europe from China. Less delicate means of threshing, or 'disintegration' as engineers put it, included treading the grain with oxen, still used in 1950 in Eastern Europe; the simple threshing stick gave way to the hinged flail, about 100 BC, and still in use; there was an especial, and violent sledge, which was dragged across the cut corn to separate the grain from the chaff; this was widely used in Mediterranean countries; in many parts of Atlantic Europe, heads of grain were scorched or burnt to make them digestible for human beings or animals. In this way, grinding the grain could be avoided.[6]

Burnt grain could be turned into a porridge-like substance, pre-toasted by the fire. Perhaps this is why no neolithic querns or threshing stones have been discovered in non-Roman Europe. Ireland, North Germany, and the Scandinavian countries all burnt grain at one time. Burning grain to make it edible is a very simple method, cheap, effective, and low-tech. Sometimes, further disintegration took place after burning the grain to 'thresh' it. The use of the pestle and mortar was widespread before winnowing techniques became widely available.[7]

At some point in every civilization in the thousand years before Christ, pounding the grain was split into two operations. The first separated the grain from the chaff. The second ground up the grain to make it more easily eaten by man or beast. If the grain was burnt, then only the second operation was required. In the Mediterranean countries, the pestle and mortar gave way to grindstones or querns.

The pestle is not to be despised. It was the first hand tool which was not only mechanized, but automated. The pestle and mortar was arranged to be operated by ropes and the return spring induced by an adjacent growing tree. This 'mechanized' the operation at low cost, and the tree required no daily food.

To automate the operation, some bright person living alongside a stream invented a device involving the pestle, operated on a beam, the end of which was arranged with a bucket. The bucket was attached at such an angle so that it filled in the stream, lifted the pestle, and then rose; at the top, it emptied; on emptying, the bucket permitted the pestle to fall. Fully

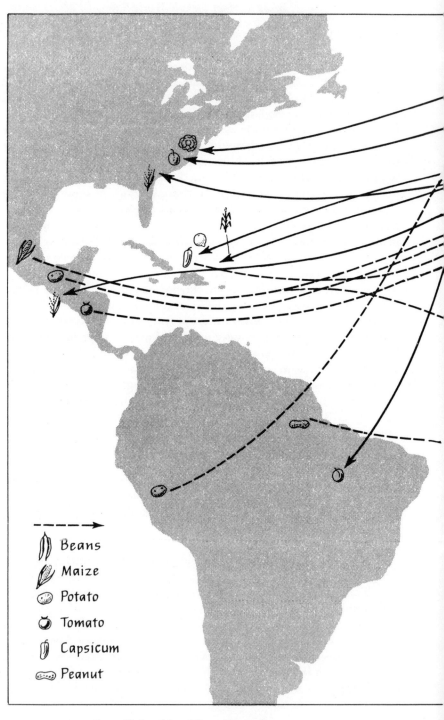

Legend

- ⫮ Beans
- 🌽 Maize
- 🥔 Potato
- 🍅 Tomato
- 🌶 Capsicum
- 🥜 Peanut

Post-Columbian Plant Transfers

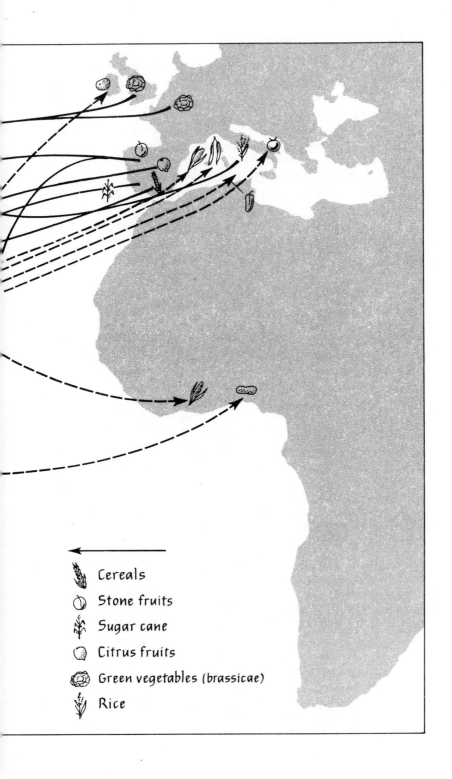

Cereals

Stone fruits

Sugar cane

Citrus fruits

Green vegetables (brassicae)

Rice

automated machines of this type were in use in mountainous districts at least as early as 500 BC. They were probably the first automated machines in the world.

Pounding was used for the staples of the ancient world: grain, oil and wine. Olive oil and wine grapes were both pounded in such a way that the stone or pips did not disintegrate and spoil the oil or grapejuice. At some point the three forms of pounding separated. Grain was ground rather than bashed. Olives were ultimately crushed in a *trapetum*, which was a rotary mill with a minimum clearance of 1.8 cm, or one Roman inch.[8] This prevented the stones being ground and entering the oil barrel attached. Wine grapes were pressed by feet, by beam presses tightened by levers, pulleys and ropes, and ultimately by screw presses, which tightened the mass of pulp between two wooden plates the size of large, square tables. The means of tightening were two wooden screws. Presses of this type for wine and cider survive into the present. They were developed about 100 BC, and in use all over Western Europe.

Unleavened 'bread' or flatcakes, baps, scones, tortillas, biscuits or wafers can be made of any cereal. Some sort of 'flatbread' can be made of wheat, rye, barley, oats, rice, millet, teff and sorghum, all of which are Old World cereals, and from buckwheat, which is a pseudo-cereal. Only of *wheat* can true leavened bread be made. Over the past five hundred years, wheat has been taken all over the world, and it has become the world's most important cereal. This position was gained only because of the unique bread-making quality of wheat. This, in turn, depends upon gluten content. Gluten is the product of cereal protein, ground up and mixed with water. When further mixed with yeast, gluten will expand to accommodate the gases produced by the yeast, mostly harmless carbon dioxide. Gluten has this extraordinary property that it expands to accommodate the gases, yet resists the expansion, and contains the gas, so that the risen bread is light, bubbly, digestible, and attractive to eat.[9]

Rye, the ancient cereal of northern countries, poor soils, and cool, moist climates, has protein which produces very weak glutens. Rye bread can therefore be made, but it rises very little. The result is dense, heavy, black or dark brown. Most modern rye breads contain wheat flour to help the poor gluten content of rye bread. Most rye is used in the developed world for hardbread, or crispbread, or for making spirituous liquor. As recently as 1956, Western Germany grew more rye than wheat, and the same was true of Eastern Germany until 1966.[10]

Rye bread is 'slimming' because it contains a high proportion of pentosan compounds which swell in the stomach, absorb large quantities of water, and take a long time to digest. All this gives an impression of fullness. Rye is almost unknown in southern Europe; it is typically the bread grain of the great European plain, running from the Rhine to the Urals. Until after World War II, it was difficult to cultivate wheat in these dry, sandy soils. Rye is now considered a poor man's bread, except for the fashionable crispbread which has been argued into the diet of every self-conscious slimmer.[11]

Barley was as important as wheat in the ancient world. Barley needs less time to grow, and has a wider adaptability, from the Equator to the Arctic Circle. It needs less moisture than wheat, and is today the preferred cereal for beer of all kinds. In the Middle Ages, barley was the staple of the southern peasantry as was rye in northern climes. Both rye and barley are less demanding of the soil than wheat, and easier to grow. Barley is a grand animal feed. The cultivation of barley on some soils in England has extended beyond what was thought possible a generation ago. One field in Somerset, England, grew continuous barley for thirty years from 1952 The average yield, on a rolling, five-year basis went up from 3,150 kg/ha to 7,750 kg/ha (2,804 lb/a to 6,898 lb/a) in the same period. Of no other cereal has such a record of continuous production of increasing output ever been made.

Barley is still the staple crop of the Middle East, but is most important in the West for its ability to produce malt. Malt in turn is the product of barley grains which have been allowed to germinate in a controlled way. Malt contains an enzyme amylase, which turns starch into sugar. This can be used to turn starch into the sugars which in turn are converted by yeast into alcohol. Alternatively, malt can be used in baking, to make a mildly sweet, nutty range of cakes and breads.[12]

Greeks and Romans thought *Oats* merely a diseased form of wheat. In Northern Europe, especially in Scotland, it became a crop which supported the people.[13] Today, only 5 per cent is eaten directly by humans. It is allegedly good for fast horses. For humans, milk, oats and herrings were one of the cheapest balanced diets in Europe a hundred years ago. This diet supported many a poor Scots undergraduate. Oats contain far more fat than wheat, together with an enzyme which digests the fat. The endosperm contains a natural anti-oxidant, furfural, which can be used as a benign preservative in foods like potato crisps, nuts, instant coffee, margarine. Some varieties of oats yield a narcotic, which was the only use to which the Romans put the plant. An excessive dose of this infusion can be lethal. Is this how the Romans used the cereal, and was this why they thought the oat was a diseased, evil form of wheat?

Rice was unknown in the Ancient Mediterranean. It was brought west from India by the Muslims after Muhammad's death. The Moors grew large quantities in Spain, and it is possible that in 1492, it was a familiar cereal for Columbus and his crew. Long before the establishment of the familiar paddy fields, rice was a dry land crop in damp, hilly districts of India, China, and Siam.

The object of the paddy culture is not primarily to flood-irrigate the crop, but to drown out the competition for the weak young rice shoots. This is an excellent example of creating an environment which favours the crop, which can survive flooding, by prejudicing the weed competition which cannot resist the developed conditions. Rice is today the world's second most important crop, nudging wheat, which is still at the top. Rice is the principal food crop for the world's poorer half. Wheat is manifestly the food of the rich. So rice is more vital. Wheat eaters can afford alternatives.

To mill rice is difficult because the food is consumed as individual grains, not ground to flour and cooked into something unrecognizable. The hulls are removed, leaving the kernel covered by the bran; this is what is known in the West as 'brown rice'. Then another process removes the bran and most of the endosperm and this is called simply 'unpolished rice'. The polishing in a vast wire-brush machine follows. This removes most of the fat in the rice, to prevent spoilage. Polished rice of commerce looks nice, sometimes even nicer because it can be shined up with added sugar. But it is not a very good food. It has lost the bran, which supplies the B Complex vitamin thiamine which prevents beriberi. Polishing also removes some of the protein and most of the essential amino acid lysine. Both problems have been avoided for 2,000 years in India by parboiling before milling. This technique is now known as 'converting' rice. It made of rice in India a food both as valuable as raw rice, and one which keeps much better than ordinary rice, because the heat of the parboiling kills the enzyme which causes rancidity in ordinary rice in hot climates.[14]

Millet has had a long history. The millets are native to Asia and Africa. Some millets have the lowest moisture requirement of any tropical food crop; some will flourish in poor soils; others require regular rainfall, irrigation and a high level of nutrient; some will keep in store for years; others have to be used within twelve months. The millets are of several families, Echinochloa, Eleusine, Papadum, Pennisetum, Setaria, but the millet of history is probably *Panicum miliaceum*, the Common Millet. This was grown by lake dwellers in Switzerland before 500 BC, and is said to have one of the lowest water requirements of any cereal. (Not a characteristic one would normally connect with lake dwellers.) It matures in two to three months, and can be grown where climates are too hot, the rain too little and the soil too poor for most other edible plants. The limit of its northern cultivation is a mean June temperature of 17°C (64°F), July of 20°C (68°F). It is widely cultivated in Mongolia, Manchuria, North China,

Japan, India, Asiatic Russia, and the Middle East. The Romans used millet bran, mixed with unfermented wine, then dried, as a form of dried baker's yeast. The remains of the grain was slave-food.

There is a huge genetic bank amongst the millets. No one has attempted to improve any of the many species. Millet has the greatest need for improvement, the greatest variability in protein level, the lowest potential yield. It is also a very boring foodstuff. Yet the potential has to be of the greatest.

Teff is a cereal unique to Ethiopia. Ethiopia was the original home of a wheat which has become essential in two most important parts of the world; it was also the origin of the grain sorghum family.[15] Both these have become commercially vital in many parts of the world. No one except the Ethiopians grows or eats teff. They have been devoted to this cereal for 5,000 years.

Teff contains little gluten. It cannot be made into bread. It is ground and mixed with water, allowed to ferment for one or two days; then the fermented mixture is used to make a kind of pancake called 'ingera'. These are elastic, slightly sour in taste, and about the size of a pizza. Unlike the pizza, the cereal portion is not filled or garnished with meat, fish or vegetables.

Teff used for grain normally has white seeds. Brown teff produces an excellent animal fodder, sweet, palatable, and excellent whether made into hay or cut green. This use of teff has made it an agricultural crop in South Africa and India. As with other cereals, there is a negative correlation between straw quality and grain quality. The better the grain, the lower the feeding value of the straw, and vice versa. Teff is a difficult crop to grow well. The seedlings are extremely sensitive to weed competition. The tiny seeds, about the size of those of the onion, are easily washed away, so it is important to sow after rain, and not before. The crop is killed by frost, and does best in temperatures of 15–20°C (59–68°F). Why with all this difficulty should teff form more than half of all the cereal grown in Ethiopia? Why should a virtual garden crop be preferred? Why should a sourmash pancake have been a unique food for thousands of years?

The Ethiopians could have tended the wheat which now dominates the Ukraine; brought from Russia by Volga Germans, it became 'Turkey Red' when introduced into Kansas in the 1880s. Within twenty years, it had transformed the hard prairie sod and made the wheatlands possible. But the Ethiopians preferred teff to both wheat and sorghum. More difficult to grow, impossible to improve agronomically, boring to eat, teff is still preferred. There can be only one answer to the question why? Teff and the Ethiopians have formed a symbiotic relationship in which both are necessary to the other. This has been going on in a closed community for thousands of years. The closed nature of the community, breached occasionally, was nevertheless sufficiently intact to survive without major modification. Ethiopians, children of Judah, with the only indigenous native Christian community in Africa, also lived with a special cereal for at least 3,000 years. Other parts of the world have been breached by botanical invaders from elsewhere. Ethiopia is unique, and worth mention on that account.

Sorghum has varied characteristics. The seed is as big as barleycorn to one quarter that size. Some of the species make for very good animal fodder, as grazed grass or as hay, and some have a considerable amount of sugar in the stems. The genus is extremely drought resistant. Sorghum is the fourth grain in numbers of people fed, after wheat, rice and maize. It is a staple food in the drier and frost-free parts of Africa, India and China. In developed countries it is used as a grain for livestock, and is grown in the United States, the Argentine, France, Hungary, Italy, Iran, Australia and South Africa. It is also grown in the East Indies and Polynesia. Some of the species contain 10 per cent sugar in the stems and these were used for sugar syrup production in areas of India and China early in the Christian era. The genus came by sea to the Persian Gulf probably about 500 BC, and arrived in the Mediterranean before 1492. It was useful in areas too dry for other grains, other fodders, or for sugar cane. It is reputed to have been first planted in the United States by Benjamin Franklin, who is said to have sown seeds picked from an imported besom.[16]

Sorghum is a great tribute to genetic variation. Self-selected over centuries by the peculiar conditions of the Ethiopian climate, relatively different populations would survive particular environments. Over, say, 500 generations, such a process would yield segregated and distinct species. Wild selection would favour small grains which disperse easily, or 'shatter' as the farmer puts it. Human selection operates in an opposite direction, and hopes to achieve large grains which remain attached to the plant for a long time, and have easily threshed chaff or glumes. No concentrated campaign has ever been mounted to make use of the great bank of available genes in the sorghum family.

An effort comparable to that applied to the breeding of wheat or maize would yield even more results. It could, for example, probably be induced to yield per acre as much as ten times its present African average.

Sorghum, of course, cannot be made into risen bread. But it is consumed as unleavened flatbread, pancakes, or as a kind of gruel or porridge. It can be made into what used to be called 'small beer' which only keeps a few days because of its acetic acid content; such 'beer' also contains valuable supplies of vitamin B. Sorghum 'beer', containing 2–10 per cent alcohol, is more interesting than the other 'mealie beer' made from maize.

It is quite clear that it was sorghum which was 'Guinea Corn' when the English reached the Guinea Coast, which stretched the 5,000 miles from the Senegal River to Angola. Besides 'Guinea Corn' sorghum has been named 'Kaffir Corn' (South Africa); milo (Europe); sorgo (USA); kaoliang (China); durra (Sudan); mtama (Kenya); and in India and Pakistan it is known as jola, jawa, or cholam.

There is one further interesting point. Sorghum leaves when young contain large quantities of dhurrin, a precursor of the lethal vegetable form of cyanide. Small plants and young shoots have twenty times the parts per million of dhurrin compared with adult, mature leaves. The poison is destroyed when the leaves are made into hay or silage. Without this self-protection, sorghum would never have survived to become an important grain or forage plant. How many other useful cultivars have been lost because they didn't survive casual grazing? How *elegant* a form of self-defence has sorghum produced, to protect itself from destruction! In turn, the same ecosystem produced a race of grazing animals which knew well enough to leave alone the immature sorghum plant. These survived. Other animals foolishly grazed on immature sorghum. They did not survive to breed.

Buckwheat is not a cereal, nor a grass, but a herbaceous annual. It is a remote cousin of the geranium. The fruit has a dark brown, tough rind, which encloses a kernel; this in turn is three-sided in form, like a beechmast, hence its German name, Buchweizen, beech-wheat. The German word has transferred into the English.

Buckwheat arrived in Europe, significantly enough, in the late, hungry thirteenth century. It is a pioneer crop *par excellence*. Planted in June, it will yield a crop before the autumn frosts. It was widely used in the Middle Ages in forest clearings and yielded another bonus. Beloved of bees, buckwheat honey is a marvellous free gift. Buckwheat today is in Western Europe a food for wild pheasants or poultry, but it was an essential crop in the past for humans.

It was widely used just before the Black Death in the Atlantic countries, to extend cultivation into forest clearings, up mountainsides, in reclaimed bogs. Because of its short growing season, buckwheat will ripen where other food crops find life impossible. So it was taken by Germans to Russia and by Russians all over that vast country and into parts of Central Asia and Siberia. Before the Revolution, buckwheat groats were part of the ration of the ordinary Russian soldier in the Tsarist Army. These were cooked with butter, tallow or vegetable oil.

Buckwheat was taken to the Americas by the Pilgrim Fathers, and it became associated with New England before the Revolution. Buckwheat cakes are popular in the USA, buckwheat crumpets in Holland, and buckwheat remains a staple in parts of Northern Russia. In Hindu countries, buckwheat is permitted on fast days. (The relative absence of protein or fat in the flour renders buckwheat a relative penance.) It is a hard crop to find as a staple; yet it has kept thousands of pioneer people alive long enough to sow a proper cereal in the following year. It would be interesting to know how much of a part it played in the settlement of the United States before the railroads made such a pioneer crop unnecessary.

By the time of Charlemagne's coronation on Christmas Day, AD 800, most of Western Europe was farmed on the manorial system. Five hundred years later, the system was beginning to break down under the stress of excessive population. In France, the country in which the feudal system lasted longest, the reverse was true. It had the lowest increase in population, by a factor of only just over three times in five hundred years, only five times in a thousand.

In the countries in which the manorial system failed at an early date, Flanders and England, the population increased by nearly five times in five hundred years and by ten times in a thousand. This was double the rate of increase which obtained in France.

In Germany and Italy, the increases between 800 and 1800 were of the same order as in France. In Iberia, the increases were smaller, at under four times. It would not be impossible to refine these crude figures and trace the survival of the feudal system plotted against increases in population. Conversely, they should be sufficient for the major thrust of the argument to be accepted.

The manorial system depended upon a manor, village or township; land was divided into five. There was the best land in arable. There was the meadow, which was mown for hay more frequently than not. There was pasture, which was grazed as common land, though individuals might be restricted as to the numbers of animals. The waste ground on outlying areas of the village would normally be summer-grazed by day only by geese, sheep or goats. The woodland would be divided so that each householder had some supply of coppice, timber, or windfall for fuel, building, and so forth.

The arable field was divided into strips, arranged so that most men had a mixture of good and bad. One third was sown to wheat in the autumn; one third to spring corn, oats or barley; one third was fallow. All the three were fenced in the growing season, as was the meadow land. Animals were encouraged to graze on the fallow one-third of the arable field, and on the meadow land after the hay crop had been removed. Thus were animal residues recycled.

Yields of wheat on most land was of the order of less than 400 kg per hectare. An English acre, yielding 6 bushels of 60 lb weight, or 360 English pounds, would be needed for each individual. There was rarely enough wheat for the cereal to enter commerce. Some northern and western manors never attempted to grow bread wheat, relying on rye, oats and barley. Mixed grain, often more reliable, was also sown, with or without beans.

The 'cash crop' of the manor was wool. This was traded all over Europe and the merchants of Flanders were already important by AD 800. The fairs of Champagne, Flanders and Germany were the annual meeting places for the wool traders. It should not be imagined that the money economy was at all widely at work. There were peasants who never saw a coin from one year's end to the next. There were many European serfs who did not know what country they lived in, only the name of their immediate lord.[17] Nor did villeins, serfs, have any more right to money, or access to the market or wages or profits than did slaves. The smallest holders of rented land were the cottiers, who held perhaps only a patch of land the size of a garden, and owned no animals beyond the universal pigs and chickens; ironically, these cottagers very often entered the market economy earlier than their larger neighbours, whose commitment to the lord for sizable landholdings made impossible the novel cash nexus. Cottiers, therefore, often became higglers, traders, marketmen for their neighbours and themselves, buying and selling on commission. They might also very early become cash tenants, the lord not bothering with the few hours' service every week represented by a mere cottage and garden.

Institutions such as monasteries, nunneries, and cathedrals, acquired lordships of manors by the death of the lord; so did the Crown, by default or crime of various kinds. During the thirteenth century, there arose in those countries whose population had substantially increased a tendency to commute labour-rents for money. By 1300, five hundred years after Charlemagne, and a generation before the Black Death, much of Western Europe had reached its Malthusian limit as far as food production was concerned. In those countries which made no change in the manorial system, output per acre did not rise. Indeed, no one today, observing the rules of the feudal system and using techniques available in 1300, could ever produce much more per acre.

It was the best guarantee for population control by hunger that could ever be devised. Nor could more acreage be brought into cultivation. The power, either of men or of animals, was simply not sufficient. The limits of cultivation were often dictated by the amount of power at hand. The only available addition to animal or human power was that derived from wind or water. It was of little assistance in cultivation.

Animal traction was limited, even in 1492, by certain inexorable facts. A horse may carry four times what a man may carry, a mule as much as a horse. A horse can pull twenty times what a man can pull. But in order to perform, a horse needs a proper harness, proper shoes and a smooth road. Harness arrived later than shoes (about AD 900 in Western Europe) but roads deteriorated after the Roman Empire. Oxen are far slower than horses, but can exert traction for long periods on vehicles which do not appear to want to move. Carts bogged down in deep mud respond better to oxen than to horses. Even with oxen, a wagonload of grain doubled in cost in Roman times in the first 100 miles that it travelled. This was along good Roman roads. Even then, efficiency was so low that each ox could only pull 70 kg (154 lb) against 2,000 (4, 410 lb) today. In areas where there were no roads, as in non-Roman Europe, the transport of grain by land was economically impossible, so local urban inhabitants, especially in large cities, adopted a carnivorous diet. Cattle, sheep, pigs, even chickens, can be walked to market.

Cities on rivers very early adopted water transport. Rivers used in the Middle Ages to transport grain long distances included the Elbe and the Vistula, which made Central European grain exportable via Hamburg and Danzig respectively. Almost every important town in Western Europe was close to some river, or built upon a river, or limited by the deficiency. The exceptions were, of course, seaports, especially Venice, and cities which built their own transport canals, like Milan.

Water-power developed early. The great Vitruvius in *De Architectura* (before 27 BC) described the then state of the art. The simplest and earliest water-wheels harnessed the flow and fall of a river to produce rotary power, usually to grind grain.[18] The simplest type of water-wheel has been found in Scandinavia, Greece, Anatolia, the Lebanon, and Central Asia, even within living memory as well as in ancient times. It consisted of a horizontal water-wheel on a vertical axle, which also drove the grind-stones. These were limited to mountain regions with fast-flowing streams. They were not efficient.

The Vitruvian mill was placed in a vertical mode, with the axle horizontal. Gearing was required to link the horizontal rotary motion with the grinding stones. The Vitruvian mill was arranged to be what came to be called 'undershot'. In this the stream of water acts upon the underside of the wheel, turning it so that the bottom of the wheel moves away from the force of the water.

Undershot wheels are less efficient than overshot wheels, which add to the flow of water the force of the fall of the height of the wheel. These can be usefully employed in a sluggish river, dammed to provide a millpond and a millrace. Aqueducts or canals can also be used to bring the water to the mill.[19] Water-transport and water-power combined to produce flour at industrial mills at Venafro near Naples (about AD 50) and later, at Arles in Provence.

The Neapolitan mills were undershot. They were destroyed by the same Vesuvian eruption which buried Pompeii, but a model has been reconstructed from the impressions left in lava. The estimated power developed was about 3 hp, and the output 1.5 tons a day, enough grain for about 4,000 people. A much more substantial plant was built at Barbegal near Arles, about AD 310. This drew water from an aqueduct, and it was arranged to pass, at a slope of 30° through houses containing sixteen overshot wheels. The capacity of this series of mills would be enough to grind 28 tons a day or enough for 80,000 people. Did the Romans export flour as well as grain from the river port of Arles, or was the flour used locally? If so, what was the density of population in Provence? At the time, Constantine the Great was living at Arles, so the addition of the court and the army to the indigenous population may have necessitated the huge milling complex. In all, it covered an area 200 metres (219 yards) long by 100 metres (109 yards) wide, or 2 hectares (5 acres). Mills of this nature must have been the largest Roman industrial enterprises. There were, however, very serious intellectual limitations to the Graeco-Roman use of power. There was no interplay between science and technology. This meant that most water-power applications came long after Rome and were typical of the Middle Ages.[20]

By the time of the Domesday Book in 1087, there were about 4,000 water-mills in Domesday England, about 1 mill to 250 people. Since this census was unique in England, no one knows whether or not this pattern was repeated elsewhere in Western Europe.

The floating mill was invented, or developed, by the soldier-genius, Belisarius in AD 537. The Goths sought to starve Rome by cutting the aqueducts. Belisarius set up a huge mill which was mounted on moored ships. Rome did not starve. The Goths failed to take Rome. Such floating mills were used in Dover before the Norman Conquest, harnessing the tide; in the Tigris, in the tenth century; in the Seine before 1200; in the Loire in 1330; and in the Yangtse Kiang before 1400. They were in use in the Persian Gulf, in the Po Valley, and near Venice. In seawater, tidal mills never really froze. Nor did the sea dry up. But in the Low Countries, no sort of water-mill could have served as well as did the windmill.

The windmill gave the flatlands of modern Belgium, Holland and North Germany, the same sort of advantage which countries with running water enjoyed. But the windmill has a more demanding technology than the water-mill.

The eastern mill, originally turning horizontally, had a set of rotary sails, like a Central Asian prayer wheel. This mill, in horizontal or vertical form, was found as far west as Southern Spain, and wherever the later Muslims took the technique. But it was not present in Palestine during the Crusades, nor can the eastern mill be said to have been copied. For once, the Western Europeans invented something for themselves. The first post-mill, wooden, with wooden sails, was to be found at the Abbey of St Sauvere de Vicomte in Normandy in 1180.

By the Black Death, there were probably 1,000 windmills, one-tenth the number of water-mills, in England, mostly in Eastern England, where river flow was too sluggish for water-mills. In the Low Countries, there were probably six times as many. In the Netherlands alone, there were 10,000 in the century of Holland's greatness, the seventeenth. Before steam, there were probably a million water-mills and windmills in the whole of Western Europe. There were probably as many or more in the states west of the Missippi-Missouri in 1900, nearly all windmills. No farm could exist without one. Even in 1900, they were not very efficient. A rather large steel structure, weighing up to 10 tons and having a wheel diameter of 7.5 metres (25 feet) could only extract 1.34 horsepower/hour. It was enough. Without the ceaseless pumping on the prairie, no settlement would have been possible.[21]

The Romans (using gravity but no windmills) tried to drain both the English fens and the Dutch Rhine district. These efforts silted up in the Dark Ages, but were reborn in medieval times. The Po Valley improvements, completed before AD 50, were more robust, and appear to have survived better. But without the windmill and the water-wheel, there can have been no general drainage and irrigation of the sort carried out by the Dutch, or earlier by the Arabs in Southern Spain and Sicily. In Christian Europe, the religious houses became identified with wetland improvement, and irrigation and drainage in turn were connected to canalizing rivers. Some of these transport improvements were in place surprisingly early. Bruges, for example, was connected to the sea by canal in 1236; Haarlem, by 1315, and Amsterdam by 1440. Milan's complex, using the flow from Lake Como, and canals to the Po, was completed earlier, in the thirteenth century.

Population growth justified bringing marginal land into cultivation; drainage and reclamation of wetlands were responses to an increased population. In the absence of cheap and efficient land transport, water was the key. Access to water was needed to trade. Any serious trade in heavy goods had to be by river or by sea. Canalizing rivers was expensive in both capital and revenue costs. So early cities tended to grow up where there was easy access to the sea, and by sea, to the world. Each town not on a river had a task even to grind the grain to make its daily bread. A town like Assisi, on top of a hill, would use human or animal muscles to grind grain before the windmill came along. If it used human power, it would have needed something of the order of one day's work for every five people fed on bread. This kind of proportion, that one man (or woman) only ground and baked enough for four other people, dominated the lives of ordinary people until steam came along to supplement animals, wind and water. For a thousand years before steam, techniques very gradually improved. There was plenty of room.[22]

In 800, Western European agriculture was low in efficiency; but the population was so low in numbers that there was little incentive to improve the position. By 1300, five hundred years later, the germ of every possible husbandry improvement which would amaze and delight the world in the eighteenth century was already present.

In the years leading up to the Black Death in 1350, Western Europe pressed upon the Malthusian constraints. In 1850, the same constraints had been met and matched in Belgium, Holland, England. The area of arable land available in 1850 in those countries was less than double what it had been five hundred years before. The population of the Low Countries was nearly four times, and of England more than five times the 1300 figure. This time, the constraints were defeated. It was a tremendous intellectual triumph for the men who had laboured over the previous century to grow enough food; there was the possibility of efficient agriculture. It would also be very profitable.

There were eight separate improvements listed[23] in the 1780s as having been adopted by English landlords in the previous half-century in order to increase profits from land – either directly for the tenant, or indirectly for the landlord, by increasing rent. It was quite clear that the initiative was expected to come from the landlord, and the improvements to be imposed by patrician and paternalist leadership upon the tenantry. The tenantry did not, of course, object provided their pockets gained as a result. Some of the tenants of larger farms became so much better off as a result of these improvements that they occupied themselves in hunting several times a week, leaving the actual supervision of the farms to their foremen. Some kind of alternative occupation was not entirely necessary, since not a single one of the improvements saved labour of any kind.

By these means England became the first country to survive a huge increase in population without massive social or political disruption. The relative success of food supply in England in the century from 1750–1850 should be contrasted with what would be the United States in the same period. A country with virtually free land had no need of systems of agricultural improvement.

Tillage Improvements. The great improver here was Jethro Tull (1674–

1741), who advocated the drilling of seed in rows, and movement of soil at frequent intervals during the growing season, by hoes – either horsehoes or hand-held hoes. He wrote that 'by frequently turning over and pulverising the soil, we not only destroy the weeds very effectively, but likewise also grubs, beetles, worms and maggots of many kinds'. Moving soil does not, of course, by itself destroy either weeds or insects. Weeds die because of lack of water – provided hoeing is carried out in dry weather. Insects are killed only if an attendant bird, following the implements, picks up and eats the insect. Nor did Tull or anyone else in the eighteenth century know that earthworms are beneficial, or that grubs, beetles and maggots all have different life cycles, or the point at which insects are harmless, or the point at which the chrysalis is damaging, or the fly dangerous, or the grub a danger, or the maggot safely ignored. All these minute observations were to follow. Of Tull's theories in general, it can be said that his advocacy did more good than harm, but no one subjected his theories to value for money analysis until at least a hundred years after his death. Then the seed-drill became important, not to kill maggots but to save seed, and to increase yield.

New Implements. The cost of cast iron came down by about half in England (but not on the Continent) between 1700 and 1750, and this enabled a very wide spread in its use. Before 1700, most implements and hand tools, shovels, even, were made of wood. After 1760, an increasing number were made by the village blacksmith using new cast iron; in the next century, the village blacksmith was gradually replaced by the agricultural machinery maker. Some of these were very local, set up in business by capitalists, or sometimes by customers, on a district basis.[24]

It is not easy to recollect, but in the same period the trades of cobbler (roughly one per 250 souls), blacksmith (roughly one per 500 souls), and wheelwright (roughly one per 1,000 souls) were as essential in the village as both the woman who delivered babies or the woman who laid out the dead. Gradually, all the functions became centralized, and the jobs moved into towns, the manufacture into factories, the midwife and the undertaker becoming professional specialists. Long before there were maternity hospitals or undertakers' parlours, the agricultural machinery makers had started to supersede the blacksmith. By 1850, rural blacksmiths had thinned out, and by 1900, just before the automobile replaced the horse, most blacksmiths were in urban areas, not the countryside. Today, the blacksmith is often mobile, travelling many miles to tend horses kept only for pleasure.[25]

Better ratio between seed sown and seed harvested. In the Middle Ages, and in most of continental Europe in 1750, there was a time-honoured belief that an increase in harvest of, say, 4–1 or 6–1 was all that any farmer could expect from his land, and that to increase the harvest it was necessary to increase the seed-rate, which would then be reflected in an automatic growth of 4–1 or 6–1, or whatever. This policy can be seen today to be scientifically absurd, but it was only generally challenged by the Dutch in the late seventeenth century, and by the English from 1750 onwards. A parallel development was to arrive, by selection, at a cultivar which gave a return better than average, and by breeding, raise the long-term average over the years.

Wheat or barley seed runs from 12,000 to 30,000 per kilo, oats rather more. A pot-sown single grain seed, properly tended, will multiply by almost 100, if the right seed is chosen; wheat multiplies less readily than barley, maize by nearly 200 times in pot-culture. Best results in the field are achieved by selecting plump seed with ample food reserves for the tiny plant in the endosperm, and by sowing relatively few of them in well-tilled soil. Today, this means 150 kilos per hectare (133 lb per acre), or one quarter of what was sown in England in 1750, and one fifth of the quantity sown in France. Miraculously, it had occasionally been noted in *ancien régime* France that, after a long winter when some of the seed-corn had perforce been eaten by hungry peasants, the subsequent harvest had been better than that of the previous year, and had yielded a return of 10–1 or 12–1. This benison was universally described as a gift of God.

No experimental work of sowing various rates of seed in otherwise identical conditions was performed in England until the 1790s, or in France until the 1850s, and only in the 1960s did true experimenters carry such a test to its logical conclusion. In that decade, full crops were grown with seed-rates of only 3 kilos per hectare, or 2 per cent of normal. In order to achieve this result, all the other conditions had to be of a perfection almost impossible to achieve in the field. Nevertheless, it shows what can be done to multiply newly bred strains of seed when such a course is necessary.

Specialization. Suiting the crop to the nature of the soil, an obvious move, became possible only when communications improved. An entirely isolated community would have to grow wheat for bread; rye for bread; oats for horses, and bullocks, the sole form of non-manual power; barley for beer; all sorts of vegetables, suitable or not suitable, for humans; trees for wood; flax for linen. The district would have to keep cows for milk; horses and bullocks for the plough; sheep for wool and meat; goats for milk and cheese; pigs as scavengers and for meat; animal skins for leatherwork of all kinds; poultry for eggs and meat; and dogs to be trained for the defence and herding of animals. Such an isolated community had no opportunity to grow and to rear what was suitable, so that better specialization of crops and livestock depended on better roads, canals, river transport. It is not surprising, when one considers carefully, that such improvements took place in the Po Valley and in the Netherlands and Flanders, criss-crossed by waterways as they were earlier than elsewhere. Improvements up and down the Seine Valley were made earlier than in the Massif Central, and the lowlands of England were improved by specializ-ation earlier than the Highlands of Scotland, parts of which had to wait for the internal combustion engine before they could safely stop growing barley for beer. Before railways, internal communications were usually less favourable than those for foreign trade. Agricultural commodities are more easily exported by river and sea from the specialist country and imported into the consuming country than they are grown in every consuming country. Yet, internally, in Greece, it would not be until late in this century that some mountain villages would safely give up growing consumables much more suitably imported.[26]

The biggest single change in the benefits of specialization probably came from the abandonment of the need to grow bread grains in every parish. There was a long-held medieval practice, almost a law, that virtually every parish in Europe had an obligation to feed itself with wheat or some substitute. There are, in fact, millions of acres in Europe in huge areas which are wholly unprofitable in wheat. This was true for much of East Prussia in the eighteenth century, where, because of the practice of growing one's own bread, Prussia ate rye bread, while next door Poland exported wheat to Holland.

Rotation of crops. The old Mediterranean-medieval 'rotation' (if it be a rotation) was winter corn, spring corn, fallow or winter corn, fallow, spring corn, fallow. (The 'fallow' was often a period during which the land tumbled down to temporary grass, mostly weed-grasses, and the resulting mess was trodden and 'grazed' by half-starved cattle and sheep.) By 1400, 'improved' temporary grasses (Italian Ryegrass) had been developed in Lombardy, and by 1700 the turnip came out of the garden and into the field, as did the carrot. Longer leys (artificial grasses sown for more than one year) were also introduced by some 'improvers' in the eighteenth century. The most productive (the 'Noble') grasses – perennial ryegrass, cocksfoot, the meadow grasses and timothy – are all indigenous to Europe, and by 1776 had been taken to North America and had become native on that continent. It was the technique of their use in the rotation which was important – the new management husbandry rather than new crops. Landlords imposed upon tenants the use of clovers – red, white and alsike – which in some form or other are native to every Western European country Clover is much more sensitive than grass to acidity in the soil.

Dung, marl and chalk. The practice of using dung and chalk (or lime) can be dated as early as 500 BC, but the application of both was very hard work, and was avoided by the less good husbandman, or when there was no immediate profit to be gained. Dung had a great chemical value as one of the few sources of nitrogen and phosphate, and urine was preserved for potash. Most of the chemical value would disappear in an uncovered heap in rain, or by nitrification in heat, and the preservation of dung in covered pits or yards engaged 'model' landlords and their agents from the sixteenth century. As with dung, so with chalk and marl. The landlord, having a longer-term perspective, again took the initiative. Landlords made their use a logical exercise, a necessity in long leases. Dung was to be preserved and used on the farm, in rotation. Woe betide a tenant who used dung produced on the landlord's farm on his own land, if he owned any, or who sold it. This was an offence against every tenet of good husbandry, and almost a crime to boot.[27]

Dung has the effect, apart from its chemical value, of making heavy soils lighter and giving lighter soils more 'body'. The actual effect in clay is to help flocculate the soil, so that it crumbles and has an easier, blander characteristic, and is easier to till, giving a soil from which it is possible to produce a good structure and a good seedbed by the action of the weather and the farmers' implements. The same is true of chalk and marl. Chalk, added to heavy soils, 'makes the strong clay rich and fruitful', wrote Defoe, of Kent chalk applied to Essex clay.[28]

Lighter land was always easier to cultivate, and it is no accident that the earliest true agriculture ('tilling of soil') took place in the sandy loams of the Mediterranean, or on alluvial bottoms in the Nile, the Tigris, Euphrates and Indus valleys. Any form of calcium applied to the clay fraction in soil makes that soil 'lighter' and easier to cultivate, since the action of calcium is to encourage earthworms and other fauna which break down organic matter into what we now call 'humus'.[29] The presence of lime in a soil is essential for nitrification, nitrogen fixation, and many other beneficial bacterial activities, including the fixing of nitrogen by the nodules on clover.[30]

At the other end of the scale, lime or chalk applied to very light or sandy soils is a waste of time and money. Since the sand does not have the necessary 'body' to hold the calcium, the added chemical material washes through the sand to the drains. So marl is employed. Marl is clay mixed with animal residues rich in calcium. There are great stories in Elizabethan times of marlpits which were found to contain hundreds of horns of dead deer. Over the centuries, the more soluble calcium in the bodies of animals, whether mammals, or sea-creatures (as in 'sedentary' limestone) or eggs (as in 'oolite') becomes mixed by natural action with the clay fraction. Marl is the end product, and it was dug all over Europe in the period following the Renaissance when various individual improvers were increasing the value of the land. The landlord's contribution was, again, to formalize the use of marl on the light land. It was an expensive business – a good dressing of marl would cost double the rent of the land manured, and sometimes the tenant and landlord shared the cost by the remission of one year's rent.[32]

Marling increased yield by a quarter, other factors being equal, and the landlord as well as the tenant would benefit, since a good dressing of marl needed renewing only every twenty years or so, other acts of good husbandry being performed in the interval.[33]

New Crops. The seventh great improvement was in the use of new crops, or of old crops put to new uses. Thus became possible the growing of cash crops in the countryside for other communities to eat in other places. This tied the farmer firmly into the cash nexus, and ultimately into a capitalist system where he was farming for the market. The list of crops grown for the first time in the century after 1700 reads like a table of contents of modern field husbandry. Sometimes 'new' crops – turnips, for example – were not as new as people thought then or think today.

A distinction had to be drawn, not for the first time in modern history, between subsistence crops, grown for man or beast, or for people within the localities, and crops for sale. Sometimes the same crop might be both a cash crop and a crop consumed at home. Wheat could be used in the village for breadmaking, or sold. Barley could be used to fatten cattle or pigs, or to fuel oxen, or horses, or to brew beer locally, or sold to brewers several hundred miles away. Carrots, cabbages, swedes, parsnips, peas and potatoes became field crops in the late eighteenth century and could be sold as cash crops for human consumption, or used on the farm whence they came for animal feed. In that event, stock might be bought in to consume and 'cash-in' the crops. Cattle would be purchased in the autumn to consume unsaleable roots of all kinds. Sheep would be finished on field-surpluses, left in rows, and 'folded' with hurdles. Pigs could be profitably fattened on peas and potatoes, though these crops had been intended for sale to humans. Poultry would be used, not only to cash in tail corn by means of selling eggs or meat, but by consuming all sorts and conditions of surplus (and boiled) vegetables. Sometimes the taste of parsnip or swede carried over into eggs or poultry meat.

The technological ideas which became much clearer in crop husbandry during the century after 1700 did not extend in the same force to the culture of animals, if only because animals are much more complicated forms of life than most plants. The aim was to shorten the time taken to produce an animal for market. In 1760, it was doubtful if most sheep or cattle could be grown to adulthood in under four years. Cattle types were indiscriminately mixed, often with unknown fathers. Sheep had been selected for centuries for wool production, and there is a negative correlation between weight of fleece and quality of wool in most sheep. So as the English made efforts to increase the fleece weight, the fineness of the wool declined. Good lowland feed was found to produce coarser wool; the demand for the finer merino-type fleeces from Spain or poor land fleeces from Ireland from the English spinners and weavers was embarrassing to a nation geared for a thousand years to the production of wool. In the end, by means of selection, the English sheep breeds were catalogued, identified and adopted for the first time in the generation after Bakewell's pioneer efforts in the 1790s. This process led inevitably to the division of sheep into meat-producers and wool-producers, which spread all over the world.

In cattle, there was a similar division into cattle for beef, cattle for milk, and (in some countries) cattle as draught animals. Economic efficiency ultimately led to the extinction of the dual-purpose, or triple-purpose beast beloved of the peasantry. The twelve-year-old bullock, having drawn a plough for most of his life, was no longer the source and provision of the beef of old England. As horses and mules replaced slower, less efficient oxen, so cattle became more specialist providers of meat or milk. In this process, the problem of winter was even more vital in cattle husbandry than in sheep production.

Cattle Husbandry. This was cited in 1785 as the final great improvement in the following way: 'the application of the foregoing to the rearing and fattening of cattle'.[34] A quick dip into the natural processes of growth in Western Europe is necessary to understand the importance of winter feed. About 30 per cent of all plant growth takes place in most temperate areas in and about the month of May, with nearly 20 per cent in June, and about 10–15 per cent in April in favoured districts. Altogether, in any area, the spring quarter of 90 days normally produces more than 60 per cent of the annual growth of any plant. The summer quarter produces about 30 per cent, leaving a mere 10 per cent for the whole winter half-year. This is an average rule, and in a country like England with no apparent 'average' weather, or in a country with no real winter like Southern and Western Ireland, or in a country like France, big enough to have regional weather, these proportions may be modified, but the principle remains true.

Even in the warmest parts of the British Isles, or in favoured Atlantic provinces of France, winter growth is much lower than in the warmer half of the year. So wintering is a major problem for all forms of animal husbandry. Without especial provision for the winter, most grazing animals left to fend for themselves, will survive but lose weight, which then has to be expensively replaced in the spring. This is as true of wild grass-eating species like deer, rabbits, or geese as it is of cattle or sheep. It was the adoption of all the principles of the new husbandry which made it possible for a meat-loving people to increase their meat production to keep pace with a rise in population of 300 per cent in one century.

It is one of the minor ironies of history that, though the period up to 1760 saw the English working class (and no other) better fed than at any time in history, that well-being would not include much fresh meat and none in winter. Outside a few 'advanced' counties like Norfolk, there were few cattle available for fresh meat in the hungry months. By the time the techniques to fatten cattle had been developed – hay or straw, turnips or swedes, some crushed grain – only the rich could afford the end product. It has been said that the poorest quarter of the population of Britain fared worse in the period 1760–1940 than they had in the previous half-century. Whether or not this was true – and it is certainly true that only government intervention brought malnutrition to an end in World War II – it was certainly never true that the poor had daily fresh meat at any time in the same period. Even families living on farms in the late eighteenth and nineteenth centuries only ultimately found meat a daily occurrence when cheap imported beef and lamb came in from the new countries after 1880. On the other hand, only in Britain was the coincidence of meat and wealth so well connected. While there were plenty of affluent vegetarians in the Mediterranean basin, no Briton was considered prosperous unless he were a carnivore. 'Beef, beer, liberty, England and St George' went the toast.

'The new agriculture', then, was seen by the people of the time to be a matter of eight techniques, worth repeating again: better tillage; new implements; better ratio between seed sown and seed harvested; suiting the crop to the soil; rotations; manuring of soil; new sorts of crops; and the application of all the above to cattle husbandry. Very few of these techniques were 'new' to anyone in Western Europe. They were brought together, interrelated, properly managed, each affecting the other, in only one country at first, England. The honour fell to the English not because of some great wisdom and nobility, but quite simply because the land/population equation, which had been so favorable to the English, compared to the French or the Dutch, in 1760, completely reversed itself when the population exploded. In 1760, the population was of the order of 6 million, and the improved agricultural sector (of 5 million hectares or 12 million acres) provided food for 140 per cent of that population. In 1850, the population was three times that number (18 million), there were 7 million hectares (18 million acres) of 'improved land', and the agricultural sector provided a much better diet for 125 per cent of the population. In the period 1660–1860, 2.5 million hectares (6 million acres) were brought into better cultivation by enclosure from common land, scrub-land, wasteland, poor timberland, and so forth. This was the ultimate extent of cultivation possible by the technological means of the time.[35] This massive achievement was not matched in any other country in the world.[36]

But it was not only food for humans that the farmers grew. The figures of 140 per cent of population in 1750 and 125 per cent of population in 1850 of course includes some export of grain, mostly wheat, for the first date, and substantial *imports* of grain, mostly wheat, for the second. Far more important, though, was the non-human food which the land of Britain supplied. In 1750, there were probably more than half a million non-agricultural horses in use, or one non-agricultural horse to twelve people. Each horse required as much food to breed, rear and maintain as ten men. Though a horse costs ten times the food of a working man, at the very minimum level of feeding the man – 30,000 K cal. against 3,000 – men cost more than just food and shelter. Even in very bad, hungry times, like the four great near-famines of 1795–6, 1800–1, 1809–12 and 1818–19, the bare keep of a working man was at least as great as that of a horse. Two contrasts exist. In 1800, in a workhouse, a man could be kept much more cheaply than a horse. At the other end of the scale, a butler, in 1900, cost as much in food and perquisites as the very best hunter. The hunter did not have a wage as well, either.[37]

Any modern farmer having to operate an open-field system would consider himself lucky to produce a net harvest of one-half that of the same land operated by a set of rules known to anyone in Western Europe in, say, 1338, the date of the *Luttrell Psalter*.[38] In other words, land tenure in common made impossible sensible rotations, manuring, fallow, culti-vations, and so forth. As will be shown, England's primacy in the eighteenth century grew from the (usually) adequate food. This was grown on land much improved agronomically by enclosure and subse-quent husbandry, only possible on enclosed land.

Yet it was not hunger or population pressure which brought about the first enclosures, but the desire to create sheepwalks. Wool was the first English crop to show a tremendous advantage as a cash crop. Wool was valued at many times the value of grain, which was sometimes in surplus, sometimes not. Wool was easily transported. Wool was the one product of England, a marginal wine-growing country, capable only of roughish wine, to equate with the finest wines as an article of commerce. Long before the Black Death, English wool was being bought by merchants from Flanders and Italy. As the population declined after the Black Death, some kind of enclosure was taking place all the time, without any overt acts on the part of the lords, who often simply seized the deserted, empty villages and incorporated them into their own estates. The major sheep-walk enclosures came later, notably in Tudor times, when commerce had largely replaced subsistence as the characteristic motive in many agricultural areas.

Men of enterprise cleared out huge districts, sometimes including a dozen villages, and turned them into enclosed estates devoted to sheep. Inhabitants were compensated by means of a formula which was less than satisfactory for families who had never before handled money. In the end, many became landless peasants and, later, when the population pressure on the land became too heavy, the same sort of people drifted into towns and became an urban proletariat. This process was continuous from the time of the early Tudors, a hundred years before Shakespeare, until enclosure came to an abrupt end in 1869. Technological progressives like the Elizabethan writer Thomas Tusser (1520–80) were in favour of enclosure. He noted in the 1560s that Suffolk and Essex were benefiting from it, while Cambridgeshire and Leicestershire were still operating the old open-field system. In general, counties with ports and feeder rivers or counties near London, the big market, were enclosed earlier than distant, boggy, or dry counties. It was transport which was the key to the cash nexus in farming, even in terms of wool, a very easy commodity to handle. Enclosure in Tudor times was the driving force for improvement, and wool was the prime export until the end of the seventeenth century, and ultimately paid for all the imported finery worn by anyone in the portraits of the time. It was wool which paid, of course, for the very pigment in the paint of the portraits, imported, as like or not, from Italy or France.[39]

There is a school of thought which says that it was population pressure which gave rise to politico-religious differences throughout Europe in the seventeenth century; in England, for example, it was the counties which had the highest population increases that appeared to have the sharpest divisions in the Civil War. It was the much smaller general increase in population (a drop in the rate of increase from nearly 40 per cent per century to the equivalent of less than 5 per cent per century) between 1700 and 1760 that made for the relative happiness of the English working class during that time; this resulted in an Augustan Age, not only in literature, but also in filling the bellies of the poor. The slackening of the increase in population pressure meant more food, more profit, and hardly any years of bread shortage in England.

Pressure to enclose almost exactly followed the pressure upon the food supply. During the fifty years before 1760, there was an annual average of only eight Acts of Enclosure: this coincided with a population increase of only about 3 per cent in the same period. After 1760, the increase in enclosure followed the increase in population: between 1760 and 1815, there were nearly 1.3 million hectares (3.25 million acres) enclosed, more than half of all the enclosures. The population increased in the same period to more than double the 1760 figure. No contemporary, of course, knew of the population increase, decade by decade, but the price of wheat was a nearly true correlation of the impulse to enclose. The change in the Bank Rate dictated the cost of the enterprise, as with all other commercial efforts involving the raising of capital. The relationship of grain price, cost of money and rental income to be expected was a powerful instrument of calculation, and graphs have been prepared to define these relationships. The peace between 1802 and 1805 saw a decline in enclosures, and the peace after Waterloo in 1815, a temporary cessation. The drop in the price of grain can be plotted against these events.

We know the price of grain in England during the period. This increase in price was driven by population growth. What we do not know is what drove the population to increase by nearly 40 per cent per century in 1600–1700, the rate of increase to fall to 5 per cent per century in the 60 years before 1760, and the rate of increase to accelerate between 1760 and 1860 to 300 per cent per century. It was this change which dictated the form which husbandry took in England, in sharp contrast to what happened in Ireland in the same period.

The process of enclosure displaced thousands of commoners. During the eighteenth century, most of what was enclosed had been the old medieval arable-strip fields, unfenced, cultivated in the summer, ranged across by every kind of animal in the winter, the strongest male fathering the most animals of his species, making improvements in animal husbandry as difficult as were advances in the growing of crops. It is entirely probable that early enclosures more than doubled the production from any given area. The process was generally seen to be desirable, even by the displaced peasants who lost their rights in the field and became wage-slaves. There were probably more jobs to be had in the new industries which arose in the period 1760–1800 than were lost in the process of enclosure. The new cotton mills and the older woollen industry were both booming during this period, as were the coal and iron twins. There was little hint of serious objection to enclosure as long as those displaced, and their children, found gainful employment elsewhere. It was a different matter in the new century.

Between 1800 and 1845, nearly 0.6 million hectares (1.5 million acres) were enclosed, and they were generally of great tracts of moor and fenland. Though fewer people were displaced in a given area than by the enclosure of strip-fields, there was also a much more difficult economic climate. In 1800, there were 50 per cent more people in England than in 1760 – 9 million against 6 million. In the next forty-five years, the population of England doubled. Wages were held down by the high birth-rate, and by the continuous ability of employers to recruit unskilled labour at short notice from Ireland. John Bull's other island in the same period increased her population by more than the English rate, and with no industrial revolution to absorb the surplus. The position of the new proletariat grew markedly worse in the years before the Repeal of the Corn Laws.[40] There were so many wholly unskilled men, women and children that employers designed systems to employ people as animals. Thus came about what we now regard as the scandals in the cotton, wool and coal industries.

Two political developments became inevitable. First, pressure on food supplies led to a curious coalition of industrialists, who wanted cheap contented workers, and do-gooders and economists who persuaded the Prime Minister, Peel, to repeal the remaining Corn Laws in 1845. Secondly, there were efforts to civilize the factories. Basically this meant designing systems which involved people as people rather than the child as a pit-pony or as an automaton in a cotton mill, or (a rare case) as a live chimneybrush-boy. The Factory Acts, as is the way, came into force a generation after the peak of the abuses they were designed to correct.

In the third period of enclosure, after 1845, there was no pressure on actual grain supplies, since imports could come from Europe or the neo-European countries, notably the USA and Canada. From 1845 onwards, and uniquely in Europe, the Irish population declined, not only from death during the Famine, but from emigration and a declining birth-rate. At the same time, the population of the United Kingdom as a whole increased at much the same rate as before 1845. English and Scots fecundity made good the losses in Ireland. But grain could be imported and, indeed, grown especially in any suitable place in the world, for the British market which became in the second half of the nineteenth century the greatest food importing nation ever known.

The Enclosure Movement reflected these changes. Enclosure after 1845 was seen to be purely for profit, not for life-enhancing food. The enclosures after 1845 were largely of the primeval manorial common rights, of all sorts of people, often near new towns, or on the edge of old towns. The benefit to the Lord of the Manor was seen to be more personal, more socially questionable than the improvements derived from earlier enclosures. At the same time, the philanthropic impulse of the age led to a decline in the automatic pursuit of economic efficiency. The idea of Malthus, that an excessive population would be automatically corrected by starvation, lost appeal. Such purity of vision was overtaken by the social movement to sanitize and purify, which became known, in shorthand, as gas and water socialism. As part of that process an increasingly polluted industrial society rediscovered the virtues of fresh air. Cheap food and fresh air put an end to any moral virtue in enclosure.

In 1869, the Enclosure Movement came to an end. This was not due to some great rural scandal which outraged public opinion. The movement came to an end in the towns, not ordinary towns, but in the metropolitan fastness of London. The twenty years after the Enclosure Act of 1845 saw more than 240,000 hectares (600,000 acres) enclosed, to add to more than 2.5 million hectares (6 million acres) enclosed since the Black Death. In 1865, an attempt was made to enclose Wimbledon and Clapham Commons, and the Downs at Epsom where the Derby is raced every year. Reformers, suburban liberals and horse-lovers joined to defeat such heinous proposals. They succeeded, and no further enclosure took place after 1869; enclosure, at least in urban and suburban areas, was to be seen as a retrograde step. The debate will continue as to its value in the country as a whole. For those who believe that feeding the people was more important than people's 'rights', enclosure was more important than Common Land.

For the mid-Victorian radical, with ample food available from anywhere in the world, the Common Lands were more important than the prosperity of English agriculture. Common Land was a place to walk, to observe nature, to breathe, to enjoy birdsong. The repeal of the Corn Laws in the same year as the Enclosure Act of 1845 had, with all the obvious wisdom of hindsight, put paid to an era in the history of agriculture in Britain. Neo-Europeans initiated, at first for the British market, an equally important age of expansion in the United States, Canada, Australia, New Zealand, South Africa, Uruguay, the Argentine, large parts of Southern Russia. All these became part of the European farm, neo-European feeders of Europeans thousands of miles away; participants in world trade.[41]

In the five years 1845–50, the population of the United Kingdom was still higher than that of the United States. The then United States contained land parcelled in thirty states, amounting to more than 2 million square miles, more than fifteen times the area of the UK at that time. Only a few areas in the north-east had a density of population approaching that of England, 350 people per sq. mile. In both England and Ireland there were districts more densely crowded than any place on earth: no one knew this at the time. Certainly, Britain was the most Malthusian problem to date: no one knew that, either. In England, enclosures met the problem for a time; then this policy was insufficient, and Free Trade and more consciously induced emigration followed. In Ireland, for a number of reasons, such solutions were not possible, and the Famine resulted, with all its grave consequences.[42]

In both the United States and the United Kingdom policies were dictated, not by politicians, but by territorial imperatives. The Jeffersonian dream was for a country of small farms, cultivated by noble farmers who would throw up local and national leaders conceived in the form of Cincinnatus.[43] Instead, there was a nation divided into slave and free states; into plantations and small farms; into ranches and ranges; capitalists and settlers. The Jeffersonian dream existed for a short time only in a few areas, before subsistence gave way to the market. Romantics in many countries have tried to create the same sort of conditions, with predictable failure. In some countries, notably Germany, the failure of the small farmer movement led directly to fascism. Today, there are many people in many first world countries trying to recreate the same sort of dream out of its time.

In England, territorial imperatives demanded efficiency in the agricultural sector. Hard on the commoners, yet enclosure guaranteed enough food, by and large, for a population grown by three times in a century. Enclosure also won three great struggles. The first, and most obvious, was the Napoleonic War, which lasted, with intermission, for more than twenty years. Secondly, alone in Europe, England's revolution was industrial and economic, not political. Thirdly, England but not Ireland went through a Malthusian experience which did not destroy the nature of the country. Enclosure helped defeat Napoleon, revolution and Malthus. This record was unique, but by 1845, it was no longer enough.[44]

Notes

1 Verse is easier to remember, to declaim, to use as a verbal teaching base. Even in 1492, there were not many books about, and not many who could read properly. Few farmers in Virgil's time could have usefully used these lines if they had not been in verse, easily remembered, competent to jog the memory. The first universally appreciated English manual of husbandry was that of Thomas Tusser, 1562. It was still being recommended for use in schools as late as 1723, by Lord Molesworth, a great educator of the time.
2 The process of partial domestication is easily understood. Men succeeded by degrees in controlling the movements of herds and flocks; they would keep them stationary at night, gather them and move them to a preferred area. Little by little, this relationship would allow for women to milk the cattle or sheep, and the pastoral system was born. This might take less than a whole human generation; the effects were rather great. A herd of cattle can support several times as many human beings as pastoralists, as the same herd supports when a hunted target.
3 A modern alternative to ploughing is to spray with a weedkiller and to

direct-drill the seed into sod or stubble. This is a contemporary answer to the age-old problem of how to save power. One ancient answer was to scratch plough in riverine soils, with minimum cultivation. Another was to use flood irrigation as a preparation, as in the Nile, Tigris, Euphrates, Indus, Ganges, Mekong and Chinese river basins. It is no accident that early civilizations often found cultivation easier in alluvial soils. Not only was power requirement lower, but returns usually greater. They still are.

4 This myth may have been based on the fact that ploughmen were usually, after the Normans arrived, too well-educated for their job. Displaced native farmers might have become serfs or slaves, grumbling away, ploughing for most of the winter, regardless of weather.

5 Two, four or eight oxen would be needed in the heavy clay. One man guided the plough, the other 'called' the reluctant animals forward. It was debatable which was harder work. One had to exhaust his wrists in trying to turn the sod, the other to walk backwards talking all the time in a threatening or encouraging way. The 'caller' was known as 'Hywell' in Celtic, and cajoled not only with the voice, but carried a long stick to encourage the beasts in a more physical way. All this was expensive in manpower. There is another point against much heavy-land grain culture by Anglo-Saxons. No purely German quern, or hand-operated grain mill, has ever been found. Anglo-Saxons learned the art of breadmaking from Celts or Romans.

6 It is not likely that straw was regarded as a desirable by-product of grain-growing before the Anglo-Saxons. It was the need to keep cattle winter-productive in inclement conditions which made straw desirable as bedding. Romans and Celts did not nurture cattle for milk, and draft oxen usually wintered outdoors.

7 To make risen bread successfully requires a degree of skill in the grinding. Battered grain, to coin a phrase, will not make any better-risen bread than burnt grain.

8 Pliny *Natural History*. This work is a wealth of information on early agricultural technology.

9 As a result of this property, modern wheat has been selected and bred for its gluten content. A high-gluten wheat is called 'strong'. The strongest wheats in the world are grown in the northern United States and Canada, several times 'stronger' than the average European wheat.

10 Lenin made a personal effort to change Russia from rye bread to wheat bread. It was a disastrous decision. Wheat is much more demanding of personal skill, and communal farms made wheat growing more risky than rye culture. 1913 production of 28 million tons of wheat and 25 million tons of rye (total 53 million tons) became 32 million tons wheat and 21 million tons rye (total 53 million tons) in 1940. This was from an area increased by 25 per cent.

11 Some wheats, but more obviously, some grasses and rye, grow a fungus in difficult years, called ergot. This poisons animals or humans who eat the grain. Curiously enough, goats grazed with other stock on ergot-infested grassland remove the ergot fungus without harm and save other stock from its effects. Ergot was derived from fungoid rye and used ethically to encourage childbirth, at least as late as 1940. Illegally it was widely used in rural areas as a means of procuring abortion. But it had to be used with care by the abortionist. Low-level ingestion of ergot leads to hallucination, see British Association, 1988. In wet harvest years, medieval people inevitably ate large quantities of ergot, and suffered from

generalized poisoning, the body undergoing gangrene as the blood-supply diminished, and there were nervous spasms. In either case, death was general. The last
widespread case of chronic poisoning or ergotism was in the hungry year, 1816,
in Lorraine and Burgundy in France. But the problem must have been serious
in the Middle Ages, and likely to act as an appreciable population control in
times of wet weather when ergot fungus growth could cause abortion and
death.

12 Barley, grown in Ancient Egypt 5,000 years ago, was less valued than wheat
in the esteem of Egyptian beermakers. Bread requires high protein, high gluten;
beer the reverse. Ancient Egyptian wheat may have been of a low-protein,
high-starch nature because of genetics, or climate or Nile husbandry.

13 The famous quotation is: 'A grain which in England is generally given to
horses, but in Scotland supports the people.' Johnson's *Dictionary*, 1755.

14 Curiously enough, this Bengali method, Europeanized as 'Patna Rice', was
apparently unknown to both the Chinese and Japanese. Though they regarded it as
of great importance that their soldiers could carry up to five days' supply of an
undemanding food which required only boiling, both Chinese and Japanese High
Commands knew, at the beginning of this century, that their soldiery would suffer
from beriberi, or thiamine deficiency. Ordinary polished rice was even carried by
Japanese soldiers in World War II.

15 Ancient Ethiopia, a distinct culture in 2000 BC, was known for both wheat and
sorghum excellence to travellers from Ancient Egypt. This makes the teff mystery
even more extraordinary.

16 Besoms (or brooms) made of sorghum straw were sold as late as 1939 in
Europe. Where that of Benjamin Franklin came from is not known.

17 In Russia, in 1905, peasants who were, at most, two generations from
serfdom, were marched towards the railhead in order to fight the Japanese. They
were wide-eyed with wonder. They passed the estate of their neighbour, then the
next place, of which they had heard little, and then the next. The railhead was still
far away, and then 7,000 miles by train. 'Where are the Japanese,' they asked, 'in
the next estate or the one after?' This replicated what must have been true
throughout Western Europe in medieval times.

18 In modern terms, the flow of a river, in weight of water, can be multiplied by
the fall of the river, in vertical distance, and the product used to calculate kg/m to
produce the theoretical horsepower available.

19 From this millstream, especially to drive the mill, it is a small intellectual step
to a pipe leading to a more efficient turbine. This had to wait for the right materials.
This took nearly 1,850 years after Vitruvius, but preceded the generation of
electricity. Low efficiency turbines were built in 1828 in France, on calculations
made by Archimedes who died in 212 BC.

20 Pappus of Alexandria (Greek mathematician, early 4th century AD) perceived
the classical weakness: 'The mechanicians of Hero's school say that mechanics can
be divided into a theoretical and a manual part; the theoretical part is composed of
geometry, arithmetic, astronomy, and physics; the manual work in metals,
architecture, carpentry and the art of painting and the manual execution of these
things. As it is not possible for the same man to excel in so many academic studies
and at the same time to learn the aforesaid crafts, advise one who wishes to
undertake "mechanical work" to use such crafts as he already possesses in the task
to be performed in each particular case.' (Pappus *Book VIII*, 1.) The interplay
between science and technology was one of the most positive factors in the

Renaissance. Leonardo and Michelangelo made all kinds of inartistic devices to perform various tasks, an activity unbelievable in ancient times.

21 Econuts who wish to replace power stations with massive windmill-farms should imagine the noise, discomfort and danger caused by such developments. The idea of having to replace, repair or renew windmills while another is cycling next door should deter all but the most enthusiastic doctrinaire. The other point is the high ratio of capital input to horsepower output. The windmill was often equivalent to a quarter of the investment on a prairie farm, apart from the cost of land itself.

22 The waste of power of all kinds has to be calculated to be believed. Even as late as 1952, two-thirds of all power 'income' from carbon fuels and water power and animal and human energy was wasted in process, transmission, poor control. In 1982, after two energy crises, the 66 per cent lost had only been reduced to 55 per cent.

23 The actual order adopted here for these improvements was that published in the *Encyclopedia Britannica* of 1790, printed in Edinburgh. But these eight factors were in every one of the six or eight 'books of husbandry' printed in the eighteenth century. The *Britannica*, Third Edition, represents a consensus.

24 A great deal of very pleasant research is required to establish just how many metal-bashing establishments were started in the UK in the eighteenth and early nineteenth centuries. During the French Wars from 1792–1815, a huge number were involved in the supply of hardware to the army and navy and the thriving export trade. All of them derived, intellectually at least, from blacksmiths. They were the contractors and sub-contractors to many industries, including the leaders of the time, wool and cotton, coal and iron.

25 More properly, the horse-blacksmith is a farrier. But a farrier was once not only a shoer of horses, but the precursor to modern vetinerary surgeons. Horseshoes were unknown in Roman Europe, and were introduced to England by William the Conqueror. The farrier, practising farriery, was an important crafts-man-expert who ministered to the health of the horses of the nobility and chivalry, with a particular knowledge of horse anatomy. At least as late as 1914, university graduates who became horse vets described themselves as 'farriers'.

26 In 600 BC, what is now modern Greece probably had a population density of only about 15 people per sq. km. Modern densities are still only about 70 per sq. km, not much by Western European standards, but still forcing many people to live in remote areas, too steep and inhospitable for railways, too far for edibles to reach them before the internal combustion engine.

27 In the days before 'artificial' fertilizers, which can increase the fertility of a farm at the tenant's expense, all fertility had to be 'made' at home. To remove the stored-up fertility in animal residues from the lord's land and credit one's own with such wealth was a form of theft.

28 *A Tour through the whole island of Great Britain*, Daniel Defoe, 1724.

29 The physical value of a soil is very much conditioned by the population of earthworms, and therefore of its lime status. Earthworms mix organic matter with the soil, prevent the formation of a mat in grassland and litter in arable conditions. They improve the soil by promoting aeration and drainage and the power of any soil to absorb and benefit from rain or irrigation. Earthworms also increase the 'workability' of a soil, making it kinder for the cultivator, and there is a distinct advantage of several days in any soil with earthworms compared to the same soil without.

30   Clover is a leguminous plant which lives in symbiosis with an appropriate strain of the nodule organism *Rhizobium*. The clover produces the carbohydrate and the organism synthesizes the nitrogen (from the air) required by the part nership. The nitrogen is used for the growth of the clover, and some may become available for the accompanying grass in the pasture. Grasses also benefit from the breakdown of the residues of the clover – leaves, roots, and the annual crop of nodules. In the days before synthetic nitrogen, clover was almost essential for the successful growth of nitrogen-demanding plants in the rest of the rotation.

31   In Ireland such outcrops were known as 'elkpits'.

32   Remission of rent was a powerful persuader in the hands of the landlord. In times of great change, it was often employed to make sure that tenants moved with the times.

33   It is worth noting that great British entrepreneurs, knowing something which the locals did not, scoured the battlefields of Europe for the bones of the fallen and the marl made by the action of time and weather upon those bones. These were exported to England, either to make bone china or paper, or to make bonemeal for manure. The marl, heavier, was sold locally. No one, before the romantic Victorians, thought such behaviour reprehensible or sacriligeous.

34   Arthur Young: *Annals of Agriculture*.

35   One of the major effects of technology is to make land increasingly possible to cultivate, less 'marginal'. No one can do anything about the climate or weather, but soils can be made less acid; more difficult conditions are susceptible to better implements; the horse proved to be much more flexible than the ox; careful breeding of livestock showed that they were more suitable for new conditions than had been the case in earlier times.

36   Nor was there any need at the time. Between 1750 and 1850 England had the largest increase in population up to then ever measured; the increase was even greater than in Ireland – a special case. This kind of increase was unknown in any other area of the world with the English limitations of land per person. In 1850, England, not Britain, had a density of population such that each individual enjoyed the produce of about 0.7 of a hectare. The next densest area in Europe (and probably in the world) was the Low Countries, where each person was fed by about 1.2 hectares of farmland in 1850. See also Sir James Caird: *English Agriculture in 1850–51*.

37   These estimates of horse numbers have been worked out without any great confidence that some worthy will not query them. Railways increased, not reduced horse numbers. There were more non-agricultural horses per million urban population than in rural areas. Horses were an index of prosperity, trade and wealth. In both 1750 and 1850, England probably had a higher horse/people ration than any other European country, probably higher than any country except what is now the United States. Horse statistics given in European Historical Statistics are agricultural, and very incomplete, non-existent in most countries before the late nineteenth century.

38   Illuminated Psalters are a good resource for medieval information, with reservations. (Psalters originated as plain collections of the psalms of David.) The Luttrell Psalter (1338) is a great illustrated tome, attractive to anyone interested in the period. It is in the British Museum, London. There is a caveat to be entered. All the processes described and illustrated were performed at a time of excessive and abundant labour. The procedures one hundred years later were quite different. The

Windmill Psalter (illuminated in Canterbury in 1270) has the earliest extant illustration of a western type windmill. But it is known that windmills were in use in Normandy nearly a century earlier. Many psalters have as illustrations the process of ploughing. But there are no surviving illuminations of eight-ox teams, yet it is known that eight-ox teams were essential in many places. On the other hand, there are several illustrations of one-way ploughs, which allow the furrows to fall all to one side, by swinging the body over at the end of each bout. Yet a swing-plough, or one-way plough, was difficult to build in terms of medieval technology. They were too difficult for most Victorian plough-builders. Equally, with wheeled-ploughs. There were probably more wheeled-ploughs in psalters than on the ground. Anyone who has ploughed knows that a wheel can be a positive disadvantage in stony soils like chalk or oolite or 'cornbrash', which constituted nearly three-quarters of the ploughland of medieval England. It is difficult to avoid believing that psalters illustrated what the patron wanted illustrating, so they should be used with pleasure, tinged with caution.

39 Lapus lazuli probably came further than any other raw material of art which Europeans ever used. The mines were visited by Marco Polo in 1271. They were in modern Afghanistan, on the banks of the River Kokcha. The stone made a brilliant blue 'enamel' and, ground up, a pigment to produce the true ultramarine, or azure blue; a sky blue colour; and a greenish tinge. No one in England probably knew it came from several thousand miles east of the Eastern Mediterranean, where it was probably bought in Levantine markets.

40 After years of efforts, the manufacturing classes, led by cotton manufacturers Richard Cobden and John Bright, joined with radicals and free traders to persuade the then Prime Minister, Sir Robert Peel (1788–1850), to repeal the Corn Laws in 1846. The laws, which covered the import and export of wheat from England, were originally introduced to try to keep the price of bread stable. They became unpopular when Britain began to import much of her corn supplies, resulting in high bread prices at a time of economic depression. The pretext for the repeal was the Irish Potato Famine in 1845, but the free traders were more interested in the principle than the circumstance.

41 Neo-Europeans were not necessarily initially interested in European food supplies. It was population pressure in Western Europe which outgrew home-produced grain, then 'Baltic' grain, then made men look to the United States from the 1780s; it would not be for another hundred years that all the neo-Europes would be in place as exporters.

42 This is detailed in the Potato Chapter of *Seeds of Change*, by the author and it is not intended to repeat the narrative or arguments.

43 L. Quinctus Cincinnatus (*c.*519–438 BC) Consul; dictator in 458 BC. Found ploughing by the messengers summoning him to office. Rescued Consul Minucius, who had been defeated and surrounded by the Aequi. Retired to his farm, after sixteen days dictatorship. A year before his death, at the age of eighty, he became dictator once more to deal with a rising of the plebs. The point of admiration was always that he really preferred work on the land to high office, and that he gave up being a dictator voluntarily. Not a common attribute.

44 As with Ireland, the whole contemporary view of Malthus in 1845–50 is reviewed in the Potato Chapter of *Seeds of Change* by the author, and it is appropriate for further reading.

CHAPTER THREE

New Worlds, New Crops, New Beasts

The exploitation of the Eastern Atlantic Islands started before Columbus, and, as is well known, Columbus victualled and repaired his ships in the Canaries, a new Spanish settlement, before he crossed the Atlantic. The Canaries are several hundred miles nearer the Caribbean than Spain itself.

When Columbus arrived in the New World, an immediately important exchange took place. As already related, diseases were given to the natives. This led straightaway to a weakening of the indigenous resistance to Europeans, a weakening which would be repeated for more than four hundred years in all parts of the world. The next act of unconscious Imperialism was European acquisition of American plants. These included cassava, yams, maize, the white and sweet potato, innumerable beans, tomatoes, squashes and capsicum. These were transferred by Europeans to Europe, to Africa, even from Central to North America. The one plant that Columbus did not find was the one he was looking for, pepper. But his discoveries were a more valuable alternative and side-effect of the search for the Spice Islands.

The introduction of European plants into the Americas is a tale with uneven endings. Wheat, long before any occupation of America north of the Rio Grande, found its niche. Wine took nearly a century to become fit to export, and then it came from Peru and Chile, not Mexico. The olive took longer to settle, and found a home in Chile after 1600, and in California much later still. Yet ever since 1492, olive oil has been exported to the Americas, one of the few staple foods of which this is true. Citrus and stone fruits are another matter. They spread and bred and succeeded magnificently in the continent. Animals, horses, cows, sheep and pigs, unknown in the New World – not only prospered but mutated and went feral. They not only changed their own lifestyles and produced a cash crop for the Iberian settlers, but their arrival changed habits in animal predators and Amerindians alike. In the North, in paticular, the horse became a force of change in the lives of both of the native buffalo and the native Indian who lived on the buffalo. There is nowhere else in evolutionary history a development to match this extraordinary tale.

The horse in North America is a great example of Darwinian forces at work; it was not a story of which Charles Darwin knew anything. Yet he visited other parts of the Americas, whose development triggered his whole corpus of writing about natural selection. The more that is known of the development of post-Columbian America, the more Darwinian the history of the continent becomes.

By 1492, the pattern had already been set. Long before Columbus's first voyage, an indication of the kind of effect which Europeans would have on the world was already available. The Americas, Australasia, most of Africa were unknown to white men: most of the world would be 'discovered' and be conquered by European crops and animals.

The first East Atlantic island to be settled was Madeira. A charter was granted by the Pope to Portugal in 1433. Earlier, it was said to be uninhabited. From about 1420 onward, Madeira and the smaller, lower drier island, Porto Santo, were colonized by Portuguese. Porto Santo was almost completely ruined by one family of rabbits, released in 1430. By 1455, the island was a desert. Whatever the Europeans did to contain the rabbits failed. They killed all the native vegetation, and the animals living on that vegetation have not survived. The island of Porto Santo, as an ecological entity, was killed by less than a dozen rabbits, one doe and progeny which were born on the voyage from Lisbon. This happened more than a generation before 1492.

This kind of ecological disaster was repeated in Hierro, one of the Canaries, in Virginia, the Caribbean, and Australia. Christopher Columbus should have been warned. The man who released the rabbits, Bartholomeu Perestrello, was to become Columbus's father-in-law.

Men who inadvertently destroyed an island were matched by those who destroyed the ecology of almost every new Europe. In the larger island of the group, Madeira itself, the rabbits were not let loose. Madeira means 'wood'. When the Europeans arrived, 'there was not a foot of ground without great trees'.[1] Timber was the first export. But some of the settlers impatiently set fire to great patches of land, to clear the forest to grow crops. There was a huge forest fire which lasted, some contemporaries said, for years. At the end of seven years, there was said not to be a native tree standing. The settlers had introduced pigs and cattle, and these went feral. The pigs alone would have prevented re-afforestation. Honey-bees were producing for export by 1460. But the colonists had sought a crop to make them rich. It would be *sugar*, they thought, a sure-fire crop with an unmeasured demand.

By 1432, the first crop of cane was being pulped. By 1470, the island was producing 70 tons a year, and exporting sugar to Antwerp, Bristol and Bordeaux as well as to Lisbon. The Portuguese also introduced the grape from Crete, and wine was exported before 1492. This wine became a cult, an especial 'Malmsey' – quite different from any Mediterranean wine. Some Madeira wine is the oldest drinkable wine, as opposed to spirit, in the world. Some drinkable wine today dates back to the eighteenth century.

It was at one time believed that European men and animals had destroyed the unique flora and fauna of Madeira. But there are still survivors which could indicate what has been destroyed by pigs or fire. There is a little wren amongst birds which is unique. There are five species of birds shared with the Canaries. The only unique land reptile is a small lizard. There is a special sort of turtle, shared with the Azores. The rest of the specialized fauna are lower animals, molluscs, not to put too fine a point on it. These snails and shellfish are divided into fresh and salt-water examples. Over two hundred species of usually flightless beetles have been found. Presumably, they survived the fire better than any larger animal. There are no unique butterflies, but more than twenty moths of a peculiar Madeiran kind.

Most of today's flora is of European origin, introduced by the Portuguese. Some indigenous plants are shared with the Canaries, or the Azores, and nowhere else. There are about a hundred plants which are peculiar to Madeira. Most of them are ferns, mosses, heaths, but more interestingly, four are laurels. These are seen nowhere else. There are six ferns common to the Caribbean and Madeira, and two small trees or large shrubs which are otherwise wholly American. The unique Dragon tree, which survived the fire, is almost extinct. Some of the introduced species have become pests, such as the prickly pear.

Madeira before 1492 was already a monocultural island. The only cash crop was sugar. By 1492, Madeira was probably the biggest exporter of sugar in the then world, and from the capital of Funchal the food (or drug) went to England, France, Flanders, Italy, South Germany; one load even went to the Levant. At that date, sugar was worth about twelve times as much as honey, and, after the spices, it was the most valuable commodity in world trade. Madeira's 1470 export of 70 tons had increased to just under 1,000 tons. By 1518, the date of the first sugar grown in the Caribbean, Madeira had reached 1,600 tons a year exported. Since there is hardly an area naturally large enough and flat enough for a pair of tennis courts on the island, this was quite an achievement.

Madeira is a volcanic ridge, pushed up out of the sea so that the mountain chain averaging 1,219 metres (4,000 feet) lies roughly east-west. The highest peaks are at about 1,829 metres (6,000 feet). The main island, Madeira, is high enough to attract rainclouds, and the precipitation in the mountains is equivalent to about 1 metre (40 inches) per year. This is measured as snow (above 610 metres or 2,000 feet) or as rain or watery vapour. Frost is unknown in the inhabited towns and villages, the mean temperature at Funchal being 13°C (55°F) in winter, 21°C (70°F) in the summer. The other islands are too dry for any crop except barley. But Madeira's average humidity is about 75 per cent. Conditions are ideal for sugar production; the moisture is in the soggy mountains and, unchecked, falls precipitately to the sea, having carved, over the ages, many near-vertical ravines. Sugar depends upon a massive redirection of this water. Hundreds of miles of channels were cut into the hillsides, redistributing the water with painstaking accuracy and back-breaking labour, to the terraces of some 10,000 original heriditaments. Today, there are still many miles of subsidiary conduits feeding individual patches of land.

Barley, a dry-land crop, can be produced for less than 1,000 tons of water per ton of grain. Wheat needs 50 per cent more, and rice four times the water needed by barley. Sugar needs more water than rice. It also needs as much or more heat. Sugar grew on Madeira, but only after many man-years of labour had made irrigation possible. Only barley grew on Porto Santo.

The people who made sugar possible on Madeira were usually servile, if not always slaves. They were convicts, debtors and delinquents who had sold themselves into slavery, or transportation, from Portugal itself. There were Guanches imported from the Canaries in chains: there were recalcitrant Jews and Muslims from Portugal and Spain who refused to abjure their faith; there were adventurers, some from northern Europe, who won their land-rights for so many years labour. This disparate labour force numbered probably as many as 15,000 in 1492. Today, there is a population of about a quarter of a million, supported by imported food and the tourist trade. Before any of that became possible, in say 1850, the population had not exceeded probably 70,000, mostly engaged in the wine trade and in victualling passing ships.[2]

Even then, and for two hundred years previously, not enough fresh fish was caught for the observance of Catholic fast days, so salt cod was imported from Boston and New York, pickled herring from Sweden, kippers and smoked mackerel from England. It was a return cargo for the ships which carried first sugar, then wine, into Europe or America.[3]

Madeira is a signpost to what would happen if the Europeans found an 'empty' island. The story in the Canaries was modified by the existence of indigenous people, the islands' closeness to Africa, and the much greater extent of potential farmland.

Like the islands of Madeira, those of the Canaries are volcanic: unlike Madeira, they are only from 60 to 250 miles from Africa; Madeira is 360 miles from Africa, nearly 500 from the nearest point in Europe, and 240 from Tenerife, the largest of the Canary Islands. At some point in the Stone Age, the Canaries had been settled from Africa or Europe, and in historical times, there has always been some sort of settlement on each of the Canary Islands, if not always a connection between them. The aboriginal Guanches, as the Europeans called the people they found on the Canaries, do not seem to have been able to use boats of any kind; nor were the Guanches of one island necessarily well disposed towards, or even aware of the natives of another island. The natives of the flat lands of Lanzarote and Fuerteventura seem, at the time of the European arrival, not to have known of the inhabitants of the other islands. These two flatter, dry, eastern islands differ very much from the much higher and steeper Gran Canaria and Tenerife. The latter, indeed, rises to over 3,658 metres (12,000 feet). This summit is the crater of an extinct volcano, from which sulphurous steam still spews; this imparts a whitish hue to the ground. This was falsely called 'eternal snow' by those who had not bothered to walk up to see for themselves. In fact, snow lies for about 150 days each year, but moisture, in the form of mist, or drizzle, heavier drops, or snow, occurs every day of the year.

Equipped with this kind of benefice, Tenerife and to a lesser extent, Gran Canaria, can grow almost any tropical, semitropical or temperature crop. The native Guanches lived on grain, and at least one sort of pea grown in a Stone Age manner; for protein and fat they had shellfish plucked from the rocks, and meat from pigs and goats, which were wild when Europeans arrived. The aborigine people in Tenerife and Gran Canaria were peculiarly well adapted to their wild, mountainous life. They were surefooted, without shoes of course, and had developed a method of calling from one hill to another, like Swiss yodellers, to warn, to inform, to reassure. In this respect, they were close to the African finches, which had also arrived some hundreds of years previously, and had developed a special method of survival in a peculiar place which was ecologically unique. Post-Darwin naturalists studied the finches. The finches of the Canaries were as interesting as the finches of the Galapagos; but the Guanches had been dead three hundred years before Darwin.[4]

If the Guanches were fierce, good Stone Age fighters, capable of defending themselves when they sought and held the high ground, those on the flat islands succumbed much more quickly. Lanzarote[5] and Fuerteventura were Europeanized by 1450. A generation later, Guanches survived on only three islands: La Palma, Gran Canaria and Tenerife. Guanches from the other islands had been killed, transported as slaves to Madeira or Portugal, or died of white man's diseases. Gran Canaria surrendered to the Spanish, after ten years of guerrilla war, in 1483. Four years previously, the Treaty of Alcacava between Portugal and Castille

Animals on the Atlantic

had given the latter sovereignty over the Canaries, and that of Madeira to Portugal. When Christopher Columbus visited the islands in the August of 1492, to revictual and refresh his sailors, there was food available only on Gomera, a flat, wooded island, green and fertile. This he had reached in only six days from Spain, a voyage apparently undertaken on one tack, all the way from the River Tinto, more than 800 miles away.

Though Guanches on Gran Canaria had only surrendered to the Spanish in 1483, there was a shipyard at Las Palmas, where one of Columbus's ships was careened and her rudder repaired. The shipyard had been there since the Spanish expedition of 1475, which had taken all of eight years to kill or capture the last Guanche. The war of attrition in Tenerife took longer.

La Palma, a small island to the west of Gomera, was invaded by a tough Spanish adventurer called Lugo, with about five hundred men. This was in the same month that Columbus set sail for the west. Lugo defeated the Guanches in less than six months, using the same mixture that similar men, Cortés and Pizarro, would use on the Amerindians – force, treachery, horses, gunpowder and the nature of Christian belief. The Spaniards introduced into the Canaries sheep and cattle, donkeys, camels, rabbits and honey-bees. These all became wild from a very early date, even before Tenerife was subdued in 1495, three years after Columbus's first voyage. Did the Spaniards also introduce that great future ally, disease? If not, how did they triumph so quickly?

An estimated population of the Guanches in all the islands was between 60,000 and 100,000. This is not overpopulation by Stone Age farming standards. The islands have enough land to have allowed each Guanche a hectare (2.5 acres) to grow vegetables or grain. This would occupy only 14 per cent of the land area of the Canaries at the highest possible estimate. Today, nearly 25 per cent of the land area is covered by tarmac, concrete, buildings, airports, swimming pools and other sterile areas as well as cultivated ground. The current population is nearly 2 million at the height of the season, largely fed from imports. In 1900, the year of the first true census, the population was about 350,000. These people fed themselves from their own land, and exported cash crops to Europe.

Before turning the Canaries into one of the first Spanish Atlantic colonies, did the Spaniards need to wipe out the Guanches? On the island of Hierro in the late 1580s, all living matter on the island was reduced to starving rabbits which lived on anything that grew. As a result, Hierro was almost denuded of plants of any kind. Nearly everything that now grows in that once rabbit-induced desert has been imported. The island of Fuerteventura was ruined by the same date by feral donkeys and Bactrian camels. Over three-quarters of both species were hunted and killed in the

1590s, and have been controlled ever since. The island of Gomera, a garden at the time of Columbus's first voyage, became a refuge for the other sort of camel, the dromedary. There were several thousand of them, eating their heads off, in 1640. No Stone Age people could resist a plague of rabbits; even a plague of camels or donkeys would wipe out Stone Age food supplies. Virgin areas free of natural enemies were so favourable to new species that European imports of animals flourished wherever they were introduced, causing a population explosion which may have starved indigenous humans.

Far quicker than imports of rabbits or rats would be disease. There was said to be an epidemic, a *peste*, amongst the Guanches in the terrible winter of 1495, during which the Spanish waited for their victory on the low-lying ground of Tenerife. The Guanches who had been driven up the mountainside starved in consequence. The strategy worked. In the spring, so many unburied Guanche bodies lay in the ravines and on the hills that the fierce wild dogs who allegedly gave the Canaries their name, were living on protein-rich carrion. Previously, the dogs had been vegetarian. Even the dogs' habits changed. No one knows the nature of the *peste*.[6]

The Canary Islands were notably healthy, to judge from remarks made by all early European arrivals. *La peste* was considered by the Spaniards, when it arrived (with the Spanish) more than a century after the first Europeans, to be a punishment for the Guanche practice of infanticide. No one would tell the Spaniards that a people without indigenous disease to control population have to practise birth control by some other method. No European Christians changed their perspective in four hundred years. In the nineteenth century, Anglican missionaries disapproved just as much of Australian Aboriginal infanticide as Spanish friars did in Tenerife.

Before 1500, the evidence was all there for anyone who wished to assemble it. An uninhabited island, like Madeira, would be exploited very quickly. The native plants and animals could be reduced to impotence by vigorous European imports. They would not be defended by native humans. Introduced European crops could be grown profitably by known methods, using human muscle in the form of easily managed, servile labour. Animal muscle, most highly developed in the Mediterranean, would be ox, buffalo, horse, donkey (to provide mules) or camel. Europeans had them all, the Atlantic islands none.

By 1500, Madeira would be the world's largest sugar exporter. An island of only 15,000 acres of land which could be easily cultivated was producing enough food for 15,000 people in 1500, and exporting at least 1,200 tons of sugar each year at that date.[7] The relationship between the gold price and sugar price in 1500 was of the order that 45 kg (100 lbs) of sugar was worth the same as 1 oz of gold. So 1,200 tons of sugar exports from Madeira were worth as much as 24,000 oz of gold. The West African gold trade was only worth half as much as the Madeiran sugar trade. No wonder the Spanish tried to repeat the Portuguese success in the Canaries.[8]

The Canaries contained a population which was killed, enslaved, sold; more died by disease. By 1525, a generation after the final conquest of Tenerife, there were few pure-blooded Guanches left. Some had travelled in Spanish ships making for the Caribbean. Others had left, voluntarily, or as slaves, for Europe and Madeira. The same pattern of conquest would be repeated in every 'new country' inhabited by indigenous, virgin populations. Having killed off the natives of most of the Caribbean islands, Europeans imported blacks who were slaves, or whites who were criminals, debtors, or indigent. In some parts of the Caribbean, whites arrived to find paradise islands free from native humans. Then the problem was much easier. 'Empty' islands offered facile solutions. Madeira was in profit long before the Canaries.

East Atlantic islands were not always profitable paradises before the tourist boom induced by jet aircraft. The Azores were an example. They were apparently unpopulated at the time of the first Renaissance voyages. Situated more than a thousand miles from the Straits of Gibraltar, the islands appear to have been visited by the Carthaginians.[9] What did they do when they got there, in the absence of anyone with whom to deal? More importantly, the Carthaginians probably never returned.[10]

The Azores, named after the native hawks,[11] are volcanic in origin. They have a mild climate, less warm than either Madeira or the Canaries, but absolutely frost free. They were fully occupied by the Portuguese by 1460, about the same date as Madeira. They were 'given' by the king of Portugal to his Flemish aunt in 1466. When they were first established in the Azores, the Portuguese attempted to grow wheat, in short supply at that date in Portugal.

After wheat, an effort was made to grow sugar, that great magic drug of the Renaissance. Yields were far lower than in Madeira, perhaps because of the extremely stormy winds in the Azores, perhaps because not enough irrigation was available to supplement rainfall. After 1540, the growing of indigo was attempted, and the making of dyes from a species of imported grass. *Indigofera*, a leguminous plant which was imported from Asia into the Atlantic islands of every sort, was the great origin of blue dyestuffs until the synthetic chemists discovered how to produce a more stable alternative from napthaline. Aniline dyes made redundant huge areas of plantations devoted to vegetable dyes. Before this, India had been found to be a better source of vegetable dyes than either the Azores or the Caribbean. After indigo, colonists on the Azores attempted the growing of pineapples, which became the favoured nineteenth-century export. Over one million fruit were often exported annually to Europe.

The Azores were never hungry, a thriving fishing industry being established before 1700, and whaling at about the same time. Portuguese fishermen from the Azores also worked the Grand Banks, more than 1,000 miles distant, but 1,000 miles closer than is Portugal to that great source of cod. The Azores are in many ways too far north, and therefore too cool; and too far from Europe, too far from the United States, to benefit as much from the tourist trade as do the Canaries. A third the area of the Canaries, the nine islands in the Azores contain only one sixth the people. Perhaps their place in history was most important when their existence helped close the mid-Atlantic gap in the days of World War II. At a time when aircraft could not cross the Atlantic in one hop, the Azores were an essential refuelling point.[12]

Columbus had taken six days to reach the Canaries, about 800 miles from his departure-port in Spain. He took 36 days to cross the Atlantic, from the Canaries to what is now Watling Island in the Bahamas, named by the Spaniards San Salvador. No one knows how far the three small ships travelled, but it is likely that the course taken amounted to more than 4,000 miles. What they took with them was the hope of reaching Japan and the spices of the Indies. In fact, they had taken with them the cultivar of a plant which would dominate the Caribbean for most of the next five hundred years. This was the noble cane – sugar.

Sugar canes were taken by many Renaissance travellers, by sea or land. The canes were cut into convenient pieces of thick cane, soft and easy to chew, high in energy, low in fibre. Some of these may have been deliberately planted by Columbus on his first voyage. On the second voyage, in 1494, cane was planted in San Domingo, and settlers left to tend the plantation: both cane and settlers succumbed to natives, but within twenty years, the sugar trade from the Caribbean had begun. It would not be until 1550 that the West Indies rivalled the East Atlantic Islands in production.

Sugar requires high temperatures, plenty of sunlight, large quantities of water. Each ton of refined sugar requires enough soil nutrients to grow 2 tons of wheat; enough water to grow 10 tons of rice; enough sunshine to grow a ton of cotton. Before 1800, a ton of sugar needed enough fuel in primitive refining techniques to produce a ton of iron; enough forced labour to equate 1 ton of sugar with the life of 1 black slave. Sugar is often said, by botanists, to be 'the cheapest form of energy-giving food with the lowest unit of land area per unit of energy produced'. By what measure?

Sugar has never been as cheap as it should, in theory, be. Even today, when new breeding programmes and new growing techniques have increased yields by twenty times over eighteenth-century levels, sugar is still nearly twice the cost of the same energy in wheat and much more than twice as much as the same energy in maize, or Indian corn. Nor is sugar a staple source of energy. No one who tried to use sugar as this would survive for long. It is used as a confection, an attractive, unsatisfying addition to the diet, an addiction for some. For the Spaniards who were obsessed by the search for gold, Caribbean sugar was much less important than for others.

The sugar trade was the most important in the world until overtaken by coal in tonnage and by coffee in value. About 150,000 tons were exported to Europe from the Americas in the early 1800s. The figure a century later was twenty times as great. Sugar was the first massive transfer of energy from colonies to advanced countries since the Roman import of wheat and barley from Egypt, North Africa, Sicily and Sardinia in the first centuries of our era.

More important than the transfer of energy was the waste of energy. In 1800 sugar cost seven times as much in economic terms as the same energy in flour from wheat, and twenty to fifty times the cost of the same energy in potatoes grown in the consumer's garden. It was, of course, a more attractive form of energy, but the waste involved has to be noted: in the Triangular Trade the huge naval resources required; in the provision devoted to trade protection and limiting piracy; not to speak of the huge number of people in Europe and the Americas engaged in manufacture or service to exchange for slaves in Africa and sugar in the Americas. It was a vast industry with great value added, except for the slave. An extreme modern economic parallel is in good wine. This commands, in financial terms, from ten to a hundred times the cost of the same energy in fruit juice. But just as wine is more fun than fruit juice, so sugar was more fun two hundred years ago than potatoes. The idea, two hundred years ago, that sugar could be addictive was wholly unimagined. Today, the first world is divided between those who regard sugar as an addiction, and those who have an interest of some sort in refusing to believe in such a possibility.

The sugar trade was never seen as a kind of energy transfer. Its importance was that it was the first modern trade in which a colonial people grew exclusively for the 'home' consumer. In the process, slaves, overseers, even owners went very hungry in the event of a blockade during one of the interminable wars of the eighteenth century. The colonial experience of a plantation product being grown at the expense of native ability to subsist on native food has been repeated all over the third world. One reason why Africa cannot feed itself is that it has lost the art of growing its own food, as has the Caribbean, because the land has been devoted to export crops. The sugar trade was the first to produce producer-hunger because of devotion to export. It was not to be the last.

Sugar was grown in southern Spain, all over the Mediterranean, and in the East Atlantic islands; metropolitan Spain had plenty of sugar; demand in Iberia never reached the French, Dutch or English levels. There may have been fifty to a hundred plantations in the Caribbean by 1592, a hundred years after Columbus, but it was the Dutch, French and English who made of sugar a great international enterprise; they also made of slavery an economic necessity and of the slave trade a social shame. By 1650, the British colony of Barbados was the largest source of sugar, producing probably 50,000 tons of raw sugar, molasses, and rum, and exporting, perhaps, one-third of all sugar in world trade. Until the eighteenth century, the statistics of sugar production and trade, and of the numbers of slaves imported with or without the Spanish 'asiento' or monopoly permission, are unreliable. But there were more plantations in English Barbados in 1650 than there were in all the Spanish colonies in 1600 – and probably five times as much West Indian sugar in 1650 as fifty years earlier.

White man's demands for labour in the sugar plantations led to the death of most of the fierce Caribs, who would not be enslaved, as well as of the milder Arawaks, who pined away and would not adapt. Europeans then turned to Africa for their labour. For nearly 350 years Africans were regularly imported, until during the peak century, that of 1690–1790, 12 million black lives were involved in the production of 12 million tons of sugar. They were captured in Africa, sold, manacled, marched to the coast, sold again, chained on board ship, sold in the islands, and then 'seasoned' to the prevailing Caribbean conditions. Africans became essential to the sugar enterprise. Slavery made the African the dominant racial group in the Caribbean. In 1950, there were more people with West African blood in the Caribbean than in West Africa.[13]

In fact, hunger in the midst of potential plenty occurred as early as the second voyage of Columbus. Finding that the stores brought over the Atlantic were spoilt or spoiling, largely because of humidity, the adventurers were driven to the only local supplies of human food – fish and cassava. *Cassava*, or *manioc*, or *tapioca*, is a shrub, the tubers of which were mashed and eaten throughout Amerindian tropical America, from 25°N to 25°S. Sweet cassava has never been found in a wild state; therefore, it had been cultivated for generations before Columbus.[14]

The sailors and buccaneers did not know how to eat the roots which derive from the annual plantings of this shrub, which can be either sweet or bitter. The bitter cassava often have a very high HCN content. This is one of the great problems of using the plant, which has many other advantages. HCN is the vegetable form of hydrocyanic acid, and is liberated when the enzyme linease (contained in the living plant) acts upon the glucoside linamarin. In sweet cassava, the HCN is usually only found in the outer layers of the root; in bitter cassava, HCN is widely distributed, and can only be destroyed by boiling, roasting, or fermentation. Stale tubers are more poisonous than fresh. One plant contains enough HCN to kill quite a large animal.

Amerindians did not have to cope with large animals in the Caribbean. There were none. At first, Columbus's sailors found the cassava almost uneatable. Yet it was the staple starchy food of the Indians. Is it possible that the Indians did not let the invaders have the (cultivated) supplies of sweet cassava, and only permitted them to eat the wild, bitter, varieties? Or did the Spanish never have access to the methods which Amerindians found best to make cassava palatable?

Cassava is quite a good staple starchy food. In the dry matter, there is normally over 90 per cent starch, and plenty of calcium and vitamin C. Nearly all the protein is in the leaves, which may contain HCN, even in the 'sweet' varieties. The boiled tubers are bland, tedious, not a food of which any cuisine can be made. Supplemented by beans or fish, they become a balanced if boring staple.

The way that subsequent generations have found cassava to be interesting enough to be used as a daily diet is to ferment the mashed, cooked roots. This is allowed to become what might be described as quarter-ale, then cooked, in flat cakes. These are then, like all fermented starchy products, nutty, sweet, more interesting than the plain, boiled vegetable. The same improvement occurs with bananas and cassava.

Fermented, cassava is also a better food as well as more interesting. If allowed to ferment fully and become mild ale, drunk straight from the mash tub becomes a product even richer in vitamins, more easily digested, far less boring. People actually enjoy fermented 'mealy beer'. It is significant that this technique was native to Africa, and employed on bananas, which are also native to Africa. These techniques owe nothing to the white man, or biochemists of any sort. Africans make use of the same techniques today on maize and cassava.

The sailors of Columbus in all probability only boiled cassava, in which case they had a pudding rather like a Victorian tapioca pudding, fed to children of every class. In the case of Columbus's sailors, manioc or cassava or tapioca was not provided with the milk or sugar without which no Victorian child would have eaten the pudding, unless very hungry. Alternatively, the Europeans may have eaten cassava raw, in which case it is even more unpalatable. Columbus's sailors were hungry enough not to grumble. Cassava was a very early import into the tropical Old World.

The great virtue of this plant, perhaps a unique virtue, is that it is the only human food which is almost entirely pest-proof. Cassava is immune, amongst all foods, to the African locust. Bitter cassava can be planted in areas where monkey, ape, baboon, wild hog, porcupine, even elephant are a problem. The same animals do not eat such crops twice. It has been interesting for naturalists to see how quickly animal intelligence associates cassava with death. What probably happens is that an ester is released by the leaves which signals to predatory animals that HCN is present. While bitter and sweet cassava can be planted at random, quite young animals know the difference. Humans find identification more difficult.

Cassava was very early taken to West Africa by Europeans, above all, by the Portuguese. The plant was in São Tomé and the Bight of Benin before 1500, and in the Congo not much later. It was not used much elsewhere in Africa until the population explosion which occurred after European rule in the nineteenth and twentieth centuries. Cassava was planted as the great reserve crop of the tropics by white governments, anxious to prevent starvation. It has one other great virtue. Certain cultivars can survive in the ground, unharvested, for several years. It is thus, literally, a food-bank, untouchable by pests, in reserve until wanted. Grown at low cost, it spread all over the tropics. If it were still widely grown, people would not complain so much of 'starvation'. Dry matter yields of over 2 tons per acre are not difficult to achieve.

The crop has acquired a more recent virtue or vice, as perspective may dictate. Grown, dried, ground and exported from South-East Asia, mostly Thailand, the crop is the cheapest form of starchy animal feed available in Europe. The industry of manioc-import has given rise to the ludicrous spectacle of European farmers substituting manioc for barley or wheat, and selling the unwanted home-produced cereal to the European Community which then has to store or sell it, heavily subsidized on the world market. This kind of folly is only, of course, made possible in the end by excessive subsidy.

In a free market, manioc would be used where cheaper. In a free market economy like that of Australia or Canada, European cereals are grown at a cost far lower than the effective cost of imported manioc. If European farmers could not meet such prices in a free market, grain for animals would give way to imported manioc.

The true Spaniard could not eat without bread, and bread needs those Mediterranean essentials, oil and wine. Early Spanish *conquistadores* used cassava 'bread' for poor people of all races. It was grown all over tropical America and in the West Indies and other hot, wet areas, it was a substitute for cereals. Spaniards, unimaginatively, sought in their first, golden century to impose upon the New World the diet of Castile: wheat, oil and wine. It would be nearly a century before all three could be produced in quantity.

Columbus had not discovered any substitute for wheat, and cassava is notably low in fat and the native Amerindians had no wine of any sort.[15] On the second voyage, Columbus took with him to Hispaniola over a thousand men and seeds and cuttings of a hundred different plants. In the Caribbean, wheat and other grains failed, as did grape vines and olive seedlings. But about half the Mediterranean imports flourished: cauliflowers but not cabbages; warm weather radishes; southern types of lettuce; melons but not marrows; oranges and lemons but not apples; figs did particularly well, and could have become a staple, as they were at that date on some Greek islands. But figs did not provide a diet for full-blooded Spanish *conquistadores*.

The Spanish, to be fair, were not in the Americas in order to repeat the hard experience which they had left at home. The idea that they should settle as colonists like pensioned Roman soldiers was not to their taste. The aim was for swifter wealth and glory: a quicker profit was intended. Quite modest settlers were given quite large landgrants, plus, of course, the necessary Indian slaves to work the land. Unfortunately, the Amerindians continued to die of white man's diseases. Nor was the wealth of the Indies to be found in the earth at low cost. By 1556, when Philip II succeeded his father Charles as ruler, most easily worked, easily stolen gold had been discovered and silver had become more important than gold. Because of death by disease of perhaps half the population or more, a labour shortage was already in evidence in Mexico. Fortunately for Spain, technology came to the rescue. It was the introduction of the mercury treatment of ore in 1557–8 that raised potential in Potosi, in modern Bolivia, for example, to become the richest silver mine in the world. It produced more than 3 million ounces a year in the period 1560–1760.[16]

In the end, the deepest mine, the thickest lode, the most concentrated ore has to give out. The only true wealth is renewable. America possessed renewable wealth, in the form of two plants which would transform Europe.

Maize today is the most widely distributed grain in the world. After wheat and rice it is the most important economically. It is able to produce more per man-hour and more per acre than any energy crop except sugar cane in the tropics and the potato in colder zones: it is more adaptable, more widespread and more easily handled than either. Maize was the staple crop of all the Americas from the River Plate to the St Lawrence. Its use gave indigenous Amerindians more leisure than growers of wheat or rice. Less than 2 days work a week suffices for maize against 4–6 days for other grains. There were seven main cultivars known to the Indians and to the Spanish after 1520, and these are still the main non-hybridized ecotypes. Hybridization in the twentieth century has transformed grain and cob size. At the time of Columbus, grain size was of the order of modern lentils, about one-tenth the volume of modern grain.[17]

Europeans took maize seed-grains with them all over the world, starting with Columbus's return to Iberia in 1493. Maize was an important food crop for both man and beast in the Mediterranean by 1550, and was certainly introduced at some early time into West Africa. During the sixteenth century, though, linguistic references in many languages to 'Guinea Corn' almost certainly refer to sorghum rather than to maize.[18]

Linguistic caution should be allied to husbandry insight. Maize cannot resist animal predators in the same way as can sorghum, cassava or millet. The important factor about maize in its original home was that there were no wild or domestic pigs, sheep, cattle, goats or horses to prejudice the growth, development and spread of maize cultivars. In Africa there are plenty of natural enemies for maize.[19] Maize was certainly a major cash crop in West Africa by 1690, and during the next century it was used as provisions for the slave-trading forts and to victual ships for the Middle Passage from West Africa to the Americas. Today, maize has transformed Africa, probably feeding, directly, up to half the population in many places.

Maize flour like cassava cannot be made into raised bread. But scone-like flat 'tortillas' were baked by Amerindians; the native tribes avoided pellagra, which plagued whites who used maize as a staple human food. Pellagra, the deficiency disease, affected people all over the world, 10 million in southern Europe in the late nineteenth century, even as many as 500,000 in the southern US states as late as the 1920s, and more than 5 million during the depression of 1929–35. The deficiency is still important in parts of southern Africa.

In industrial countries, pellagra was cured by the addition of vitamin B_4 (niacin), discovered in 1934. Amerindians had used three methods to avoid the disease.[20] White men arrogantly ignored that part of maize culture when they arrived in the Americas. They took maize seed all over the then world but failed to avoid pellagra.

The influence of maize throughout the world has been immense. Maize is now the staple food of millions, cooked as a thick mush or dough, as a gruel or porridge, as a mildly fermented beer, as 'bread' mixed with wheat flour. In the first world, immature cobs are eaten 'sweet'; the more mature cobs are roasted; dry grain can be used to produce hominy grits, corn-flakes, popcorn and cornflour for thickening of all kinds.

After maize, the most valuable plant transferred from the Americas to

Europe was the *potato*. The history of the potato is well documented. Brought by Europeans from the Andes, Peru and Bolivia to various countries before 1600, it was of no economic importance anywhere except in Ireland before 1700. Though species of tuber-bearing solanum have been found as far north as modern Colorado, and wild tubers were, and are, eaten in parts of Mexico and the south-western United States, there were no 'potatoes' cultivated except in the Andes, and no solanum species with edible tubers existed outside the Americas.[21]

Neither maize nor cassava (manioc, tapioca) will grow in the Andean highlands. It was the potato culture that permitted human settlement there at the end of the last Ice Age. At the end of the pre-Columbian period, the Inca culture evolved, and this necessitated, or was the outcome of, a centralized government. When the Spanish arrived in the 1520s, Inca agriculture involved irrigation, terracing, artificial reclamation of land, the use of guano brought from the coast, and the planned, directed colonization of mountain districts to grow the potato. The town of Cuzco, the centre of Inca culture and wealth, lies at an altitude of nearly 3,500 metres (over 11,000 feet). There is a mass of Inca artefacts relating to the potato, the only staple food that could have served the population. At the time of Pizarro's capture of the city in 1533, it is likely that the inhabitants of the valley numbered about 100,000, all of them basically dependent upon the potato, or upon maize brought from lower altitudes.

Protein was short in the diet, and potato-dependent Incas could not usually, like the maize-eating Mexicans, supplement starch with beans. There were few sources of animal protein, except guinea-pigs. Since the Inca dictatorship was not noted for cannibalism, it is possible that the potato was then of a higher protein content than the European examples of today, or that the guinea-pig culture was highly organized.[22]

The potato became of world importance in the peculiar circumstances of Ireland after 1650. The population multiplied and multiplied, until there were nearly 9 million people by 1844, despite twenty years when the potato crop failed and at least 15 per cent of the population died in each of twenty separate famines.[23] Such a horrifying failure of a staple food occurred because of six diseases which diminished the yield of potatoes from 10 per cent to 50 per cent in various parts of Ireland.

Before 1844, there had been no total failure of the potato crop in the whole island. In 1845, a new disease, Blight,[24] appeared, and changed the course of history. Arriving from the United States by steamer in June 1845, the new plague killed every potato field in the United Kingdom, and vast areas throughout Europe. This disease was caused by a fungus, the control of which was impossible until the 1920s. The fungus killed the potatoes. Resulting famine killed more than a million Irishmen, caused perhaps another million not to be born, induced another 4 million to emigrate in the following half-century, and reduced the population of Ireland from 9 million in 1841 to less than half that figure in 1941. The rest of Western Europe had more than doubled its population during the same century, despite considerable emigration.

On the European continent, the use of the potato was not normally monocultural. It took a very long time for the tuber to be accepted by the peasantry, and it was not really until after the Napoleonic Wars that the vegetable became a staple food for the poor. Ironically, it had been accepted as a curiosity by the rich a century previously. From 1820 onwards, the acreage of potatoes increased throughout Western and Central Europe, both absolutely and as a percentage of total arable and garden crops. In the last case, peasants were never driven to the Irish expedient of total reliance, but the potato as a source of human and animal energy was of great importance in all the major European continental countries. There were significant national differences. In Germany, potatoes were more important than wheat, and rye was an essential, with potatoes, on light sandy soils before the post-1950 agricultural revolution. In France, with better soils and a warmer climate, wheat was more important as a staple, but potatoes were more widely grown than rye. In Italy, maize was more widely grown than anything except wheat, but potatoes, at one-quarter the arable area of maize, were also widely grown in gardens and plots. Many authorities consider that Germany's nearly threefold increase in population in the century before 1914 was largely fuelled by the tonnage of potatoes grown, which rose from about 1 million metric tonnes to about 50 million in the same hundred years.[25]

Potatoes were of great importance in countries further east, but statistics are not wholly reliable. It is obvious, however, that potatoes in Eastern Europe were of cardinal importance in saving life in both world wars, and their aftermaths. Without this Columbian addition to the diet, so easily cultivated on a cottage basis, life in Germany, Russia, Eastern Europe and the Balkans in the period 1919–22, and 1945–50 would have been even more savagely unpleasant than it was. Perhaps the potato prevented 20 million deaths from starvation in these years. It remains a staple standby today in every kind of kitchen-garden, allotment or patch of ground in any troubled country with an incompetent government.

There is a certain amount of confusion about early references to potatoes. The name was given to the white potato, or *Solanum tuberosum* which only reached Europe in the late 1570s. It did not reach North America until the white man brought it west. Indeed, it was known as the Irish potato in Virginia in the early 1620s. In turn, the white potato stole its name from the sweet potato, or *Ipomea batata*.

The Carib word *batata* was taken by Columbus when he took the sweet potato to Europe in 1493. From Europe, the Portuguese took it to West Africa. The Spanish took it from Mexico to the Philippines in about 1550, and the Chinese obtained it in 1590. It was seen growing in Japan in 1698. Meanwhile, it had been taken by the English from Europe (or the West Indies) to Virginia before 1650. This was later than the Irish potato, which by then had had a score of harvests in the new colony.

Sweet potatoes have a nutritious tuber which can be baked or boiled. They are drier than white potatoes, with 90 per cent carbohydrate in the dry matter, more protein at 6 per cent, and they are rich in vitamin C. As its name implies, it is, like most tropical vegetables, high in sugar. Like white potatoes, they have to be ridged, and are harvested as required. The tubers store poorly out of the soil. The crop is seventh in tonnage of world dry matter, following wheat, rice, maize, barley, cassava and white potatoes. It is ahead of oats, sorghum, sugar cane, the millets. Since the sweet potato is easier to cultivate than yams, acreage is growing at the expense of that vegetable; while cassava has an easy culture, and can be stored with ease, so the sweet potato is easy to grow, but harder to store than cassava. The sweet potato has been cultivated in almost every tropical and subtropical country. In one country outside the Americas, it was present when the whites arrived.

A New Zealand form of sweet potato, Kumara, was the staple food of the Maoris when the first Europeans arrived. They were the crew of the two ships commanded by Abel Tasman; some of the crew landed in what is now called Massacre Bay in the South Island, on 18–20 December 1642. Four or five of the Dutch were murdered by the Maoris, and Tasman reimbarked; not before he found the Maoris using sweet potatoes as a staple food. It was also found as a staple all over Polynesia. How had the cultivars reached New Zealand? This has puzzled botanists, geographers, ecologists ever since.

To start with, mankind had to assume that *Ipomea batata* was taken by men from South America to the South-West Pacific. This 6,000 mile journey may or may not have been made. If so, it was the only voyage made to or from pre-Columbian South America. This was linked together by Thor Heyerdahl with the remains at Easter Island, and the superiority of the Polynesian voyagers led many white researchers to plot pre-Columbian voyages of great importance. The only problem with these theories is that, if the voyage was ever made, why was not much more than the sweet potato brought over? There are a hundred vegetables which would have been useful for settlers to take from South America to the Pacific. But the sweet potato is unique. To believe in the intervention of mankind, the searcher after truth has to believe that the sweet potato, either in tuber form or as seed, was brought, alone, across the Pacific. There is an alternative.

The sweet potato is today usually propagated by cuttings, not by seed. If these are allowed to become too dry, life departs the tissue. This was observed by the early Spanish returning to Europe. Cuttings left soaking, even in salt-water, would live on. So it is entirely possible that the sweet potato, like some of the coconuts, reached the south-west Pacific on their own, by sea.[26]

It is likely that the sweet potato was brought to New Zealand by the Maoris when they arrived in AD 1200–1300 from Polynesia. The Maoris also brought with them a small dog. This was their sole source of tame animal protein. The dogs were also seen in Tahiti, Fiji, and elsewhere in the Pacific at the first white contact. The Maoris were also cannibals at the time Captain Cook arrived. This would seem to indicate a protein shortage, as anyone would indeed expect from a diet largely composed of sweet potato. The Maoris had few vegetables high in protein.

Despite its boring nature, the sweet potato offers more return for less work than almost any other staple plant in any climatic zone. As a result, it had spread, by 1800, to every part of the world where the white man had to be responsible for feeding people. It grows from 40°N to 32°S, in the tropics from sea-level to 2,200 metres (7,000 feet), but it needs a temperature of about 23°C (75°F) and lots of sunshine. It needs an annual rainfall of at least 762 mm (30 in), and this should be well distributed, since sweet potatoes do not stand drought at all well. They are a short-day plant, and long days – of more than 12 hours daylight – inhibit flowering. It is wrong to confuse the moist, jelly-like flesh of some of the varieties with yams, and Americans are apt to do so. The flowered members of the tribe are called 'Morning Glory' by subtropical gardeners. The sweet potato does not travel well in commerce; it has not entered world trade.

The Irish or white potato has undergone a profound and almost incredible mutation in the years between its 'discovery' by Pizarro's ruffians and its adoption as a staple European food. In the Andes, it was a short-day plant grown almost on the Equator at a great height, in relatively dry climatic conditions. In Ireland, it became a long-day plant in a notably high-humidity climate at low altitudes.

Some of the best quality potatoes in the world are now grown in the Arctic Circle, in Northern Norway, Sweden, Finland and Russia. In the Americas, the best modern potatoes are grown in the north of the United States, or at altitudes in northern Ontario and in southern Argentina or the Falkland Islands. Whatever has happened to potato cultivars, they remain divided, after thousands of years, into mealy types and waxy types. The mealy types contain more starch. The difference can be discovered without cooking. A brine solution of 10 per cent (10 parts water, 1 part salt) will act as detective. Waxy potatoes float, those with mealy interiors sink. No potato buyer ought to be without a 10 per cent brine solution. The reaction of the average friendly shopkeeper may be imagined.

The Americas had no native animals of any agricultural consequence, but they had a great many available plants besides the four staples which have been treated at length. These were used by the Iberians to make up Latin American cookery. They were taken back to Mediterranean Europe. From the Mediterranean they spread all over Europe, and then all over the world. The food plants are a formidable list, but they include everyday vegetables which Europeans now regard as their birthright as well as extraordinary exotica like vanilla and 'allspice', which took many years to find a place in European cookery. The most important group, nutritionally, were the beans.

Beans, amazingly, were hardly known in Europe before Columbus. The broad bean (or horse bean, field bean, tick bean, Windsor bean) is the only European variety; it suffered in antiquity because some Greeks and Romans thought that this then unique vegetable contained the souls of the dead. There is a peculiar genetic sensitivity in certain Mediterranean people to the toxin *vicine* which occurs in broad beans. The toxin causes anemia. Did the Ancients know about the danger? Was the genetic condition commoner in Ancient Greeks and Romans, perhaps only 5 per cent of the gene-bank of the modern Mediterranean? Are there other peculiarities of this kind, now swamped by the genetic change in people? This anemia is called *favism* in people, because the broad bean is also known as the *fava* bean.

The 'French' bean was grown in Mexico for nearly 7,000 years. Brought to Spain it developed best in France, hence its European name. Europeans in turn took it to North America, where it became a staple legume, together with peas, and other beans. The French bean, in England before 1592, has spread all over the world. It is very old. Recognizable uncharred pods have been found in Mexican caves and carbon-dated at about 5000 BC.

The scarlet runner bean was grown by Amerindians in maize sections, and allowed to take over for a couple of years after the maize harvest. The ground was thus rested, and restored. This is a long-day plant, killed by frosts, but specimens have been found from as long ago as 7000 BC. Has the scarlet runner changed since that date? As a garden cultivar, this bean is more successful in cool, moist Atlantic climates than the French bean.

The lima bean, or butter, or Madagascar or Burma bean is grown for its shelled seed, like a broad bean. Some cultivars contain hydrocyanic acid, like cassava (manioc, tapioca). Other cultivars, as with manioc, are harmless. The more dangerous lima beans should be soaked or boiled before eating; in practice this means all.

Every other garden bean known has been developed from genetic material brought from the Americas, including the special bean, grown in Michigan, which is used for Boston baked beans. In Mexico, one plant biologist has identified over seventy varieties of beans, white, black, red, green and yellow. It is probable that, like maize, beans contain a huge bank of genetic material, which is even now not yet fully exploited.

Like maize and potatoes, beans became important in Europe as 'break' crops. Instead of fallow, alternative crops can be planted which make different demands on the soil, and so 'rest' it by using different nutrients. For example, the cabbage family, the brassicae, require certain qualities in a soil which potatoes do not; both beans and peas are legumes, so that their growth not only demands different nutrients to those taken by cabbages or potatoes, but the action of the nodules on the roots makes nitrogen (from the air) available to soil and the plants. This process was not, of course, known in the Ancient or Middle Ages, but beans and peas were regarded as 'restorative' crops.

In Europe, potatoes and peas and beans were not grown on a farm scale until they could be properly mechanized in the eighteenth century. Maize was a peasant alternative to fallow by the eighteenth century in a broad swath leading through Portugal, Spain, Southern France, Northern Italy, to the modern Balkans. Arthur Young[27] writing just before the French Revolution said: 'Where there is no maize there are fallows; where there are fallows, the people starve for want.'

For Arthur Young, the cause and effect were quite clear. For the French landlord of the *ancien régime*, cause and effect was less certain. For the peasant, as for the peasant in Russia as late as in 1913, agricultural method came from above. In England, in Arthur Young's day, this was also true, but in England there were landlords who imposed upon their tenants both land tenure and good farming methods which made for profit for the landlord and plenty for the tenant. The improvements in England described in Chapter Two were not in place anywhere else in Europe before about 1850. Nor was the use of fallow crops systematized. If the French peasant grew maize in the 1780s, he was lucky, and ate better than his neighbours.

Out of maize, too, grew many modern French meat dishes, including pâté de foie, the goose being overfattened by the force-feeding of maize, and thus given fatty liver.[28] Maize was known as *'blé d'Espagne'* in France, and similar names were in use in Italy, Greece and Turkey. It was almost universally used in North-West Europe as a feed for fattening animals whether home-grown or imported from the Americas. Thus it has remained. Some efforts to use maize directly for human consumption were not successful.[29]

In Eastern Europe, matters were very different. Maize 'bread' is a tradition in the Balkans, Hungary and Romania. Hungary has become one of the great modern maize-growing countries; but right up until the eighteenth century, while most of the population were inert victims of warfare between Turk and Christian, the Magyar peasantry may well have been kept alive by the use of maize. The crop has three advantages on a peasant basis over wheat. It produces much more per unit area on a small, unscientific scale; it is easier to store, in cob; it is in many ways easier to render palatable by cooking. In Romania, a production pattern grew up in which the natives grew wheat and maize. Wheat was exported: maize supported the people. Wheat, a centuries-old staple, became a luxury. If maize helped Southern Europeans, then potatoes were slower to catch on in the north and in the mountains.

There was in places an almost religious objection to the potato which is related to the poisonous belladonna or deadly nightshade. There was also an objection, semi-religious, semi-naturalistic, which claimed that mankind should not eat what grows beneath the earth. This prohibition was in force at a time when Jerusalem artichokes, turnips, swedes and radishes were all new ideas for human food. It was sheer necessity that drove Europeans to eat the potato, led by the Irish in the seventeenth century. Frederick the Great (1740–86) forced the tuber upon his subjects a century later with limited success. There was hardly any considerable area of potatoes grown on farms in pre-Revolutionary France. In contemporary Russia, it was considered weird, strange, evil, underground, unnatural. In France, Germany, Poland and Russia, the potato took off in the nineteenth century, and while never becoming the staple diet it was in Ireland, nevertheless became as important a primary source of energy as wheat or rye. Potatoes were seen as a staple, easily stored, cheap accompaniment to meat at a later date, when meat could be afforded. Since World War II, it has been 'chips with everything'.

A cousin of the potato was adopted in the Mediterranean much earlier. The tomato, now in every kind of Italian dish, was available widely and only in Italy before 1600. Other Europeans were highly suspicious. It was considered poisonous, like the potato. (Perhaps Europeans had had bad experiences with cooking and eating the foliage: in which case, they would have suffered indigestion, serious poisoning, even death.) It was called, by one English herbalist, a love-apple; others thought it a form of mandrake. Like the white potato, the tomato was introduced into North America by Europeans, and at some time after 1750, a century after the potato.

Tomatoes, squashes, the capsicums, even potatoes all increased the amount of vitamin C available in Europe, thus assisting the cure of scurvy, which was a recurrent problem.[30] The beans very greatly increased the protein level of the food of the poor, and indeed they became known as 'the poor man's meat'. It is difficult to see how, without beans, any vegetarian could find enough protein, of a high enough quality, to raise a considerable family. The soya bean was, of course, not available in Europe before the twentieth century, but other beans must have had a profound effect on European diets. The use of potatoes has been fairly well documented. The effect of the crop on Ireland was in no way beneficial, but the rise in population in Middle and Eastern Europe in the nineteenth century was almost certainly largely helped by the potato. West German peasants had been exported to Pomerania after the Black Death to settle the sandy wastelands. Six hundred years later, Pomeranians were imported by the Ruhr coal and iron undertakings. This surplus peasant labour came from the use of the potato. There was simply not enough rye and wheat grown in the middle of the nineteenth century to account for the increased population.[31]

As for maize, it was primarily a southern European crop for humans. But it was imported for animal feed from the 1850s in a steadily increasing tonnage. Maize became the fuel for the animal-protein explosion of the twentieth century, in Europe as well as in the Corn Belt. Today, grain maize is grown as far north as northern France and southern Germany. Whole maize for silage is grown over most of southern England, northern Germany, southern Scandinavia. The line creeps northwards every year. The effect upon animal nutrition of unripe maize cut green has been as profound in post World War II Europe as grain maize was in the first half of the twentieth century. There is another point.

Maize is the only crop which can benefit from saturation application of animal manure upon the ground. A cow will eat the 10 tons of maize silage in a winter that can be grown upon a quarter hectare, properly manured. The total detritus from the cow during the winter can be spread, all 50 tons of it, on the quarter hectare chosen for next year's maize crop. The cycle is beneficial in the sense that the cow has become self-supporting as a plant nutrient. There is, of course, a great input of energy in the form of horsepower into the virtuous cycle, but there is far less need of pest control, and no need at all for artificial fertilizers. The same process can be established with pigs or poultry and grain maize, and has been in parts of West Germany, especially with pork pigs. The problem arises when the surplus organisms from the manure reach the water table.

It is entirely arguable that pre-Industrial European populations 'took off' only because of the important additions to the diet which came from the Americas. There is one exception to this truth, if truth it be. In England, as opposed to Ireland, Scotland, or the maize-eating countries, agricultural husbandry and capitalism were insufficient alone. England was capable of feeding the huge increase in population without any important use of American cultivars. Everywhere else, the European increase in population, proportionally the highest in the world in the years 1500–1900, could not have taken place without Amerindian plants. In England, it was imports of staple European foods from neo-European countries which fuelled the doubling of population between 1850 and 1914.

Finally, in examining the effects of New World crops upon the Old, it should be remembered that many New World crops were removed and grown elsewhere. These will be noted in due course. What happened to the condiment which started it all? Whatever happened to pepper? Did the Europeans forget pepper when all the lovely new plants were available? Far from it. There is no doubt that pepper, like sugar, is a habit which can easily become addictive, in the sense that the use of either becomes habitual, and the habit is difficult to give up.[32]

Pepper was only one of the 'essential' Renaissance spices. The others were ginger, cinnamon, nutmeg, cloves, mace and cardamom, in no particular order. All these spices and others, were important in cookery and as constituents in Chinese, Indian and Arab medicine. Before Columbus, pepper was first in importance and ten times as valuable as any other spice in world trade. It is assumed, with considerable justification, that pepper formed about half the total Eastern spice trade in 1500. Today, it still forms a quarter of the spice trade.

It was also of universal application. Historically water was of doubtful quality. Vegetables, by themselves, and boiled, are boring in the extreme. The only preserved meat or fish in many areas was salted. Water to wash out this salt may not always have been available, or clean enough to perform this duty, or close enough to the cooking pot for the water to be changed frequently. Oatmeal, spirits of wine, even throwaway vegetables were cooked with salt meat to reduce salinity, but often this was not enough. Pepper is a safe way of making oversalted meat or fish edible. Once used for this purpose, it became difficult to persuade the natives of Europe to return to pre-pepper cooking. It was also widely used to make less boring a mass (or mess) of boiled vegetables masquerading as stew.

Pepper was in use in antiquity, in Greece rather than Egypt. Pre-Muslim Arabs were not exactly in charge of the pepper trade since time began, but there were two ancient Arabian routes. One was from the Indian south-west coast to the Gulf of Hormuz, then to Basra, Baghdad, and Syria, and on, in Greek and Roman times, to Antioch; after Alexandria was founded in 322 BC as a Greek city, there was an alternative route via the Red Sea.

Both routes later led, of course, to Rome, and Rome consumed an unimaginable tonnage of pepper and spices.

Prices to the Roman Empire were somewhat reduced by the Graeco-Roman discovery, in the first century BC, of the Monsoon Route, from the Red Sea to India, outward in the south-west winds, from April to October; back to Egypt in the north-east airstream in the northern winter. The Egyptians had founded, in about 260 BC, Berenice, a port just north of the Tropic Line in the Red Sea. From Berenice, a road, provided with watering-holes, led to a point near modern Aswan on the Nile. On the Red Sea, trade was carried out for five hundred years, until the port silted up and the later Romans returned to the use of Suez. A land-route, via Attock in the Indus Valley, joined the Silk Route from China in Central Asia, at a later date.

Silk, spices and pepper came to an end as normal items of East–West trade during the years between the Arab Muslim explosion into the world (632–732) and the resumption of East–West trade by the Venetians and the Genoese, which was the chief long-term result of the Crusades. During the pepper dark ages, to coin a phrase, meat was relished redder and redder, often hardly hung or seasoned, as in some periods of Texan cowboy history. What happened in the winter, in the absence of both fresh meat and of pepper, no one knows. It is possible, however, that pepperless barbarian northern Europeans taught the Mediterraneans to smoke meat and fish, not to salt it. Certainly, smoked viands of all types are more characteristic of the cuisine of the northerner. Even Vikings preferred smoking and the smoked cure to salting – witness smoked herring, cod and salmon.

The pepper trade is always assumed only to have become very difficult after the Turkish occupation of Constantinople in 1453. But this was not necessarily the case. After the failure of Byzantine traders in India in the sixth century AD, the pepper trade reverted to the Arabs, shortly to become Muslim. Demand picked up very strongly as Europe returned to some sort of east–west intercourse after the Crusades, and Venice, in particular, grew rich on pepper, which is largely responsible for the Venetian Golden Age.

It was not the Turks who destroyed the Venetian–Turkish–Arab–Indian pepper trade, but the Portuguese, rounding the Cape and finding their way to India. The Arab merchants on both sides of the Indian Ocean reacted in two ways. One was to plead with the Turks to fight the Portuguese at sea. This was partially successful. Aden was retaken by Muslim forces, but successfully blockaded by the Portuguese. Hormuz (Ormuz, or Ormes) had become a Portuguese colony in 1514, after Albuquerque had established the Portuguese in Goa and Malacca. Ormuz, as the Portuguese called it, remained an entrepôt for the spice trade. Some cargoes would go round the Cape to Lisbon. After 1560, some trade would be allowed to return to the Arab–Venetian pattern and route, but only after the Portuguese had extracted a sizeable 'tax' upon every ton. This was a mistake. An easily levied toll or tax offers too much temptation to sticky local fingers, and little of the proceeds arrived in Lisbon. The Lisbon pepper trade dried up, and the tolls from Ormuz, which were meant to replace it, did not materialize in any substantial form. Venice was very much on the ascendant again in the second half of the sixteenth century.

The second reaction of the Arab and Muslim Indian merchants was to move the cultivation of pepper further east, to what is now Malaya and Indonesia. There was probably an oversupply, since *Piper nigrum* is an easy plant to grow in the Indies. The Portuguese at Malacca were not successful in controlling this traffic, and their monopoly was broken.

From 1600 onwards, the Dutch drove the Portuguese out of the East Indies – the Spice Islands – and established a monopoly in nutmeg, mace and cloves; later they controlled the world supply of cinnamon, but not of pepper. Pepper ceased to have the glamour of a commodity worth as much as any other edible, at times nearly as much as saffron in Europe, vanilla from Central America or gold dust from the Sudan. An end to the European distribution monopoly revealed also that there was little magical about the production of pepper. From the European necessity which paid for, even produced, the genius and glory of Venice, pepper became a dull, rather pedestrian commodity, on a par with salt and vinegar and not much more expensive.

Piper nigrum is one of over 1,000 species of the genus pepper. They are nearly all climbers. Its original home was Travancore and Malabar, but it is now grown commercially in Indonesia, Malaya, Thailand, the Philippines and the Caribbean. Black pepper is the dried fruit of *Piper nigrum*: white pepper is the dried fruit, further treated, with the outer black skin removed by chemical or physical means. In modern plantations in the original home, Malabar, yield is more than 5 tonnes of dried pepper per hectare (2.5 acres). At this yield, in the Middle Ages, 300 hectares (740 acres) would have supplied the probable annual import into Venice. Even if the yield was only a fifth of modern yields, then a mere 1,500 hectares (3,700 acres) would have supplied Europe in, say, 1400. No wonder the Arab and Indian Muslim merchants pretended to a skill and hidden magic which never existed. No wonder there was a conspiracy of silence between Arabs, Turks and Venetians. No wonder the morality of the pepper trade was no better, no worse, than that of the modern drug trade. Even in the 1790s, without any kind of 'improved' European husbandry – without modern fungicide, insecticide or fertilizer – dry yields were of the order of

(1 kg (21 lb) from each vine, 1,000 plants per acre, nearly 2,300 kg per hectare (2,000 lb per acre). Pepper was of the same order, as a conspiracy against the consumer, as a harmful drug. Every outsider tried to break the monopoly.

One East Indian alternative to *Piper nigrum* was, and is, long pepper, known to Greeks and Romans, and said by them to be better than black or white pepper. Rarely cultivated today, its roots are used in Indian medicine, and the fruit is appreciated in India, for pickles and medicine. Little Long Pepper is today exported from the East.

The first true alternative, exploited by trans-Saharan traders in the thirteenth and fourteenth centuries, was the Ashanti pepper, *Piper clusii*. Arriving on the Muslim camel-train at Tunis or Algiers, it was distributed by Genoese merchants all over the Mediterranean in rivalry to the (largely) Venetian *Piper nigrum*. It reached France and England at some point after the Black Death, in the 1360s, and a century later the Portuguese for a short time tried to break the Turkish–Venetian monopoly by following the Genoese and using *Piper clusii*. After the Portuguese installation in the black pepper trade, little was heard of Ashanti pepper, which was not cultivated but the wild plants 'hunted' rather than farmed. It still is.

The other early, pre-Columbian substitute for the expensive true pepper used to be known as guinea grains, or grains of paradise. These are the exceedingly pungent seeds of a member of the *meleguetta* family, a sort of ginger. It was carried by caravan overland to Tripoli as early as the thirteenth century. Queen Elizabeth I was very partial to its use in her cuisine; it was also used at the time for disguising poor wine and flat beer. Later it was prohibited as an additive to beer. In the eighteenth century a brewer was subject to a fine of £200 if he had guinea grains in his possession. The seeds form part of the spices of the North, Central and West Africa because of their very great strength and, therefore, economy. It is a reed-like plant, and today is regarded as a substitute for cardamom, not pepper.

On the beach in Cuba on 4 November 1492, Columbus showed the natives a peppercorn which had come from Malabar, via the Arabs and the Venetians, to Seville, and with the explorer across the Atlantic. 'Ah, yes,' said the natives, 'we have lots of those.' Or words to that effect. What Columbus was then shown was *Pimento officinalis*.[33]

Pimento is indigenous to the Caribbean and was found wild by the Spaniards in 1494. After 1509, the fruits were 'hunted' by Spanish settlers, like everything else. The British, from their capture of Jamaica in 1655, cultivated fields of the smallish, evergreen tree, exporting more than 200 tons in 1755, and a record of more than 10,000 tons in 1908. The Jamaican pimento, or allspice, as it is known, is not a pepper, and does not taste like a substitute, though it has been employed as such by the Spanish, the French and the British. It really tastes like a mixture of cinnamon, clove and nutmeg. Pimento has been a relatively unsuccessful transferred plant. Nowhere has it done as well as its original home. It is widely used in meat-processing, canning, fruit preservation and jam and marmalade manufacture, in pharmaceutical products and in perfumery, especially for men. World production today remains steady at about 10–12,000 tons.

Finally, there is cayenne pepper, which was also 'discovered' by Columbus, who must rank as one of the most pepper-lamented people in history. Cayenne pepper comes from an extremely hot member of the capsicum family. There are thirty of these, ranging from the hottest Mexican chilli to the mild green, yellow or red salad plants. Cayenne pepper, which comes from *Capsicum frutescens*, is more pungent than paprika, which comes from a European cultivar, developed or 'discovered' in Hungary in the seventeenth century. The paprika type of capsicum came possibly via Turkey, in which case the cultivar may have come round the world, from Acupulco in Mexico, to the Philippines, then to India, Persia, Syria and Turkey. Capsicum plants were in cultivation in the Philippines in the 1570s, and there were seven species in India by the 1580s; they were found in the Eastern Mediterranean before 1600. The cultivars also travelled eastward, with Columbus and with later sailors. The seeds remain viable for a very long time, and the capsicum has a huge gene-bank of potential cultivars, not all of them explored.

In Baroque Europe, flatulence from onions, cabbages and beans was reduced by the use of capsicum. It also reduces hysteria. It is today an essential ingredient of various curries, and India and Thailand export the hotter sorts of capsicum all over the Eurasian landmass. Curry powder, or something like it, is in use in every country east of Italy. It is difficult to see how curry (Indian *Kara*) could have reached its current power without capsicum. The powder may contain from 3–30 species of spices; few Eastern people eat anything without spice of one sort or another. The curry smell is permanent.[34]

Pepper today is a condiment taken for granted, cheap to produce, medically less important than salt; the alternatives to *Piper nigrum* are mere addictions to the diet, luxuries, just options, however attractive. Pepper has had, however, three fundamental influences on history. First, after a long, hard fight, Venice became rich and glorious on the trade in the late Middle Ages. Secondly, the whole history of the backing for Columbus's voyages depended upon the prospects of pepper profits. Thirdly, two other countries, Portugal and the Netherlands, became rich and important because of the trade, which was as significant in the sixteenth century as the grain or drug today. As an aside, it can be claimed that the Americas were discovered as they were and at that particular time, as a by-product of the pepper trade.

There were no imports of American animals to compare with the transatlantic transfer of syphilis, maize, or the potato. No Spanish entrepreneur made much use of the llama, the vicuna, or the guinea-pig. It would be many years before the North American turkey became 'useful' in Europe, and the American bison, the so-called buffalo, the moose and the caribou have never been tamed or transferred. Nor has the coyote.

Rich in wild game which could be easily caught and eaten, much of Amerindian North America was well suited to support a relatively small human population without farming. Some of the North American Indians, however, lived as semi-farmers before the white man came, and they lived happily for centuries on maize, squashes, beans of many kinds, supplemented by flesh from birds and fish. There was, however, no domestication of any animals north of the Rio Grande; few tamed animals on the continent. Many thousands of years would be needed to turn the American buffalo into a transatlantic version of the European ox.[35]

Very, very ancient America seems to have been a veritable park of wild horses, dogs, cattle, sheep, pigs and so forth. They were apparently killed by the early human arrivals who walked across what is now the Bering Strait. Travelling south and east, early humans killed and ate everything that they found.[36]

These humans must have been extraordinarily successful as a species. They are said to have obliterated all trace of any of the animals which Europeans have since domesticated. Whether this is credible or not, the fact remains that there are plenty of fossil remains and absolutely no native American horses, oxen, asses, sheep, goats or pigs.[37] More significantly, there are no native American species of grass or graminae out of which a true mixed farming pattern could evolve.

Since European plants and animals came over concurrently, and since, by selection, grazing animals can 'create' their own pasture, plants and animals must be examined together. Hay for horses and cattle contained seeds which spread. Seeds which spread conquered the continent before Europeans. Animals, released by mistake on the Caribbean coast, reached Lower California before the Spanish. Pigs escaped on some Caribbean islands, killed all the native flora and fauna, made re-afforestation impossible, as rabbits did on the Madeiran island of Porto Santo.[38] So animals and plants, introduced on purpose, or by mistake, in the New World, have to be examined together. It all began very early. The Iberians, when they had to, survived on manioc and maize. But the preferred staple, the bread of life, was wheat. With wine and the olive, these were the traditional foods of

Iberia, indeed of the Mediterranean. Iberians tried to grow wheat wherever they could. It failed in the hot, wet Caribbean, the ocean provinces of Brazil, the Amazon, of course. But there were places where it succeeded, and before too many years of Iberian occupation.

Wheat was successful, as would be imagined, in the drier lowlands and in the highlands, wherever a temperate climate could be found. In Mexico, it was grown in the highlands as early as 1525; ten years later, Mexico was exporting wheat to the Caribbean; by 1556, wheat flour in Mexico City was cheaper than in Madrid; by 1590, it was even suggested that wheat might be exported to Spain to make good the fourth quarter of the century which produced so much hunger, misery, famine even, in the home country. As the metropolitan Spanish problem was due to landholding contradictions, agricultural husbandry incompetence, and almost incurable transport difficulties, such imports would not have solved many shortages except immediately round Iberian ports.

In the sixteenth century, wheat was to become the staple energy food for the Spaniards, not the natives, in the valley of the Rio de la Plata, in what are now Colombia and Ecuador, in Chile, and in the Central American highlands. Wheat was often grown by Amerindians as a tribute-crop, which replaced rent or service. By 1592, any of the 50,000 Iberians could obtain wheat flour, and therefore bread, unless they were both too poor and living in a non-wheat area. Some Amerindians were weaned from the staple maize, potatoes or manioc. Perhaps risen bread was also used, in larger volume than the wafers at Mass, for the conversion of the Indians. If so, wheatbread became a status symbol, but not universally. Even today, wheat is not the staple food of more than a third of the inhabitants of Latin America.

Nor was wine a substitute for maize ale amongst the Amerindians. To begin with maize requires much less skill to ferment. When the Spanish started growing wine grapes, if only for the household of the *conquistador*, the Indians quite rightly pointed out larger, sweeter and better grapes growing in many places. Although there are many native American grapes, there is no known American cultivar out of which wine can be properly made. Mexico is not good country for wine because European grapes do not ripen properly. In Peru and Chile, it was a different matter. The first Peruvian vintage was in the 1550s, and export commenced in the 1570s. The first good Chilean vintage was in the 1580s, the first export in the 1600s. The Mexican experience, however, was ecologically important for what would happen more than three hundred years later.

Despite the fact that wine was no longer necessary for the lay mass, because of the Council of Constance in 1415, and the Council of Trent in 1562, the Roman Catholic clergy are historically connected with viticulture in the Americas. The word 'mission' used to be a great selling ploy. There was one great lay exception to this rule. Hernando Cortés (1485–1547) was the *conquistador* of Mexico. Among his more peaceful traits was his residual inherited interest in agriculture. His father was a minor landlord, a keen yeoman fruit and wine grower in the Estremadura.

Cortés Senior became the hero's agent for the transmission of hardwood cuttings of apples, pears, peaches, apricots and so forth, from Europe to Mexico. Vine cuttings sent from the Canaries, and acclimatized to the no-real-winter, perpetual spring of those islands, failed. Cuttings from the continental uplands of the middle of Spain, with harsh winters and baking summers, succeeded.

In Mexico, the *conquistador* caused it to be ordained that every landgrant, the usual semifeudal way of rewarding the adventurer, and to which natives were attached as slaves or serfs, should be conditional upon a quota of vines being planted. Landgrants were for about 50 hectares (124 acres) of land, depending upon the quality of the soil, aspect, drainage, irrigation, and so forth. There were allotted 100 slaves to work the land, and 1,000 vines to be planted on each *repartimento*, or grant of land. Many of the slaves died, perhaps up to 90 per cent in places, of disease, but the vines flourished.

This was one of the few recorded Spanish cases of relating land, serfs and crops. If there had been more husbandmen like Cortés, Spanish occupation of the Americas would not have resulted, as sometimes it did, in hunger in the midst of plenty. Sometimes, hunger was as bad as in Spain. Not that the hunger, in Old or New Spain, was ever allowed to hurt the ruling classes.

The grape in the Americas went on spreading northwards from Mexico, and westwards to California, where it became indelibly connected with missions. North of modern Arizona, and east of the Rockies, grape vines from Europe never performed. It was not for 250 years that anyone diagnosed phylloxera.[39]

The third element in the ancient diet, olive oil, was more difficult of achievement than wheat or wine. How many transatlantic attempts were made to grow the olives before the first successful efforts in Chile in the 1560s? Olive seedlings are with difficulty transferred without a Wardian case,[40] and with more difficulty acclimatized. The olive, a native of Syria, loves a dry, Mediterranean climate, with winter rain and summer drought. In the right places, typically the Levant, Greece and Italy, trees of very great antiquity survive. Edward Gibbon (1737–94) was shown a tree near Rome allegedly planted at the time of Virgil (70–19 BC). Whether modern scepticism imitates that of Gibbon at the time, it is certainly true that trees of well over five hundred years of age are still yielding. Carefully pruned and tended, olives improve with age.

Olive oil was the regional alternative to butter and goose-fat in the traditional tricorne cookery of France, long before cuisine became intellectual. It was universally used, inside and outside the body, in Ancient, Medieval and Renaissance civilizations, from Afghanistan to Portugal. Long before Christ, the olive became a symbol of peace, abundance and goodwill amongst peoples. It is no accident that the olive is such a metaphor in the writings of Ancient Greece, Rome, and in Hebrew and Muslim holy texts. Live olive trees are more than that today; they are an indicator of faithful husbandry over the ages. The first act of a barbarian conqueror, ignorant of the benevolence of the olive, has always been to cut down the tree for fuel. Survival, in the olive, indicates at minimum an invader whose savagery is mollified by knowledge of the plant.

The olive, however mystically regarded by the husbandman, is not happy throughout the world. It was unsuccessful in the Canaries (insufficient frosts). It died of new parasites in the Caribbean, which was also too hot and had no winter. The first ideal place found in the Americas was in the dry valleys of the folds of the Andes in Chile, irrigated, or watered by winter rain. Later, it transferred successfully, in about 1600, to Peru. Much later, it found a home in California. Less generally successful transfers were made on the East Coast, after the founding of the United States, in Florida, South Carolina and Mississippi. White men introduced the plant to China, and it is a feature of Queensland, South Australia and the Cape of Good Hope. The Mediterranean remains its chief home, and despite all the efforts of those involved in plant transfer, over 95 per cent of the acreage is still in the Mediterranean. Olive oil was exported from southern Spain to most of Latin America at one time or another after 1492. It still is.[41]

The stone fruits and the citrus trees, planted in the Caribbean, prospered with unaccustomed vigour. Not all of them ever became of economic importance in the island of first lodging. They were often more successful as feral escapes from man's orchards. Citrus and stone-fruit trees were to be found, in suitable places, all over tropical and temperate America within two hundred years.

Citrus fruits bred new 'sports' for themselves in the Caribbean, including the grapefruit (eighteenth century) the ruby variety, a genetic Texan 'sport' of 1926, and the Ugli, in the West Indies in the 1950s. The lime of modern commerce is a natural hybrid of the European lime and the Chinese citron both carried to the West Indies by Europeans. There are other hybrids, the 'temple orange' which is a cross between the ordinary orange and the mandarin, the tangelo (mandarin/grapefruit), and numerous crosses and sub-crosses between various mandarin/tangerine/satsuma cultivars. It appears that citrus fruits only have to be loosed in the Caribbean to set up an intensive biological hybridization programme. In this respect, citrus fruits do not differ from humans.

Citrus fruits were not followed by stone fruits to commercially profitable hybridization. There are no great number of peach/apricot hybrids, nor of cherry/peaches; but cherry will cross with plum, and nectarines and peaches can hybridize with ease, or create 'sports'. Nectarines, fuzzless peaches, have become several times bigger since the Renaissance, though the hairy peach remains genetically dominant. Some peach sports are so hairy as to be unsaleable.

All the fruit tree members of the rose family, apples, pears, apricots, cherries, peaches, plums, were introduced into the Americas before 1500, as were citrus fruits. They wandered far and wide. They were found up the Orinoco, down the Mississippi, on islands on the Parana River, on the shores of the River Plate before the white man was in any of these places as a farmer or fruitgrower. Feral fruit trees became a feature, particularly, of South America. There were perhaps areas as large in all as an English county covered by escaped and much modified citrus trees or stone fruits or apples and pears.[42]

The other members of the rose family, the creepers, the berries, the *rubus* genus, are native on both sides of the Atlantic. Blackberries and raspberries are multiple fruits, the strawberry, a false fruit, an *achene*. Wild Chilean strawberries have had a distinguished role in improving bred strains of European strawberries.[43] The most interesting *rubus* 'sport' is the loganberry, named after its discoverer, an Oregon medical doctor.[44]

The chief impact upon the Americas of the Iberian immigrants is not remembered as an invasion of microbes, still less of plants which were transferred, or moved themselves. Nor is European fauna considered important. Most history books tell us about gold and silver; most economic historians tell us of the impact of gold and silver upon Spain and Europe; most conventional historians ignore the natural world altogether. But gold and silver in great amounts could not have been mined without three animal products; without them, the ore would have remained underground.

The first was meat. Without meat, and plenty of it, the hard work of the miner would never have been done. There has never been a vegetarian mining community which achieved the output of carnivorous men before the advent of power. Modern attempts, in the Soviet Union and elsewhere, to use underfed humans as miners, merely killed the miners. This may have been the Soviet intention; but, despite Spanish brutality towards the Amerindian, they were always short of labour after the first few years; and the huge losses occasioned by disease made getting output per man out of the miners vitally important. It was not until the nineteenth and twentieth centuries, in Mexico, that there was a large enough population for the ruling class to be brutal in its demands upon labour. By that time, the ruling class was of Mexican stock.

The second mining commodity essential in a sixteenth-century mine was tallow. Millions of candles a year were in use in Latin America by 1600. There was no other form of lighting available underground. Perhaps by that date, as many as 100,000 cattle a year were being slaughtered for tallow alone.

The third piece in the jigsaw was the ox, used for transport and for ploughing. The ox-cart was the only heavy transport available in those areas where roads could be built. Without roads, it was a question of pack-horses, mules or donkeys.

Most metal which reached the coast after 1557 was silver. In the first century after the Spanish management of the great silvermine of Potosi, production was over 3 million ounces a year – or 10,000 tons in the century. This would require the mining and transport of a million tons of ore, the feeding of a total of nearly 100,000 people every day for a century; the transport of supplies inward to the mine, and of gold, heavily defended, to the coast in the Caribbean, over 1,500 miles away. None of this could have been performed without the animals that the Spanish brought with them. Nor could Potosi have functioned until animals and plants had modified themselves to survive in the new land. Potosi was only half the production of the mines of Mexico in 1600, one-tenth the production of Mexico in 1800, on the eve of independence. How can animals be ignored, or their existence be assumed?

There were huge cattle numbers in four places in Latin America. These places had been found by accident, or more properly, by the animals themselves. Cattle had been ranched in Spain for generations: the only part of Western Europe of which this was true. The nearest non-Spanish ranches were in Poland, Hungary and the Ukraine. Spanish cattle were fast and scraggy, fit to run or to defend themselves with their long horns. They were the ancestors of the modern cattle bred for the bullfight. They were in huge numbers in Hispaniola in 1520, in Mexico, and their slaughter forbidden, in the next year; by 1540 they were in such quantity in Mexico City that beef was cheaper than anywhere in Europe. Cattle found their great home on the ranges south of the Rio Grande. By the end of the century, they had expanded north and occupied what is now Texas. By 1592, over 200,000 a year were being slaughtered in New Spain (Mexico) alone.

The second great place for cattle was in the so-called *llanos* of Venezuela. In the flatlands of this hot country, with a temperature far higher even than the Spanish summer, with both drought and flood, it took some time for Iberian cattle to adapt. Production did not build up for at least fifty years after the first large-scale introduction in the early 1550s. As in Mexico, the cattle moved inland, ahead of the human 'owners' and a vast number of feral cattle filled the land. These longhorns were fierce, and well able to defend themselves from jaguars and snakes.

The third and fourth great natural cattle regions were the hinterlands of two great modern cities. The first was the plain inland from Buenos Aires, first 'discovered' in 1535. The second was in Portuguese territories, inland from São Paulo, and permanently settled in 1532. Buenos Aires, abandoned by the Spanish between 1540 and 1580, was so favourable an environment for cattle that by the time of permanent Spanish settlement there was a 'crop' of nearly 100,000 a year to be taken from the descendants of the few hundred which went wild in 1535–40. These cattle bred every year, for at least ten years, and they grew and grew and grew. What was true in Buenos Aires was also true in São Paulo. In this great empty land, one day to be a giant coffee plantation, there were so many cattle that they could not all be eaten. Slaughtered for hides and the tallow derived from suet, the rest of the body was left to rot in the semitropical sun. How many parasites also had a population explosion to deal with the carcasses?

Cattle produced a 'cash crop' – hides, which could be exported to Europe. From Latin America in 1600, hides were more valuable an export than anything else except gold, silver and diamonds. Even in 1650, hides were more valuable, American use included, than sugar. To our modern age, sated with plastics, rubber, both natural and synthetic, and paper, the importance of leather is generally decorative. Before about 1900, it was essential for boots, clothing, harness, saddlery, buckets, washers, seals, pumps, bellows, belts, boxes, and a hundred and one other uses. In some areas of America hides produced the best (and cheapest) ropes.

Sheep were brought over to produce wool. In the end, outside what would be Chile and Mexico, and in parts of Brazil, there were not enough people to shepherd the sheep. So they ran wild, and took their chance in areas where the native or introduced predators were not too thick on the ground.[45] In those areas where they did well, the superb merinos were valued more for tallows and hides than for wool or even meat. They also had a devastating effect upon the native wool-bearing, camel-like creatures – guanaco, alpaca, llama, vicuña. These four animals shared about twenty sheep diseases with the European intruders. As with humans, the native immune system was incapable of dealing with the novel parasites. As with humans, the new settlers, unconsciously or not, killed off the natives. As with humans, it all happened so quickly that it was over before the full story was recorded or quantified. As with humans, perhaps 90 per cent of the natives were killed off by imported disease.[46]

If sheep were downgraded from being producers of wool to mere carcasses, from which hides and tallows were removed, it explains why sheepmeat has been considered only fit for the poor and shiftless in most of the Americas. American cattlemen inherited from the Spaniards their contempt for sheep-raisers. This is entirely a Spanish-American experience and development. Pigs were also deflated in esteem by mere numbers. They were landed on every island. They preceded mankind across the Continent, arriving in Pacific Guatemala ahead of the whites, in Massachusetts before the Plymouth Brethren, in Virginia (complete with peach trees) before the English brought pigs from the home country. They also met the same sort of Englishman when he arrived in Barbados or Bermuda. The English found the islands 'uninhabited' by humans, and thought the wild pigs native.[47]

Pigs were poor man's meat in all the Latin American countries, and remained so in the United States. Next came the sheep, still a poor man's meat, but slightly upmarket from pigs. Next came the beef animal, bigger, more expensive, but still one-tenth the price of the same animal in Europe: relatively far cheaper in producing areas, in the days before refrigeration than in the last one hundred years because of the difficulty of transport. In every future neo-Europe, meat would be far cheaper than in the old Europe: one reason the new countries had a birth-rate three times that of the old. The Americas set the pattern about animals. In Cuba, cattle went wild; Mexican pigs arrived in Lower California before the white man, thus mightily confusing the contemporary naturalist; sheep were found in the Rocky Mountain foothills before any white shepherd had arrived; modified and evolved, cattle were settled in the Amazon basin when the first whites arrived to settle. Of all such developments, that of the horse is the most causative of evolutionary change in wholly unexpected directions. The evolution also goes full circle.

The horse (*Equus equus*) was apparently native to the Americas, and died out about 6000 BC after the initial onslaught when men crossed over the Bering Straits and killed a large proportion of American fauna. The first Old World horses were brought to the Americas by the Spaniards in 1494. Both Iberian countries had had experience of the value of the horse, used as a weapon of war against horseless warriors, both in the Canaries and in West Africa. To have the use of the horse, even by the individual man at arms, was at the time believed to multiply the power of Europeans against horseless natives by a factor of eight or ten to one. This was the first time that Europeans had fought with a weapon of this order of advantage, and it was comparable to the effect of firearms against 'natives' armed only with spears or bows and arrows. The horse in the sixteenth century was a greater asset than firearms, since firearms at that time were not much more efficient than most good bows and arrows. Both Cortés in Mexico and Pizarro in the Andes relied on the military effect of horses which, together with gunpowder and religion, were the contemporary explanation of Spanish success.

Cortés originally set forth from Spain in November 1518 with not many more than thirty horses. Until reinforced by the troops sent by Velázquez to 'arrest' him, Cortés had fewer than a dozen horses by the time he reached Mexico City. In the end, in 1523, after the successful second siege of Mexico City in August 1521, Cortés had still fewer than a hundred horses. Two years later, five or six, necessarily including both genders, escaped. This flight (and others after 1530) produced the feral horses of the North American continent, and from these accidents were derived a complete change in the habits of the Plains Indians, and in turn, because of the new habits, the inevitable destruction of millions of American buffalo.

Horses multiplied in Mexico and Texas in numbers which cannot be more than estimated. In most of the New World, horses were without natural enemies; there were neither the macro-parasites of wolves or lions nor the micro-parasites of the score or more diseases which afflicted horses in the Old World. If the experience of the human increase in the temperate New World at the same time is translated into equine increase, then the five or six of 1530 could have become several thousand by 1600. After that time, geometrical increase would show up as significantly more powerful than mere arithmetic. If the wild horses of America increased in number twice as fast as the wild horses of the steppes of Eurasia, then there could easily have been several million horses in favoured places in the great plains of North America, in the pampas of the Argentine and in many discrete parts of Brazil, Uruguay, Mexico and California.

Three Darwinian processes took place at the same time. First, the horses themselves were selected for the characteristics of survival in their new environment. 'Mustangs' (anglicized from the Spanish *mesteno*) became a distinct type of range-horse – hardy, capable of long distances without horseshoes, sure-footed and with great courage, of a frontier type. The wild horse of North America redefined, once again, the relationship of horse and rider, not necessarily to the rider's advantage. Often the horse knew the job better than the rider. Certainly a wild horse was often wiser than a 'dude' rider.[48]

Secondly, the horse altered the ecology of the plains' grasses. By the 1780s there were so many horses in Texas that the earth around waterholes was carrying European species of grass. The horses had killed the native grasses – which had previously supported a much thinner population of buffalo, or no herbivores at all. Horses made their own new pasture out of European seeds which had travelled either within the alimentary system of the imported horses, which had been sustained on hay during the voyage, or as passengers clinging to their coats, the horses concerned having been bedded on board ship. There are many stories of this kind of accidental import. What is not documented is how the original imports crossed the continent so quickly that Kentucky Blue Grass, for example, was found in Kentucky before the white man arrived there, but after the first feral horses and cattle. Before Kentucky, its more modest name was, and is, 'smooth-stalked meadow grass'.[49]

Thirdly, the horse changed the habits of the Amerindians who were parasites of the American buffalo. How many buffalo were there at that time? Five million? Ten million? Nearly 2 million sq. miles were originally occupied by American bison or buffalo in Canada and the United States. That makes 500 million hectares (over 1,000 million acres). Ten million animals in the US and Canada would have resulted in a density of one buffalo per 50 hectares (124 acres). In 1900, when the killing stopped, there were fewer than 1,000 wild buffalo, and 1,119 in parks and zoos.

Horses were found by Amerindians who had never seen a horse; many may have been eaten before the Indians learnt to ride them. When first seen by whites, mounted Indians, like some of the Asian invaders into Europe at the end of the Roman period, and like the Romans themselves, had no stirrups. They often had no bridles or saddles either. Amerindians never made horseshoes.

By 1800, most but not all Indians encountered by white trappers were equipped with horses, bridles, saddles and stirrups. Then the Indians had to teach themselves to shoot arrows from horseback, often from moving horses. This was a key problem in Eurasia for hundreds of years. It is a difficult art, and was much admired in Persians, Mongols and, above all, Parthians. How did the Indians teach themselves to become so expert in such a short time – perhaps a hundred years at most?

On top of all this, there is a further Darwinian possibility. Did the arrival of the mustang increase the birth-rate amongst what might be called the buffalo-Indians, which is not quite the same thing as the Plains Indians? Horse ownership could have led non-Plains Indians to adapt to a dependence upon the buffalo. Logically, the possession of the horse – a multiplication of mobility of the order of between five and ten times – would have increased the range of operation of a hunter-gathering tribe by a significant amount, and led to increased intertribal conflict, before any friction with white neo-Europeans. The key to this was not land use, but water, wintering grounds, sites to grow the essential Indian corn, and the habits of the buffalo which had themselves become much modified by the Indians' possession of the horse. The buffalo, of course, evolved to respond; the animals were divided into the quick and the dead. None but the quick could survive the mounted Indian with bow and arrow. Many agricultural Amerindians became hunter-gatherers again because the horse made it possible and profitable.

What the arrival of the horse and its explosion of numbers certainly did was to seal the fate of both Indians and buffaloes. Without the horse, the Indians would have been more settled than they became, once mounted. It is entirely possible that because of the opportunities offered by the horse, the Indians reverted from farmers who had an annual buffalo kill, to hunters who followed buffalo all the year round. Whether or not this is so, they became so identified with the buffalo that the animals were deliberately exterminated by whites in order to drive the Indians into the reservations, so that the range would become available for graziers and farmers. As a by-product, buffalo meat fed construction gangs on the railroads.

Without the horse, the argument runs, the Indians would not have become so dependent on the buffalo. Had they had the horse since time began, on the other hand, instead of from only about 1750, the Plains Indian, the buffalo, the horse, and (presumably) some sort of ox and sheep and goat would have worked out some sort of self-renewing, sustainable ecology. As it was, the ecology of the mounted Indian was too fragile to survive the white man, the white man's diseases and the white man's greed. In these years, the descendents of half a dozen Spanish riding horses escaped from Mexico City in 1523 had changed the habits of Amerindians in one-quarter of what would be the United States. And the change killed the culture.

At no point before the present would Europeans question the means of their victory over the world. This victory was won by the inhabitants of only 2 per cent of the Earth's land surface. These inhabitants – diseases, plants, animals – conquered most of the temperate and subtropical regions. Europeans transferred and improved the performance of plants from the Americas. The pattern of biological dominance is so markedly favourable to the European historical case that it has been largely ignored. Europeans have invented all sorts of political and intellectual theories to account for their success. In few cases can non-biological explanations for the Triumph of the West prove to be as convincing as the more earthy, the more visible, the more palpable. Because every action in history provokes reaction, or inhibits other actions, or can be examined only in relation to other events, there can be no certitude. But there can be recognition.

Notes

1 Quoted in *Ecological Imperialism: the biological expansion of Europe*: Alfred W. Crosby Jr, Cambridge, 1986.

2 At that date, Madeira could probably feed itself. Today's capability is probably not much higher than in 1850, since the land is difficult to mechanize. Large areas still have to be cultivated by hand, which is acceptable for wine, not so acceptable for wheat.

3 The fisheries of Madeira are neither as productive as those of the Canaries, nor as those of the Azores.

4 Finches, *Fringillidae*, are an adaptable, widely disseminated race of small songbirds with hard bills, often parasite on mankind, and capable of changing their habits with man-induced changes in the environment. The finches of the Canaries are the songbirds called 'Canaries', more properly *Serinus canarius*. They are native to the Azores and to Madeira, but not to the mainland of Africa, near the Canaries. The native stock is of olive-green, darker above, and mottled below. The yellow colour is produced by selective breeding in captivity. The native stock, though, differs greatly in each group of islands. See Charles Darwin, *Animals and Plants under Domestication*, London, 1868.

5 Lanzarote, named after a Genoese, Lanzaroto Marocello, who discovered it in 1325, has become yet another tourist paradise since the jets made for easy access.

6 Dogs in Tahiti were fed meat by white sailors for the first time during the late eighteenth century, at the time of the first European visits, by Bougainville, Cook and Bligh. Previously, the dogs had been vegetarian, and eaten by the indigenous natives. The same metamorphosis probably occurred in the Canaries.

7 The total land area of the Madeiran Islands is less than 80,000 hectares (200,000 acres).

8 The relationship today is that 1 kilo (2½ lb) of gold is worth the same as 70 tons of sugar.

9 Carthaginian coins have been found on the island of Corvo.

10 Favourable N.E. trade winds make possible the westward voyage of a crude sailing or sailing and rowing ship. There was not enough room on board to feed the crew of a pure (rowing) galley so that any return to Europe would require a ship to discover the eastward winds north of the Azores, which, incidentally, Columbus knew about and used for his return to Europe in 1493. The Carthaginians, as far as is known, did not return.

11 *Acor* means hawk in Portuguese.

12 The Azores have joined Bermuda, Shannon and Goose Bay, Labrador, and Gander, Newfoundland as once-important refuelling stops. These were all vital for ten years after World War II. Today, most people would not know of their one-time fame.

13 In 1950, people of African descent (all Negro) in the Americas numbered as follows: USA, 20 million plus; Caribbean-washed countries, 20 million plus; non–Caribbean Iberian-America, at least 30 million. Total 70 million plus. In Africa, from Senegal to Nigeria inclusive, excluding non–Negroes, 45 million plus; from the Cameroons to Angola, excluding non–Negroes, 20 million minus, probably no more than 18 million. Total 63–5 million. Since 1950, West African population censuses have been very suspect, for a number of political, not demographic reasons. See R. M. Protheroe, *Geographical Magazine*, London 1974.

14 The words 'cassava', 'tapioca' and 'manioc' all come from three different

Amerindian languages describing the same plant. The botanical name is *Manihot esculenta*, and it was found by Europeans cultivated between 25°N around Southern Florida, and as far as 25°S in Southern Brazil.

15 According to one Jesuit, in about 1550, natives who knew neither leavened bread nor wine could not be Christians by nature, and therefore, were logically not able to be pagans either. Such a doctrine, widely adopted, might have saved much misery.

16 Mexican mines reached their pre-Independence peak about 1810, just before the successful revolutions. The production of the Mexican mines alone was of the order of 5–6 times the silver mined in the Americas in, say, 1550. It is fair comment that if the Spanish Crown had had access to all the silver which was annually exported in the early 1800s, financial management would not have been enough developed to have dealt with the wealth. In other words, management was the problem, not precious metals. See Braudel, *The Mediterranean in the Age of Philip II: American Silver*. Fontana/Collins, London, 1975.

17 These seven cultivars are:

Pod maize, a primitive form of the corn, not commercial, turns up as a freak; was sometimes preserved by Amerindians who thought it had magical virtues.

Popcorn Grains small with hard outside; small, soft, starchy centre. On heating, steam generated inside the grain causes it to pop or explode.

Flint Northern type, used by Pilgrim Fathers in 1619. Predominant ecotype in Europe, Asia, some parts of the Americas and tropical Africa. Early maturing.

Dent Southern type. Principal natural hybrid of Corn Belt in USA and of Mexico. Origin of most grain improvement in twentieth century. Late maturing.

Flour Maize Dryland grain type. Easily chewed when uncooked. Used to make Amerindian beer *Chicha* and mealie beer in South Africa. Easily ground. Used by primitive Amerindian tribes.

Sweet Corn Recessive prevents conversion of some sugar into starch. Used sometimes in conjunction with flour maize to make *Chicha*. Internationally used, cooked on the cob.

Waxy Maize Has different starch composition from other cultivars. Found mainly nowadays in Eastern Asia, particularly Japan. Useful as a source of industrial starch.

These are ecotypes, or cultivars, not botanical varieties. Maize has never been found growing in a wild state, and much work has been done by one man to uncover the origin of maize in historic terms. Maize going back to 3600 BC (carbon-dating) was found in the so-called Bat Cave in New Mexico, in 1948–50. Further excavations in La Perry Cave, North-Eastern Mexico (1949) and the nearby Swallow Cave (1954) are to be compared with the Bat Cave discoveries. In 1954, maize pollen was discovered in a drill core, 70 metres (300 feet) below Mexico City. This was carbon-dated to 80,000 BC. This is before mankind reached America, and proved that *zea mays* is an American plant, unknown elsewhere. Work has been best described in *Corn, its Origin, Evolution and Improvement*, P. C. Mangelsdorf, Cambridge, 1974. There are many technical papers by Mangelsdorf, MacNeish, Galinat, Kelley and Lister. Maize is a fast-growing crop which requires a frost-free period of at least 120 days; the grain yield is very variable. In Israel and New Zealand, crops of over 6,000 kg/ha 5,340 lb/a) have been recorded; average, in New Zealand, over 4,000 kg/ha (3,560 lb/a). In peasant Africa, the yield is of the order of about 500 kg/ha (445 lb/a) one-twelfth what has been achieved in Israel or New Zealand, and one-eighth the New Zealand average. The average in the

United States is about three tons per hectare. This, in some places, fell to less than 1,000 kg/ha (890 lb/a) in the drought year of 1988.

18 Changes in the meaning of crop names are plentiful in the early post-Columbian period.

19 Elephant, lion, leopard, giraffe, hyena, buffalo, many kinds of antelopes and gazelle and innumerable monkeys. In the rivers there were rhinoceros, hippopotamus and crocodile. More types of birds larger than pigeons than exist is Europe. These were the animals reported within 50 miles of the coast of the Bight of Benin before 1500. How could maize survive such predators? No wonder immune cassava caught on.

20 The three methods were first to interplant beans, which produced enough vitamin B_4 to provide against pellagra; secondly, the Amerindians had used ashes, lime or naturally occurring soda, or mollusc shells to process the grain by boiling for one hour, then washing, drying and grinding the corn. This breaks down the cell walls, making the main storage protein, *zein*, less available to the human body. This in turn increases the availability of lysine by 2.8 times and of tryptophan by 1.3 times and releases B_4.

Other tribes allowed the corn cob to rot under mud for two–three months. This has the same effect as adding beans, or boiling with ashes, lime, etc. None of these three techniques were taken by Europeans to Europe. As a result, pellagra (*rough skin* in Italian) became a common complaint in the Mediterranean. Pellagra is a deficiency disease of poverty, absence of alternative foods, and of winter, when home-grown vegetables are scarce. Ironically, the disease retreated during the Depression in the Deep South, since unprofitable cotton gave way to subsistence vegetables.

21 The *Solanaceae* include tomato, potato, aubergine, capsicum, the tree tomato, Cape gooseberry, tobacco, belladonna, thorn-apple, henbane, mandrake; only belladonna, henbane and mandrake are native to Europe. The rest come from the Americas, though there is some suggestion that thorn-apple is indigenous, in some forms, in tropical Africa as well as America.

22 Apart from cannibalism, the Incas had almost every attribute of which modern liberal democrats disapprove. It was a dictatorship, illiterate, but highly numerate, with a statistical obsession expressed in knots of a decimal nature and akin to a crude computer. The central records were called 'Quipu'. The people by birth below the Royal Incas were all equal, all servile, and all working for the greater glory of the rulers. There was no money, no written record except statistics, no slavery, in the European sense, no form of exchange except through state barter; marriages were controlled by the state; social security was from the cradle to the grave; famines were abolished by great storehouses of several seasons' food; the central government controlled the amount of land allotted to each person, and denied all any real private ownership, except perhaps, in some places only, the peasant's house.

23 The full story is told in the Potato Chapter of *Seeds of Change*, by the author.

24 See E. C. Large, *The Advance of the Fungi*, Jonathan Cape, 1940.

25 German potato-production increased from 7 million tonnes in 1846 to just below 50 million tonnes in the years immediately before 1914. In the same period, the population increased from 30 million to nearly 70 million. As recently as 1935–50, a greater tonnage (by dry matter) was grown of potatoes than of wheat or rye in what used to be Imperial Germany.

26 The only other plant common to New Zealand and the Americas is the cotton plant, *Gossypium*, several varieties of which have been floated in sea water for up to two years and the seeds remain viable. It is possible that cottons, coconuts, and the sweet potato floated from the Americas to the South Pacific.

27   *Travels in France*, 1794.

28   Fatty liver is the human condition, usually attributed to too-good living. There is, however, a cottage industry in inducing the same condition in geese through forcible feeding without choice. A goose liver in epicurean condition may weigh as much as one fifth of the entire plucked and clean carcass. This condition of the liver was encouraged as early as the time of Justinian in Constantinople, sixth century AD. But maize made the job much easier. More digestible than any Old World animal food, maize permits a very rapid overfattening of the goose, usually by force-feeding.

29   Starving Irish peasants were given uncooked, whole maize without being told how to deal with it. Not surprisingly, they continued to starve. This cruel folly was first committed during the Famine of 1845–6, but repeated at later moments of shortage.

30   Scurvy was an annual familiar in pre-Columbian Europe, during the late winter and spring, before the fresh vegetables first appeared.

31   The population of Pomerania and East Prussia, where the peasants came from in the nineteenth century, remained fairly static, while that of the Rhineland and Westphalia increased by more than any other part of Germany in the fifty years before 1914, with the sole exception of Berlin, the capital. *European Historical Statistics, 1750–1975*, Macmillan, 1981.

32   The alkaloid, *piperine*, creates its own demand in the system. Demand is inelastic. When supply was a problem in the years immediately after World War II, the world price rose by over 16 times, and attempts were made to naturalize the plant in the United States. See *Journal of Economic Botany*, 1955.

33   *Christopher Columbus, Mariner*, S. E. Morison, London, 1956.

34   One effect is that, in second-hand aircraft of the so-called Curry Airlines, an appreciable sum has to be discounted for refurbishment. It may cost nearly a million dollars to tear out the curry-infested furnishings and replace them with new. Curry Airlines therefore have to depreciate aircraft at a higher rate than other airlines. There is no means of ventilation that can cope with the olfactory burden.

35   Caribou have been tamed in more recent times.

36   Certain very vulnerable animals survived, like the passenger pigeon.

37   There may or may not have been domestic poultry.

38   See page 96.

39   *The Great Wine Blight*, George Ordish, Sidgwick & Jackson, 1987.

40   See description, Quinine Chapter in *Seeds of Change*, by the author.

41   Certain fish oils and olive oil, uniquely amongst edible oils, actually reduce cholesterol in the human bloodstream. Animal fats, of course, increase the level.

42   Charles Darwin noticed one such phenomenon in 1833. By 1870, this had become an important industry. The orange groves of Paraguay produced millions of cases for export before 1914, and millions of tons of *floating* oranges and lemons, and crosses, were netted from the rivers downstream and fed to pigs and beef cattle, and the carcasses exported. As far as is known, there were thousands of acres of citrus fruits before the white man arrived in force in Paraguay in 1620; none of the early citrus orchards were planted by humans.

43   A French engineer named Frezier (no pun: the French for strawberry is *fraise*) was in Chile in the early eighteenth century. He brought back the large berried native Chilean strawberry. It was crossed with the *fraise du bois* in about 1720, and modern strawberry culture began. The American cultivar had the size, the European the taste.

44 The loganberry is named after its breeder (or discoverer) Judge Logan; this Californian is said, by some, to have bred the cross between a raspberry and blackberry. That was in 1881, and dispute still rages as to whether the hybrid was a natural 'sport' or developed with judicial cunning.

45 There cannot have been many wild dogs, or wolves, or the sheep refused to panic. Almost any European breed of domesticated sheep today refuses to stand up to dogs when attacked.

46 Ironically, however good merino wool may have been in the sixteenth century, it can never have been of the same quality as fibre from the Andean ungulates: alpaca, llama, vicuna and guanaco. Alpaca wool is supreme in the world for length, sometimes stretching to 304 mm (12 in). Vicuña is soft, fine and very supple. In fact, none of this wool could find its proper market until Titus Salt (1803–76) invented a method of machine weaving, using a cotton warp and an ungulate weft. From the date of this invention in 1836, imports into England from Peru and Chile rose from £10,000 a year to an average of more than £250,000 a year in the last ten years of the nineteenth century. In 1853 Salt also built a model manufacturing town, on the River Aire, named Saltaire, inspiration for Cadbury and Lever towns built later in the nineteenth century.

47 How quickly can wild pigs multiply? How long is a piece of string? De Soto, in Florida, in 1539, brought ashore 13 pigs, sex unspecified, and killed them with careful restraint only when very hungry; three years later, there were seven hundred. Hodges & Lewis, *Spanish Explorers in the Southern United States*, Scribner, New York, 1907.

48 There have been innumerable instances of horses warning their riders of hostile humans, or dangerous snakes like rattlers, or bad paths ahead. The wise rider makes use of this information.

49 Within a few years of the English arrival in Virginia, the plantain was known by Indians as 'The Englishman's Foot'. It was meant to grow only where an Englishman had trod. A hundred years later, it had reached the Mississippi, long before more than a few Englishmen, if any.

CHAPTER FOUR

Challenge and Response

This chapter treats in detail with the development of the United States, both before and after Independence, and in such a way that the physical is accentuated. The primacy of disease and food supply in an almost 'empty' country, and the important truth about the New World is contrasted with ideological explanations of American success. The important truth for the time was that this was the first country in the world in which it was unnecessary for a man to be hungry. The effect of this fact upon the future has never been properly measured. But there were still challenges in the young United States, and American responses have proved valuable in every other new country.

The story of the neo-Europes outside the earliest – the United States – are mainly told in the next chapter, since most of the important relationships between the new countries and Western Europe have grown up in the last hundred years. But the pattern followed in the United States has been an ambition of many other countries. Canada has developed economically in juxtaposition to her big neighbour; Australia has been conscious of the American example for a century; New Zealand, once so interlocked with England, is now more of a Pacific country, as is the United States.

In Russia, old challenges have become insoluble problems, without responses – walked away from. This is as true today as in Tsarist times. An astonishing nineteenth-century birth-rate produced no more food, nor has the last half century. In Japan, the challenges have been accepted and triumphantly answered. A country with only 20 per cent of its main island potentially agricultural against 75 per cent in England, maintained a glorious isolation for two hundred years, with an increase of population during that time of only 28 per cent – against 400 per cent for England. During those two centuries, Japan was self-sufficient, much more crowded than England. She still is. This space-challenge has produced a response which is unique in the world. It is not properly understood. It is the prime cause for Japanese success.

The American experience is so profoundly different to that of any other country that Americans today are apt to ascribe their history to especial factors. Many speak with a tinge of sanctimony, a hint of holiness, of the unique nature of the United States of America. Freedom from the arbitrary rule of kings and nobles was obviously important; escape from the tyranny of some church or other was at least as significant; even the all-important change between the medieval meaning for the word 'liberty' (privilege) and the modern meaning (natural rights) has been ascribed to the American Revolution. In fact, all three of these desirable elements in a modern free country were held to be essential by John Locke (1632–1704) and nominally in place in England by 1715. Largely because the Founding Fathers had to appear to be anti-British, the credit for these vital ingredients in the Constitution were related to Greece rather than to England. To be fair to the men of two hundred years ago, it also appeared at the time that King George III was trying to abrogate what the Glorious Revolution of 1688 had done to the rule of kings. Eternal vigilance is the price of liberty. Many Englishmen supported the Americans, whom they regarded as fellow citizens, suffering for liberty and justice. The loss of the American colonies was the price which the English paid for their lack of vigilance about their King. There is another physical scenario about America, which is an alternative to 'Man's arrogant insistence that he alone has been the principal player'.[1]

Neither in Spain nor in England were there insupportable increases in population in the two hundred years before the American Revolutions.[2] Spain's population increase in the eighteenth century was less than that of the European average (44 per cent instead of 50 per cent). England's was more, 60 per cent, but most of the increase was in the last third of the century, by which time the troubles between London and the colonies were already important. There was not much British emigration into the thirteen colonies or states between 1770 and 1800. In fact, the total emigration from Spain and England across the Atlantic was about the same before 1800, one million from each country. What happened when they got there was what was important.

In 1650, there were, perhaps, 50,000 Spaniards south of the Rio Grande. They were an élite. They did no manual work; even plantation managers were usually half-breeds.[3] There were huge losses from disease in the Spanish Caribbean colonies, and some in other parts of South and Central America. Only in certain areas did the absence of disease coincide with massive food supplies. There were three principles about the Spanish Empire. First, all power centred in a provincial viceroy, usually a grandee from Old Spain, who went home, if he survived, at the end of his period in office. The 'captaincies' or viceroyalties were, from north to south: New

Spain (Mexico); Cuba (the Caribbean); Guatamala (Central America); Venezuela; New Granada (Colombia); Quito; Peru; Charcas (Bolivia); Chile, and Buenos Aires, which included modern Argentine, Uruguay and Paraguay.

Secondly, it was the function of Spanish colonies to furnish the mother-country with precious minerals and tropical products. The strictest mercantilism was implicit. There was little trade between colonies, or between Spanish possessions and those of another country, and no approved trade with Europe other than between Spain and the colonies. Inevitably, the rules were honoured in the breach, not the observance.

Thirdly, since Spanish whites could not hope to occupy Central and South America, less the three Guianas and Brazil, an area bigger than Europe, interbreeding was encouraged. Red and black should be made more Hispanic. The *conquistadores* should spread their seed throughout the continent. This philosophy was even approved by the priests. Was it before or after the connection between Spain and *machismo*? The result is that Latin America is an extraordinarily complex mixture of red, white, black and, ultimately, yellow genes. The pure Spanish did not multiply very greatly.

The English, of course, had no 'philosophy'. The colonies just grew up. But they were of vigorous stock. They lived in a paradise, compared to England. Shakespeare's England was no more, no less crowded than the Continental United States of today. The England of the time of the French Revolution was as densely occupied as is the Eastern seaboard today, but without railroads, with less coal and water power, without any cheap steel, or the internal combustion engine or electricity. The early English emigration during the eighteenth century was mostly to the Caribbean, and that was even truer of the seventeenth-century movements. Most of those who went to the Caribbean died of disease – yellow fever, *falciparium* malaria, enteric disorders. In 1700, there were about 250,000 people in the colonies running from Maine to South Carolina. In 1800, the same colonies, now states, east of the mountains, contained nearly 4 million people.

There have been great arguments among demographers and historians about how this increase came about. Was it all natural increase, in which case it would be about 3 per cent per year, about the same as in Ireland at the latter end of the period? How much was immigration – 400,000? More or less? Politics are mixed up in this argument. If Americans in 1800 were 60, 70, 80 per cent, derived from the 1700 stock, then the Americans of 1800, Washington, Jefferson, Madison, Adams, Hamilton, and the rest were all special people, not just overseas Englishmen. And what about that quintessential American, Benjamin Franklin, born the seventeenth child of poor parents, self-educated, an FRS, the discoverer of the lightning conductor, of the course of the Gulf Stream, of the heat-absorbing quality of different colours; signatory of the Declaration of Independence. He crossed the Atlantic on four missions, fought the English but retained their respect and made peace with them. No one could call such a man anything but an American. He was more uniquely American than Washington or Jefferson. He was one of the first able to make good.

This, then, was the quality of America on which the hope of every subsequent revolution has been, in part, floated; from France (1789) and the Spanish colonies (1809–23) to Russia (1917) and even to the Iberian Revolutions of the day before yesterday (Portugal, Spain). Every free man or woman living today believes that he has the right to make the most of himself. The Parable of the Talents takes new form. It was previously the law, the inaccessibility of education, the unfairness of autocracy, the unbridled privileges of the nobility, the corruption of the Establishment that prevented men making good. Whether this was true of the England whence came the inhabitants of British North America, the important point was that people were able to believe it. This sort of freedom meant that people had to be allowed to forget the past as well as to look forward to a prosperous future.

If there is no structural reason for economic inefficiency, people get rich. Americans in 1775 were richer than the English. Poor Americans, even ex-convicts, were very much richer than poor Englishmen. If men believe there is no limit to the gross wealth of this world, they are more likely to increase that wealth rather than attempt to share it. If men believe that anything is possible, some part of that possibility may be realized. If economic freedom, without overmuch regulation, and true competition exists, there is more chance of efficiency. If the market is more important than politics, then there is less likelihood of corruption. There was an implicit belief in the Constitution that economic freedom was part and parcel of the total freedom of mankind, part of his birthright. It is an intriguing possibility in history that, if the Americans had not been there pointing the way, in the 1790s, as in the 1950s, Europe would have reverted to the cosy restrictive practices that those in positions of power and privilege regard as 'normal'. Guilds, combinations, cartels all have the function of reversing the word 'liberty' from its modern meaning to its ancient, an acceptable form of 'privilege'.

By 1592, a century after Columbus's first voyage, mercantilism had already been perceived by a few to be a fallacy. The received opinion is that it was Adam Smith who proved that mercantilism was damaging to everyone who traded. In fact, English Elizabethans had included men of sufficient vision who saw that the mere pursuit of gold was not as valuable as the creation of wealth. The earliest, truest creation of wealth was the growth of food in a hungry world. 'That is the richest land that feeds the most men,' said Sir Humphrey Gilbert, brother-in-law of Sir Walter Ralegh. Gilbert drowned in 1583, homeward bound on the Atlantic, having failed to find the fabled North-West passage, but having taken possession of Newfoundland for Queen Elizabeth. Ralegh died on the scaffold in 1618, having been in turn the quintessential Elizabethan: courtier, poet, wit, explorer, historian, soldier, lady's man, a survivor into the subsequent, dark, ungenerous reign. It was Ralegh who had a vision of planting an 'English nation' in North America which would be an outlet for England's surplus capital and surplus people. In 1584 a full-scale expedition had planted people on Roanoke Island near Cape Hatteras. The 150 colonists did not survive; perhaps they were massacred. After Ralegh had spent most of his fortune on this and other expeditions, there was no result, except for the well-known introduction of the potato and the tobacco plant to Ireland. Both had momentous, unforeseen consequences.[4]

Ralegh, broken in fortune as well as reputation, was succeeded by a chartered company. In 1620, the London Company became two, the Virginia Company, and the Council for New England. The Virginia settlers were mostly well born and did not welcome toil; starvation was a familiar, friendly and supportive Indians notwithstanding. Like Spanish 'aristocrats' the British gentry preferred to find gold; if gold was not forthcoming, others worked; after 1619, there was a slave trade to cure the shortage of labour.[5]

In 1623, after the massacre of 1622, there was an inquiry. Five thousand five hundred whites had emigrated to Virginia; 300 had returned to England; 4,000 had died; only 1,200 had remained. The next year, it was judged that the 'democratical' colony had failed. Virginia became a Royal Colony. By 1642, when Sir William Berkeley became the Governor, there was already a self-sustaining corn-based colony, with tobacco as a 'cash crop'. Gradually, other crops were grown. Apart from maize, the legumes and tobacco, they were all introductions. Squashes came from the Caribbean, brought by the Spanish. Peanuts, taken from Brazil by the Portuguese to West Africa, came over with the slave ships. The Irish potato was brought over by Englishmen, and went wild, and was adopted by the Amerindians. Onions had gone feral, having been introduced further south by the Spanish, and spread by the fauna, perhaps pigs, also left by the Spanish. Tomatoes, Jerusalem artichokes, capsicum (peppers) and sunflowers were introduced from the Caribbean. The stone fruits had been introduced by the Spanish missions further south, had gone wild, and travelled north, also with the pigs. This was true of figs as well as peaches, both of which thrived in Virginia.

Wild fruits and nuts prospered as distinct American cultivars, and included grapes, wortleberries, cranberries, huckleberries, gooseberries, strawberries, certain apples, persimmons and mulberries. The last excited exaggerated hopes for a significant silk industry, which never materialized. Maple sugar was the standard sweetener of the North East, and was extended south by the English. Amongst the nuts, pecans, butternuts, hickories, chinkapins and chestnuts were indigenous. Few fruits or nuts were domesticated, though their genes were used in improving European varieties. It is not clear whether anyone could survive without agriculture. The only form of native livestock discovered by the original settlers were turkeys, some sort of 'peacock' and 'guinea fowl'. There may have been a domesticated hen, but the settlers' poultry crossed with the natives, so no one could tell, by 1650, which poultry were indigenous. Pigs had migrated from the southern tidal country before the establishment of Jamestown in 1607–8.

The cultivation of tobacco soon boomed. Under Charles II, the colony became the monopoly supplier to the United Kingdom, in exchange for which the colony's entire trade had to be with London. The brave vision of Ralegh did not survive the mercantile bureaucrats who took over his legacy. The Dutch had broken the mercantile system during the English Civil War and Interregnum, while Cromwell in turn broke the Dutch and introduced the Navigation Acts. These locked the English and their colonies and trading 'factories' into a rigid system from 1655 till the 1840s. The British Empire prospered in spite of these Acts, not because of them, but they formed a point of grievance for every enterprising American from the very earliest days.

Tobacco is a very demanding crop. Three plantings in ten are sufficient for the poor land of coastal Virginia. Small farms did not have, by definition, enough land to fallow or to grow restorative, rotational alternatives. So tobacco exhausted small farms and impoverished the farmers. Poor men left the tidal water and went west. Joining them was an average crowd of 1,500 'redemptioners' who had worked out their term of service. In 1676, a hundred years before Independence a complicated, populist revolt was led by one Nathaniel Bacon (1647–76), who challenged the long, apparently wise rule of Sir William Berkeley. Charles II pardoned all the rebels except Bacon (who, fortunately for reconciliation, died of fever) and Berkeley was recalled. The latter refused to return to England until he had hanged a score of rebels and illegally sequestrated the property of those who opposed him. The consequences were important.

Poor whites identified with the frontier. From 1676, for at least two hundred years, the east became more and more Establishment, ruled by men who did not work with their hands. Jamestown, burned in 1676, was replaced by the grander, more urbane Williamsburg. The executive and the judiciary was under control of the Crown; but the Crown was at least a month away; perhaps three months was required for an answer. So the governor, burgesses and judges, drawn from the same educated classes, or from England, or educated there, represented the Eastern Establishment. On the frontier, a moving line, were the enterprising, the discoverers, the men of the future. On worn-out tidewater plantations, magnates employed black slaves, white criminals, or indentured servants or redemptioners, all of whom had to work seven to ten years to pay for their crimes, or their sea passage.

The frontier was peopled by those who had to make good: the coast was occupied by those who already commanded wealth and position. One way to divide the growing colony would be to say that on the tidewater, there were the territorial: in the Piedmont and in the mountains, there were the entrepreneurial. That was to use divisions which exist in the majority of European countries to this day. The important point to remember is that it was population density which brought it about in America.

However well farmed, the coastal regions, from the Potomac to Key West, could only support so many people in comfort before the Industrial Revolution. When life became too difficult, the poor whites moved west, if free to do so. If there was Indian trouble as a result, so be it: there was 'Indian trouble' as early as 1622, with 347 white deaths; no one thought twice about the causes, then or later, whites and Indians competing for the same land. Because there was always more land to the west, Americans, from the first, did not farm 'well'. The shortage was not of land, but of humans. So output per man became more important than output per farm. Even if labour was in the form of black slaves or white indentured servants, it still cost money; even if a free paid labourer was not to be found in Virginia in 1750, and the only workers were blacks, or tradesmen, or indentured servants, there was still a labour shortage. It would, in the end, lead to an important sort of freedom. Its origin was confused with some especial kind of intellectual or spiritual cause. In truth, the agent which produced this form of freedom was a shortage of people compared to a bonanza of 'empty' land.

The New England colonies had a different youth. There were vague traces of European fishermen and traders spending winters (before 1607) in what is now New England, perhaps with ships damaged in the Grand Banks fishery; there was an abortive 'Popham Colony' near the mouth of the Kennebec in the winter of 1607–8. The *Mayflower* arrived in September 1620 near Cape Cod, with 102 passengers. They survived, with Indian help. The Pilgrims undoubtedly took white man's diseases with them to the Americas, but they found that other whites had already given the Amerindians of Massachusetts 'a raging mortal disease'. This was smallpox. The Indians kept their distance, and did not mingle with the Puritans, who met little resistance. This they ascribed to Godliness, not bad Indian experience with the red plague. The death-rate amongst Indians in New England appears to have been as high as the death-rate a hundred years earlier in Mexico, and higher than in Virginia. This may well have been because smallpox is a disease of density. This would suggest that Indians were settled densely in Hispaniola, Mexico, Peru and New England, less densely in Virginia and the Carolinas. Or had the Spanish already spread smallpox along the coasts of the South, from Florida northwards, before the British arrived?

It is suspected that smallpox had been taken, by some infected person in a boat, to Florida before the Spanish, and up the Mississippi before the Spanish or the French. It was endemic when George Vancouver arrived on the island named after him.[6] So why should it not previously travel to Chesapeake Bay? In any event, the existence of smallpox in New England brought by Amerindians from the French further north is almost certain in 1620, and to that accident can be ascribed some of the Puritans' success. John Winthrop said of the Indians in 1634: 'They are all neere dead of small pox, so as the Lord hathe cleared our title to what we possess.' The Puritans benefited from the disease in two ways. It emptied the land for them to fill: it proved, by striking the Indians, that God was on their side.[7]

Smallpox, of course, hit European populations very hard at the same date. But it killed children, not adults. Survivors were inoculated, at least against death, for life. Attacks in later life, if any, were mild and innocuous, except for disfiguring the face. But almost every living Englishman in the seventeenth century would have been exposed to smallpox, as were most other Europeans. Death-rates amongst children were very high. Perhaps as many as 75 per cent of the victims were under four years of age.

In the Americas, wherever the white man went, smallpox killed indiscriminately. Instead of having to replace a baby, biologically and economically not too difficult, the Amerindians had to replace people of every age. Demographically, this was impossible. The Algonquin were hit in the middle 1620s.[8] The smallpox slaughter went on: Cherokees, Catawbas, Hurons, Iroquois, culminating with perhaps half the population of Indians in the Mississippi–Missouri basin in the great plague of 1837–8.[9]

Assured of God's favour, the Puritans marched forward to the tunes of success. Success on this earth would ensure heaven in the next. New England, ill-suited to become a Plantation Province, became instead, and very early, a much more urban place than Virginia. The South had, within a generation, acquired the characteristics that would still pertain in 1860. A broad, flat land of magnificent horizons, it was sparsely populated. Immigrants had arrived, not as complete 'congregations' or even as families, but as individuals. In the South, there were few Indians organized in tribes against which whites had to huddle in self-protection. The rivers and sea-inlets lent themselves to a direct trade with England. The English county was easily transferred as a unit of jurisdiction. A court was established in each county, usually of eight justices. These made the rules, enforced them, and acted as the petty judiciary, as they did in England until 1889. The Common Law obtained as far as serious crimes were concerned. It was shared with England and still is, and decisions of the courts remain vital. [10] There was a governor, usually appointed by the Crown, and the Church of England was the established religion, ultimately, even in tolerant Maryland. Throughout the South though, there was far more religious toleration than would have been possible in New England.

In New England, the settlements were formed by the facts of population density, disease and food supplies. Because of the Indian population, the unit of settlement was the town, laid out around a square common, with a place for church, school, and town hall. The town gave protection from the Indians, and easy access to church and school during the savage winters. Frontier towns acted as forts against the Indians, and before 1700, it was illegal for settlers to abandon their lands and move north or west. Because of the rigorous climate, broken terrain, poor communications, rocky soil and a shortage of potential arable land, no system involving plantation crops grown for Europe would have provided a decent standard of living. Subsistence crops were grown, but wealth was otherwise generated.

Fish were a major export from the first, dried, smoked or salted cod for Catholic Europe. Timber and timber products were obvious and even as early as the 1650s and as late the 1850s, New England built wooden ships cheaper than anyone in Europe. The region challenged the Baltic for masts and planking, and England for the ribs and knees of the wooden walls, and for tan bark for the curing of the essential leather. Barrel staves, hoops, and whole barrels were exported to the South, to the West Indies, and all over Europe. Timber was burnt in huge tonnages to make charcoal and potash. Fur remained important long after most furbearing animals had been driven from the other Atlantic colonies. Trade of every sort was essential for poor New England.

By 1700, New England had over 1,000 trading vessels, in a population of not much more than 100,000. A triangular trade grew up between Africa, the West Indies and New England, which involved slaves, rum, sugar and the products of New England manufacture. Earlier than any colony of any White Imperial power, New England developed manufactures and became independent of the home country for leather goods, and ironwork and pre-industrial craftwork of every kind. Earlier than any other colony of any European power, New England demonstrated an ability to live without depending directly or indirectly on the home country. These characteristics were ascribed, then and now, to superior Puritan virtue.

In fact, they were the effects of geography, climate, disease, food supply, population density and so forth; they were exactly mirrored by the absence of slavery which was due to the same factors. In 1700, Massachusetts and Virginia probably had the same population of whites. Virginia, with eight times the total area, had more than twelve times as much agricultural land. Against those imperatives, what position can ideology hold?

It was chance which made the Pilgrim Fathers land on Cape Cod. It was the circumstances of their new life which made the Puritans what they were. In 1700, with Salem, Boston, Newport, New Haven, and more than 200 other towns, there was as much urbanization as in any comparable area in Europe of that day. Is it not idle to speculate what the Puritans would have been like three generations later, if they had landed on Long Island or near Cape Hatteras instead of Cape Cod?

The Middle Atlantic colonies had a much more varied history before 1700. In 1609, Henry Hudson, an Englishman in the Dutch service, arrived in what would become New York harbour in his ship, the *Half-Moon*. The local Indians of the Delaware tribe, were offered Dutch gin. The island on which this historic exchange took place was henceforth known as Manhattan, or 'the-island-where-we-all-got-drunk'. The Dutch very quickly established trading posts, not settlements, at New Amsterdam (New York), Fort Orange (Albany), Fort Nassau on the Delaware River, and Fort Good Hope on the Connecticut River. The whole of Manhattan was purchased in 1642 for $40 worth of trade goods.

The region was not much cherished. Furs and wheat (established by the Dutch in 1625) were less desirable commodities than tea from China, the huge East Indies spices trade, gold stolen from the Spanish, or the slave trade between Africa and the Caribbean. Even the salt trade from the island of Aruba in the Caribbean was considered more valuable than the products of New Netherlands, as the Dutch settlements were called. When the Dutch were defeated in North America in the 1660s, and title passed to the English, there were probably only 8,000 people in New Netherlands, not many Dutch amongst them. There had been, for a generation, an autocratic, corrupt Dutch rule ill-supervised from Amsterdam, ill-supported by the directors of the West India Company, ill-regarded by the native Netherlanders.

New Sweden was an interlude, allowed by the Dutch, who were temporarily in alliance with Queen Christina. From 1638 to 1655, a Swedish settlement was permittd at 'Fort Christina' on the site of present-day Wilmington, Delaware. In the latter year it surrendered to Peter Stuyvesant, the authoritarian, peg-legged 'director' of New Netherlands. Nine years later, Stuyvesant surrendered to the English. [11]

As is well known, the Quaker William Penn acquired title to what is now known as Pennsylvania in 1681. The feu-rent payable was two beaver skins. An aristocrat by birth, Quaker-democrat by conviction, Penn drew up a form of government which gave franchise to all landowners and taxpayers, with freedom of worship, and treason and murder the only capital offences. The Penn family remained in a quasi-landlord position for nearly a hundred years. Meanwhile, the city of brotherly love had developed into the most American city, larger than any other in 1700; the next city then in population was Boston, its rival New York always having a more commercial, more cosmopolitan air. The Middle Atlantic colonies prospered exceedingly, growing grain, producing butter and cheese, beef, pork, and exporting these all over the Caribbean, and to many parts of Europe. In 1700, there were British colonies all the way from Maine to South Carolina, and inland to the 'fall line'. [12]

Inland from the fall line and as far west as the mountains was the Piedmont, a gradually rising plane. Below the Piedmont land was easily brought into cultivation, easily approached by ship, and useful for the primary production of cereals and tobacco. Though unable to withstand the improvidence of plantation monoculture, the tidewater lands below the fall line were never a limitation in those areas which were farmed so badly as to cause exhaustion or erosion. [13] The feckless just moved on. In those areas of New England whence the early settlers were unable to emigrate, the population either earned its living from non-agricultural pursuits, or treated the land with the same sort of respect they would have shown at home in England. Emigration from New England to the West was not a general option before Independence.

In Virginia, westward movement was popular with those who had worn out the land of the tidewater and for indentured servants who were free of obligation after their redemption. In the South, redemptioners received fifty acres of land, plus the usual tools, clothing and livestock. The land tended, of course, to be in the West.

In Pennsylvania and New Jersey there were opportunities in the Piedmont. It is narrower than in the South, but a rolling countryside of higher than average fertility. West of the Blue Ridge, and of its northern extensions, lies the 'great' Appalachian Valley, the Kittatinny Valley in Northern New Jersey, the Allentown-Lebanon-Cumberland Valley in Pennsylvania and Maryland and the Shenandoah in Virginia. These areas are the most fertile, the most moderate in climate, the best watered, in the Eastern United States. Because pre-railroad transport except by water was so expensive and difficult, the parts of these valleys nearest the rivers became influential in eighteenth-century America. They were more than that. They were the main reason that Americans ate, on average, twice as well as Europeans of the same class. These valleys not only fed Americans. They also provided food exports for the Caribbean and Europe of great economic value. These exports, according to figures published at the time, were far less than recorded imports except in the South. There is not, however, quite the faith in colonial statistics as there once was. For example, New England statistics reveal a deficit over the fifty years before 1776 larger than either New York or Pennsylvania. Common sense suggests that exports were either undervalued or underrecorded. How could the coast be watched by a body of officials with whom the population had scant sympathy?

There was an independence bred in most Americans which derived not from politics or religion, but from the effects of the natural circumstance. The sheer scale of the landscape in North America, dwarfing in 1600, 1700, 1800, even today the works of man on the same continent, rendered most men conscious of their humble gratitude. To this was added the tendency of Europeans to eat far better in America than at home, to rear many more children, to lose far fewer neighbours to disease, to live longer themselves, to surprise each other. Not only of the English was this true. Scots came as families or small congregations and became prominent in America as merchants, lawyers, schoolmasters, and ministers of religion. Their influence on America before Independence was profound. It could never have happened if the same men and women had had no more chance than they had at home.

The same is true of the Scots-Irish, or Ulstermen, who came over in large numbers when the English restricted their woollen and linen industries after only a century of settlement in Ireland. A people planted by James I in the middle of largely Roman Catholic natives, the Ulstermen were of pioneer stock at home. They imported these qualities to America, and they settled in the Susquehanna Valley and in the Carolinas. The flood of Ulstermen coincided with large numbers of peasant Germans who settled in the so-called 'Dutch' counties of Pennsylvania.

These Pennsylvania Dutch were encouraged by William Penn himself, and he attracted many settlers from Switzerland and the Rhineland. By 1776, there were probably more than 150,000 of these peasants, immensely hard-working, thorough, thrifty, patient, industrious, and with large families. They had a mystical love of the soil (and of real estate) combined with an intellectual and intelligent application of new methods of husbandry. What is so notable about these Germans or Ulstermen or Scots, is that each group developed positive characteristics which were only obvious in a minority in their own homes. The full potential of all these people only occurred in the new Europe which they called, in time, the United States of America.

At the bottom of the success of the new country was a simple fact, often ignored. For the first time in history, the poorest person in America had enough to eat. Of the poor in Europe, still less of Asia or Africa, that could never be said before 1776. It has only been possible to claim that there is enough food of enough quality for every Western European for the last generation and a half. This truth is not yet in place in Eastern Europe, or Africa or Asia.

The effect of such circumstances upon mankind in the seventeenth and eighteenth centuries was to unleash the full physical potential of human beings. Europeans were 'restricted' by religion, constitution, politics or feudal custom. In fact, is it not time that an alternative be considered; is it not more important to eat properly; to rear most children born, instead of

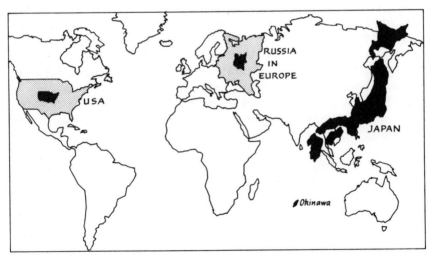

Three Superpowers Redrawn to Show Density of People in Cultivated Area

a minority; to live ten years longer; to see large numbers of grandchildren at a time when descendants looked after the old? Is it any wonder that Americans, even before Independence, were regarded with ill-concealed envy, tinged by the kind of patronizing superiority exhibited even today?

The key tools to make market agriculture possible were the children of steampower: the railway and the steamship. It is true that there had been a market agriculture in the United States, operating by water. The land serving the trade necessarily had to be beside a river or the sea. At Independence, such a system existed in the river valleys east of the Alleghenies. The Connecticut, Hudson, Delaware, Susquehanna and Potomac all gave easy access to the sea, and small ships had sailed almost directly from the wharves on these rivers, and those of the south for a hundred years before Independence.[14] Northern farms found markets in the Caribbean, the South, and in the growing American cities, long before the first railroad was built.[15]

The loss of the British West Indies as a preferential area after Independence led to a change in a market which had taken over 20 per cent of all Northern farm production in 1776. When the young United States became – for the British – a foreign nation, the British navigation laws excluded American ships from the trade of the British West Indies. Trade between the United States and the West Indies did not cease; American merchants were hampered, English merchants helped. Fortunately for the United States, the war between England and France which occupied most of the years from 1792 to 1815, led to a relaxation of the Navigation Acts. But the war, which was waged with one short interval with increased success by the Royal Navy, led in turn to a short war between the United States and the former mother country. Through all these alarms and excursions, American food production and the American food trade expanded at a rate whose volume meant a doubling of trade every twenty years. In the years between 1783 and the Wars between the States (1861–5), food trade in the United States increased by more than eight times. The population, meanwhile, increased by only three times in the same period.

Most of the reasons why the food trade grew so greatly were domestic, not foreign. First, the South was a deficit food area, partly because the more suitable Southern grain crops were not bread grains. The South grew more than half of all Indian corn, or maize, in the Union, even as late as 1860, but less than a third of the wheat; a fifth of the oats and rye, and a twentieth of the barley and buckwheat.

Secondly, the South grew a great many cash crops for direct export, or export to the North – cotton, tobacco, rice, indigo, sugar. Of these crops, only the unexported portion of the sugar and rice crops directly increased food supplies. Thirdly, labour organization in the South, dependent as it was upon slavery, did not assist in the economical use of food. Slaves were given land to feed themselves, or so many bushels of corn per family per week. There was little incentive to use either land or labour properly. Finally, the urbanization of the North was an important factor in the food trade, long before railroads. The urban element in the whole United States population increased between 1790 and 1860 by three times the national average, or nine times altogether. In the North, the increase of urban population was of the order of fifteen times the 1790 figure. Urban growth in the whole of New England and the Mid-Atlantic States, except for Vermont, was greater than the rural increase by 1850. In that year, urbanization was greater in Massachusetts, Connecticut, Rhode Island and New York than in Old England. Before the railroads, foreign trade, usually meaning trade with England or the English colonies (still 80 per cent of the whole) was the chief function of all cities; after railroads, cities had a primary function outside foreign trade and they were often only enabled to practise that function because of the railroad.[16]

In 1790, 80 per cent of all gainfully employed workers were in the countryside. In 1860, more than half were outside agriculture. In 1790, 95 per cent of Northern farm production was consumed in the Northern countryside. In 1860, the figure had fallen to 50 per cent. Only 4 per cent of farm production was exported in both years; the difference was the greater proportion eaten in Northern cities and in the South. The United States had become one of the world's first market-driven agricultural economies.

There had been, of course, many colonies in the past which grew food for the Home Country; the Greek city-states, for example. There had been empires such as Rome which had taken tribute from colonies in grain. There had been, and were in the nineteenth century, many places where peasants paid their lords in kind, who then sold the produce on the national or European economy. This was true, for example, of Russia, Poland, Prussia, parts of Italy and France. But the United States would be the first *free* agricultural economy. She would be followed, by 1914, by Australia, Canada, New Zealand, and to a certain extent, the Argentine and South Africa. These neo-Europes became part of the European economy.

There are two favourite 'truths' about the American population. If immigration had ceased in 1776, the population of the United States would probably have been at least as great in quantity as it is today.

Secondly, in that case, half of all Americans would be descended from those who had been transported as criminals, debtors, or indentured servants.

Even as early as 1700, some non-Establishment people like Quakers would support transportation over imprisonment at home, seeing in the New World the possibility of a fresh chance for 'misfits', in return for the provision of labour for an area which was almost 'empty'. Humane people increasingly tended to regret the death penalty for the theft of objects worth about a month's wages: in the absence not only of detective methods but also of almost any effective policing, transportation was therefore to be favoured.

The original impulse for transportation was not the result of a need for an alternative to the death penalty; Elizabeth I's Vagrancy Act empowered magistrates at Quarter Sessions to banish vagrants to some place overseas, as should be directed by the Privy Council. This was extended by acts in each of the next reigns, so that by 1666 perhaps two-thirds of those sentenced to prison or death had their sentences commuted to transportation 'for life'. These people, rescued from jail or the gallows, were not treated with any degree of gentleness. There were also 'vagrants', or those shipped out as surplus by their lord, or volunteering to work as indentured servants for so many years in exchange for the passage money. Today, no one knows the sum total of those 'transported', nor do figures exist for the total of criminals, vagrants or volunteers who crossed the Atlantic for many and complicated reasons, some with great hopes. Such cargoes included eighty-one 'maids' sent from Liverpool to Virginia in 1683.

Transportation meant that thousands were sent out to the Caribbean Islands, to the mainland colonies, to Bermuda, and at least one cargoload to Newfoundland, from about 1620 onwards, and more than 1,000 were sent out to Barbados after Monmouth's rebellion in 1685–7, a shipment exceptional, and thus recorded for posterity, only because of the circumstances.

Between 1493 and 1846, probably fewer than 7 million people had travelled long haul from Europe. Some went across the North Atlantic. Some went on down the South Atlantic, across the Indian Ocean, and finally, all over the Pacific. Of the 7 million, at least 2 million died prematurely; did a million return to Europe, leaving barely 4 million to settle long enough to produce progeny? In 1846, those progeny amounted to more than 50 million, 25 million in the USA alone. That was the result of three and a half centuries of emigration and 'transportation' from Europe.[17]

Between the repeal of the British Corn Laws in 1846 and the outbreak of World War I in 1914, Europe increased its population by 100 per cent. Of that increase, a quarter emigrated to the 'new' countries, including the USA, then in the prime of life. In those 68 years, in other words, probably 50 million went abroad, and settled permanently.

These new emigrants were the more enterprising of their kind – or the more desperate, opportunistic, or fickle, or they were the more entrepreneurial, or those with fewer territorial ties at home. There were always more men emigrating than women, more poor than rich, more unskilled than qualified. But despite the apparent shortage of social virtue among them, they nearly all did far better in the new countries than anyone, including themselves, could have imagined as they arrived as poor huddled masses on Ellis Island, or wherever. Even the surviving convicts in Australia surpassed and surprised themselves.[18]

The health of the immigrants was improved on landing. Quarantine was carefully enforced in most ports in the United States, from about 1819. There was a by-product to this sanitary prudence. Because ships had to be less crowded, in order to avoid the disapproval of the Health Inspectorate, transatlantic fares rose. Because they rose, the quality of immigrant, or the wealth of those paying for the passage, rose. But fares came down rapidly in the last quarter of the nineteenth century, from $50 to $10; neither figure included food, which the immigrant usually carried and cooked on board. Once arrived in the United States, the immigrant enjoyed better food, cleaner air and water and less disease than in most European cities. Ordinary workers in the United States ate far better than Europeans of the same income group. American cities had usually little smog, and supplies of clean air and water were expected. It would not be until after 1865 that places like Pittsburgh or Birmingham, Alabama, or the mining towns in the East, or the manufacturing cities would have serious pollution problems. Those of Los Angeles, and other places, had to wait for the motorcar.

Immigrants were attracted by brokers, who were acting for railroad companies, or for New England mill owners or for companies running coal mines or steelworks. So German peasants, overburdened by fees and rents due to feudal landlords, and often in debt, sent some part of their family to the Middle West; this happened both before and after the 1848 revolutions. The Irish almost everyone knows about: 100,000 a year for 15 years after the Famine. Scottish mill girls were imported, sometimes for a few years only, to work in the textile industry of New England. Welsh coalminers came to Pennsylvania, Ohio and Western Virginia. Slavs from every point of the compass staffed the steel and metal bashing industries. Greeks formed colonies all down the Eastern seaboard. Italians flocked into the large cities. Sweden sent 1 million – a quarter of the population – because of insufficient food at home. Finns, fearing a repetition of famine,[19] left in nearly as large a proportion as the Swedes. Jews, especially later in the period, left Eastern Europe in droves, and by 1914 formed a quarter of the population of New York City.

Of the 25 million Europeans who came to the United States in the years 1846–1914, more than a third came across the Atlantic in steerage. The contrast with the luxury of the first-class section in the same ship made the conditions even more startling.

Arrived ashore, the immigrant was still at risk. Did the ignorant immigrant speak English? More than half did not. Did European ignorance lead immigrants into grave trouble? Well, there was always Tammany Hall to bail them out, or equivalent organizations in other cities. Ignorance, misconceptions, romantic views of the opportunities undoubtedly existed, but the conditions were so much better than those left behind that most immigrants prospered. About a quarter went on to the land between 1846 and 1914; three-quarters went into the cities. An unsuccessful European farmer could sell up, buy passage for himself and his family, and still have enough left to establish himself in the new states close to the frontier. There was a difference in spirit to still-feudal parts of Europe. There were no kings, no nobles, no extortionate taxes, rents, tithes, no master to be acknowledged. Farmworkers sat at table with their masters; there were no large estates with a 'ruling class'; there was no danger that the arm would be worn out doffing the cap or touching the forelock. Rural America was unbelievable for a European farmer.

For any European the most incredible feature was the cheapness of land. For most of the century, land could be bought for $1.25 an acre. A section (260 hectares or 640 acres) therefore cost $800, or £160 at the prevailing exchange rate. Each section, half-section or quarter-section would require water, usually pumped by windmill, costing at most about $500, and a house, from a sod-cabin, to a log cabin to a wooden-frame house, and costing anything from a few dollars to, say $800 for the materials for a frame house with four rooms. Every house had to have a stove, from $12–$50. The requirements for an arable farm, in the period after the Civil War, and after the railroads were in place, would be for horses, cultivating equipment, harvesters, and so forth. These might come to between $500 to $2,000 for a farm of a section-size, depending on the quality of the land, soil aspect, whether fencing was required, and the nature of the neighbours. The first three harvests of grain off prairie soil, broken for the first time, might average $20 per acre.[20] If the farmer-immigrant spent $800 on land, $2,000 on windmill, house and furnishings, and $2,000 on live and dead stock on the farm, all outside figures, he would have invested less than $5,000. His harvest would come to over $10,000, allowing for an appreciable proportion in fallow each year. The balance was represented by hard work, and on the debit side, there was the cost of keeping farmer and family for a year between harvests. The whole equation depended upon cheap land, healthy demand for grain, and cheap transportation.

If the putative farmer had to buy from the railroad, rather than from the Federal Government, he would have paid more for his land. If there were no water on the section, the land would have been useless, or water would have been expensively bought from next door. If he had 'bad luck' or if he were incompetent, or broke a leg, or contracted some lethal sickness on his way West, or if he were cheated, the immigrant would fail; there were not a few. Those responsible for the farmers' 'bad luck' were often said to be the railroads.

Unregulated before the end of the century, the railroad mileage increased by four times between the end of the Civil War (1865) and 1900. They were led by buccaneers of whom their victims said: 'When they speak, they lie; when they are silent, they are stealing; while they sleep, they sin.'[21] The 'sinners' included Dillon and Sage, who were operating before the Civil War, and their younger colleague, Gould, who was the most spectacularly successful and outrageous. This is not to say that the actions of Morgan, Vanderbilt, Rockefeller, Huntington, Stanford, Cooke, Villard or Harriman would prove to be legal at a later date. But for their times, they acted within the law. Government help to the railroads west of the Mississippi was given to provide an impetus to open up and populate the West. Nearly 210,000 sq. miles – an area almost exactly the same size as France – was given to help get the railroads built. It included wasteland, mountains, deserts, unfarmable areas, range unfit of grazing. But cheap or free land had been the only way to make sure of the railroads.

It was, in fact, the railroads which gave the land any value. Land and railroads formed an elegant syndrome. The lands in Minnesota, with 40 per cent of the state area granted to railways, were originally sold for $3–$5 an acre in the 1890s; in the 1910s they were worth perhaps $25 an acre in big blocks of arable. By the 1920s, the wheat price had risen (through World War I), then fallen, so that Minnesota became much more of a land of mixed farms. The land was then worth more than wheat farmers could afford to pay. Farmers, or the original farmers' sons, changed their husbandry, or new people moved in.

The process was more rapid in Iowa. It has one of the naturally richest soils in the world, comparable to that of the Ukraine, and with a better climate. Iowa had the highest percentage of 'improved land' as defined by the Department of Agriculture. Even in 1900 the proportion was nearly 60 per cent. In that year, Iowa's agricultural production was greater than that

of any other state. Iowa was a child of post-Civil War railroad construction. In 1860, there were only 655 miles: in 1900, more than 9,000 miles.
The state became a network of railroads. Fifty per cent of all farms were
within 5 miles of a station, and only 10 per cent were said, in 1900, to be
more than 10 miles from a railroad. In this respect, Iowan farmers were
better off than their equivalents in Europe. In 1900 the agricultural
production of Iowa was worth about $20 per acre, and nearly $1,000 per
man-year. The first figure was below the equivalent mixed-farming area
of Europe, the productivity per worker far higher. The Iowan farmer was,
of course, a beneficiary not only of good soil and an unsurpassed railroad
network, but also of the most efficient agricultural implement industry in
the world.

This industry had, before 1914, and before any internal combustion
engine had been applied to agriculture, alone produced the potential for a
grain-growing system. In essence this machinery was identical to that
which every child in the Western world can watch with awe in the field
today. The system included high-speed ploughing, high-speed cultivating
and sowing in the spring, and high-speed harvesting. The speed was an
answer partly to climatic conditions, partly to the cost problem. It was
practised in the wheatbelt of the United States, in the Canadian prairies,
California, and parts of Australia. The system was described at length in
many publications before World War I, and would have been the answer
to grain-growing in Russia, France and South America. It depended not
only upon cheap land which was flat and lent itself to mechanization, but
also upon the necessary infrastructure. The railroad was vital, of course,
but also what the railroad brought – all the necessities of modern agriculture. The railroad, of course, was also essential for cheap marketing of the
main product, grain, animals, or whatever.

By 1900, the spring wheat 'Scotch-Fife' had begun to rival the winter
variety Turkey Red, and 40 per cent of the breadmaking wheat in the
United States was of this ecotype. Hard spring wheat was sown throughout the Northern prairies, in the Dakotas and in Minnesota, and the total
product in Minnesota in 1900 was more than 2 million tons, more than the
UK produced (of wheat of all sorts) and twice as much as Australia
produced. The wheat could only be produced in such profusion because of
the low cost. The low cost, in turn, was due to an effective system.

First, in August, the straw of the previous crop was burnt – a great
labour, unrewarding, but one which limited plant disease. Then began the
ploughing. At these latitudes there are only about eight weeks in September, October and November when the year's ploughing can be done.[22]
This was managed at the time by putting in teams of ploughs, each to
cover 100 hectares (250 acres) in 50 days, or 2 hectares (5 acres) a day, five

times the contemporary English rate. A team of five horses drew two furrows of 41 cm (16 in) each. This compared with a pair of contemporary European oxen or horses each pulling one furrow of 19–20 cm (7–8 in). The American team was also required to move faster. An hour with the American plow produced nearly an acre plowed, while the European plough of 20 cm (8 in) turn-furrow would have to pass through nearly 12.4 miles to plough an acre. There was more wastage in the European field, since the fields were smaller, and the plough was not in useful work as long as it would be in a long field. One 'field' in Saskatchewan at this date, alongside a railroad line, was so long that ploughing outwardly took all morning, and ploughing back to the starting point took all afternoon. Such fields were exceptional, but gangs of 8–10 ploughs, moving in echelon, shifted a great tonnage of soil. That is the function of ploughing.

After ploughing, the land was left in furrow for the frost and snow to act upon the soil. This was wholly beneficial. Less beneficial was the habit at this time of dismissing most of the men, casual workers, who went off home for the winter. When in work, they were paid a quarter as much as Henry Ford would be paying similar men in 1914 – $25 a month, instead of $100. The ploughmen also received their board and lodging, just like cowboys. Board and lodging cost farmers in those days about 50 cents per head per day, and was of great importance. [23]

Much of the year's moisture on the prairies and in the Midwest falls as snow in the winter, and the snow must not only melt, but sink into the earth as water before spring cultivation can begin. That depends upon latitude and season, but it is usually April before the ploughed land is dry enough. Ground which has been set up in furrow, can be very quickly 'knocked down' ready for sowing after the winter frosts. In the early 1900s, chain harrows had already grown huge: 7.5 metres (25 feet) or even 9 metres (30 feet) wide, drawn by 4–5 horses, capable of working down 24–30 hectares (60–75 acres) a day, with one man walking behind.

The seed-drill, throughout the world, has always traditionally followed the harrows. This was to conserve moisture, and to prevent one part of the field being harrowed, but not sown, while another part would be sown and not harrowed. A good manager of any farm, regardless of size, would arrange the 'bout' for the day, harrow once, drill the corn, and harrow again to cover the seed to the correct depth. Harrowing is no problem. Drills require more time than harrowing, being narrower, and having to stop to be refilled with corn. At that date, there was no fertilizer sown with the seed. Thirty acres would be a good day's work for a drill, involving a walk for horses and men of nearly as many miles.

The spring sowing was carefully tailored to an elegant equation. Time involved, say 25–30 days, dictated the number of workers in ratio to the acreage sown. If the sowing took only 15 days, too many seasonal workers had been hired. If the sowing took 35–40 days, too few had been found. After the spring sowing, the workers were 'let go' again. Too much social indignation should not be developed about this practice, since seasonal workers, who valued their independence and freedom, often returned, year after year, to the same farm.

While spring warmth encouraged the young wheat, the permanent staff of such a farm would be sowing oats for horses, Indian corn for man and beast, and millet or barley as a fail-safe measure; there was little work for horses in high summer, and they were left out in a grazing paddock. By the end of June, the earliest grain, sown only 90 days before, would be ready for cutting.

At this date, about 1900, the reaper-binder, invented by Cyrus McCormick (as the reaper) in 1837, had developed into a reliable machine used the world over and built by hundreds of makers. In Europe, machines with a cutting-bar of 1.5 metres (5 feet), would be typical in the small fields, often as small as 2 hectares (5 acres). These machines cut, assembled into sheaves, and dropped off the corn in groups of sheaves, usually five or six. One man drove the team of two horses, and another man sat on the back of the machine, watching out that everything was working properly, the twine moving smoothly and so on.

Such a relaxed and bucolic picture did not obtain in the new countries. Teams of 6 to 10 horses would draw a huge reaper-binder, with a cut of 5 metres (16 feet). In a good crop, the sheaves would pop out of the carrier-deck, which held them after they were tied, like chocolate bars popping off a conveyor-belt. These large machines, each with a team of horses far more difficult to drive than a coach-in-hand, would be tended by two men, just like the European example whose output would be no more than 20 per cent of the American, Canadian or Australian equivalent. In California, Canada and Australia, combine-harvesters, which cut and threshed the grain, were already in use, with as many as 24 horses pulling a machine whose whole rumbling interior was driven by the forward motion of the vehicle. In Australia, there were combine-harvesters drawn by as many as 32 mules. This must have been one of the most demanding tasks in the age before internal combustion, and a fit challenge for the young men of the young nation.[24]

The reaper-binder/thresher combination was more general than the combine-harvester. Both cleared fields with great rapidity, but the advantage of the combine was not only in the actual harvesting. Straw came out of the back of the machine, as it does today, in a continuous stream, which made for much easier burning than when huge heaps were left by the stationary threshing machine.

However threshed, the grain was carried in bulk from the machine in the field to the silo, which was characteristically by the side of a railroad siding. Tipping box-wagons would be as close to the modern truck or trailer as can be imagined, except that they were horse-drawn, usually by three horses. The grain was lifted to the top of the tower-silo, confusingly called an elevator. From the elevator, grain was shipped in bulk all over the world, without any manual labour being involved. All this bulk-handling was common in most of the wheat states by 1910 at the latest.[25]

The bottom line in, say, 1910, was of vital interest. Assuming a land-value of less than $25, including all buildings and improvements, the cost per acre, allowing 10 per cent interest on the capital employed, would be about $9. If the yield per acre was 20 bushels (544 kg, 1,200 lb), the cost per bushel would be 45 cents. The average price at the railhead in the fifteen years before World War I, was between 56 and 60 cents, allowing a modest profit of between 11 cents and 15 cents a bushel. This does not sound much, but 10,000 acres of wheat at 20 bushels to the acre would yield a profit of between $22,000 and $30,000, clear of all expenses, land taxes and interest. This was equivalent to twenty times those figures in today's situation, and a respectable yield from a middling-sized business in 1910. By such industrial methods did the new countries compete with the old, assisted by cheap steamship transport.

Not everyone could make this kind of money. Yield in the north-west wheatbelt averaged 18 bushels, not 20, in the period 1899–1913.[26] Planting could be less than timely. Insufficient labour at harvest might risk the early autumn rains. Incompetent selling might not achieve the optimum price. Each and any of these, and other, aberrations might well destroy not only the 'profit' of 15 cents a bushel, but also the ability to pay interest on the money employed.

The selection process, applied to farmers, was as harsh as any applied to plants or animals. Failure in times of excessive production was common enough; farm workers, often without wives or children, might have arrived with little, and moved on, usually to the west, with less. Failures in times of scarcity proved to be more incompetent. Iowa, and the older settled states east of the Mississippi–Missouri were not as subject to climatic changes at those in the shadow of the Rockies. Drought was rarely an excuse in the true Midwest. Failure was always cushioned by the rise in land values. Bought from the railroad at less than $5 per acre, perhaps, in 1880, the farm might well be worth ten times as much a generation later. In the absence of progeny, such a capital sum would provide capital for retirement in a warmer state, and in an age without federal pensions.

The corn-kings, wheat-viscounts, barley-barons, producers all, were not, of course, true farmers. They were primary producers, very efficient primary producers. But they were monoculturists. It is, of course, one of the minor ironies of all environmental argument that the phrase 'monoculture' is used pejoratively about growing cotton, or grain, or tobacco; there is a long history of the dangers and tribulations of soil-erosion and self-induced poverty as a result of such practices. No one ever complains about the 'monoculture' of indigenous timber or grassland. These are the crops which shield the land. In the case of the United States, it would be more than three centuries before any efforts were made to encourage, nationwide, the use of restorative crops like legumes and grasses. By then, much damage had been done.

It has been reckoned that in 1492 only 7 per cent of the United States was wholly useless by reason of soil condition (i.e. desert). By 1910, half the natural forest of the United States had already been destroyed, and between a quarter and a half the topsoil of the Missouri–Mississippi basin had been shovelled into the rivers and washed downstream. Vast areas of the eastern states had been abandoned by early farmers who had moved west.

Throughout the nineteenth century, agricultural prices tended to fall over a long period, and it was often commercially only possible for the farmers in the New countries to skim the cream from the situation and pass on. The 'cream', of course, was the topsoil, a precious commodity made by man in the Old countries and by God in the New. When it was destroyed, or blown away in the wind, or eroded into the rivers, the farmer moved on. One old man, surviving into his seventies in Nebraska, is said to have claimed that he had worn out as many farms as he had had wives: four of each. He was proud of his manhood.

The farms of post-Civil War America were also made possible by one further factor: cheap, efficient machinery produced by the ancillary industry which had replaced the local blacksmith. John Deere, McCormick, Massey-Harris – all these names are now connected with tractors, involving internal combustion engines. In the period 1900–14, there were virtually no tractors on any such farms. The motive power here was the horse and the steam locomotive on the railroad. The technology consisted of ploughs from Iowa, harrows from Indiana, harvesters from Illinois, seed-drills from Pennsylvania, barbed wire from Ohio, horseshoe nails from Delaware, horseshoes from New Jersey, harness from New York, human shoes from New England – and when these objects were worn beyond the ability of the farm staff to repair them, there was no point in seeking any other solution but to replace them. Farms were littered with the dumped, scrapped hardware from industrial America. Anything that would not burn would be left to rot in the field.[27]

Slightly modified by patterns of trade, climate and communications, exactly the same symbiotic relationship between industry in the town and industry in the countryside had grown up in parts of Canada, California, Australia, the Plate basin and Southern Russia at the same time. By 1914, the only way to compete in the world market for grains was to industrialize the growth of the crop. The mixed farmer, the trustee of the soil, the true husbandman could never compete with the economy of scale. It is a mistake to imagine that grain monoculture is a modern phenomenon.

The Eastern United States, the small farms of old Canada, the traditional holdings of Europe, were all turned into something quite different. They might still grow rather than buy feeding stuffs, but their most profitable enterprises were those based on animal husbandry.

Milk was becoming desirable to consume, as hygiene improved. Meat became cheaper, more of an everyday occurrence, not reserved for Sundays. Chickens came down in price, and continued, all through the century, to cheapen in relation to red meat. [28]

The conversion of grain into the more appetizing and higher protein meat, milk and eggs became, in the end, just as specialized as the monoculture of grain. It would not be rare to find a European farm 'importing' far more energy value in the form of cheap feeding stuffs than it 'exported' in the form of human food.

Nor were the underdeveloped nations as badly off in 1910 as such a waste of resources would suggest. There were only a third as many people in the whole world alive then as now. There were fewer than 300 million in the Indian subcontinent, against twice as many now; in China, fewer than 500 million against more than 1 billion; in the hungriest area of all, Africa, there were 110 million at most in 1910, against nearly four times that figure today. It is arguable that the peasant in the village in the underdeveloped world of 1910 was better off than the poor in cities today, in Calcutta, Cairo or Mexico City. One of the great lost virtues of villages is the possibility to be poor with dignity: that, too, is a part of husbandry.

Between 1846 and 1914, Western European population doubled. The rate of increase was uneven, and depended, as always, upon disease and food supply. In the sixty-eight years to 1914, 40 million people left Western Europe, many times the number who had emigrated in the previous four centuries. Most of the whole population increase, from about 130 million to 260 million, was due to better food supplies. These in turn were the result of better technology, in the field, on roads and railways, and at sea. There was very little scientific biology or chemistry applied to agricultural problems, and little physical science involved in transport, the design of farm implements, or to the application of power to field husbandry. Practical men using what came to hand did much to make money and educate their competitors. 'High Farming', limited at first to England and Scotland, involved farmers and landlords. Peruvian guano, Chilean nitrate or superphosphate were all available from the 1840s as a direct result of a shortage of bone-based fertilizers. Plant breeding was not in the heads of geneticists and biologists but, in a pre-Mendel age, in the hands of practical farmers, as were animal improvements.[29]

Drainage was improved by the use of steam-drawn mole ploughs and British Government subsidies encouraged tile drains from 1846 onwards. Steam was used in the form of 'stationary' engines to draw ploughs, cultivators, even harvesters: truly stationary engines drove stationary threshing machines, and this last activity went on until after World War II. There were numerous severe animal diseases unrelieved, as were human diseases, by science. Then there was a succession of wet summers, before and after the disastrous year 1879.

In the succeeding twenty years, the consumer suffered little. Grain, meat and animal feeding stuffs were available from all over the world. Cultivation in Europe declined, pastureland increased proportionately. Liquid milk became a 'cash crop' taken by fast, cheap, efficient trains to the large cities. By 1900, European agricultural systems had been much modified. Cereal growing had been reduced. Meat, milk and eggs were produced to exploit grassland and cheap imported feeding stuffs. New crops included the mass field production of potatoes, green vegetables and root crops which were formerly grown in the townsman's own allotment or garden. Farmers who adapted, survived.[30]

In Germany, the best English practices were introduced by up-to-date landlords, and German biochemistry under Liebig and Hoffmann and their pupils was ahead of the British.[31] Fallow as a proportion of total arable fell as new crops came in. Tile drainage systems were imported from England, including, at first, the tiles themselves. Chalk, marl, artificial fertilizers were applied to the poor soils of the German plain. The tonnage of potatoes grown increased by eight times between 1846 and 1914, while that of rye increased by six, wheat by four. Germany was much better fed in 1914 than in 1846, even if there were more than twice as many Germans, and much of the potato crop was used for industrial purposes. The German population had grown from 33 million in 1846 to nearly 70 million, while that of France only increased from 35 million to 40, a mere 12 per cent against more than 108 per cent. More Germans had emigrated too.

The very low population pressure in France compared with Germany combined with better land, better climate, and twice the area per head to produce a curious circumstance. Urban intellectuals were interested in improving agriculture. But drainage was so expensive relative to increased output that it did not appeal to peasants. Early plant breeders found their barley more appreciated in England and their sugar-beet seed sold better in Belgium and Germany than at home. Animal breeds were established in herd-books, on the English pattern, after 1880; but this was the action of the same sort of gentleman-fanciers as bred racehorses. Seed-drills, mowers, reaping machines replaced hand labour on the bigger farms. But much of France was so subdivided by the *Code Napoléon* that it was not always possible to apply modern techniques to small areas. Potential output per hectare increased, but the gross national production of wheat did not alter, nor that of rye, while potato production only doubled. In one area, that of wine production, France remained supreme, surviving losses engendered by phylloxera. These were reckoned to be three times greater than the cost of the Franco-Prussian War.[32]

The Low Countries were still farmed as well as anywhere in Europe. Though their population increased by less than in England or Germany, the primacy of rotations, root crops and heavy horses and cattle were still notable. Dairying became more important in Holland than in Belgium. In the Netherlands, too, an increased demand for foodstuffs could always be met by land reclamation and polderization.[33] Drainage throughout the Low Countries was vital and essential even for ordinary, non-agricultural purposes, as army generals discovered in Flanders after 1914. Grain was imported from overseas to maintain the standard of life of the average townsman, while farmers were encouraged to adapt.

In Italy, the sixty-eight years provoked the least positive reaction. With an increase from 22 to 36 million, population pressure at first glance would not seem to have been critical. But the political changes involved in the Risorgimento (Unification) from 1860–70 did nothing for the post-feudal system of landholding. This was a form, usually, of sharecropping, onerous to the peasant.

There was a general decline in the productivity of most commodities except for liquid milk for towns and sheep for wool and meat. Peasant poverty led to large scale emigration, not only to North America, but also to the Argentine. The challenge in Italy was not only not answered, but in many cases not recognized. The only product which really improved in manufacturing method and quality was wine, which benefited from the post-phylloxera revolution. The rest of agriculture was in a poor way to meet the conditions of the modern world. Agricultural stagnation remained largely true until after World War II despite an occasional flashy improvement such as the drainage of the Pontine Marshes.[34]

The management of food between producer and consumer in the sixty-eight years affected everything eaten. Stonemills gave way to roller-milling; breadmaking became an automated, industrial process; the curing of fish, bacon and ham was transformed; milk was 'pasteurized'; butter was standardized by centrifuge cream separators, whey removers and, above all, by refrigeration; cheese became a factory product from neo-European countries; Borden invented evaporated milk (1853); vacuum drying of milk followed; canning and refrigeration were applied to meat of all kinds; vegetables and fruit were bottled and canned. Refrigeration before 1914 was not generally applied or even available in the home; so daily shopping was still a necessity in towns. European governments became anxious to ensure a higher standard of hygiene and purity in food supplies. This was often difficult in the absence of modern packaging, whose influence has been at least as great as refrigeration in the urban environment. Only since 1914 have the many subacute forms of enteric disorder been reduced so that stomach-trouble is an occasional misfortune worth noticing rather than a common occurrence. In the same area, attention should be drawn to improvements in dentistry. No longer did 'civilized' man, teeth made rotten by diet, have to suffer from unchewed food.

Extraordinary, luxurious vegetables and fruit which are taken for granted in every first world supermarket today had to wait, in general, for further technological improvements to make their everyday consumption possible. There was probably no one alive in 1914 who had eaten litchis, kiwi fruit, avocado, mangoes and kumquat. Certainly, no living European could have eaten all these fruits of the earth if the European had not been a great traveller.

These exotica had to wait for packaging, transport even faster than refrigerated steamers. Improvements to diet due to the import of tropical and semi-tropical products were limited to what could be called 'bulk staples'. Sugar was one-fifth the price it was in 1846, resulting in serious medical problems. Imported oils of various kinds were challenging butter in the United States and Europe, margarine having been widely introduced about 1880. Market penetration depended upon the political clout of the butter lobby. Sweden and Switzerland were notable opponents of margarine before 1914. In the United States, the Federal Government refused to buy it for the armed forces, and it was illegal, bootlegged in the state of Wisconsin before 1965. Today, three times as much vegetable margarine as butter is consumed in the United States, twice as much in Europe. Ice-cream, another largely fat product, was an important semi-luxury in 1914, reaching its peak about 1950; it is now in decline, for obvious reasons.

Meat became much cheaper in Europe in real terms by 1914, but consumption per head was still only one-third that of the United States, one-fifth that of New Zealand or Australia. Meat is today under the same sort of cloud as other fatty products. Fish was a considerable social cut below meat in 1914, even the most expensive fish being one-third the price of the most expensive meat. Today, fish is dearer, retail, than meat. Bread was white in most countries in 1914, having been almost wholemeal everywhere in 1846. Again, fashion has reverted to the former practice.[35]

Railways made possible rapid transport of perishables on land – broccoli from Cornwall to London, winter vegetables from California to the East Coast, fresh fish all over Europe. But between continents, the improvements between 1846 and 1914 were much less significant than the developments in the future. The combination of airfreight, deep-freezing and hygienic packaging would prove to be more dramatic in their effects after 1945, than the improvements after 1846. These would not have been possible without the transformation of the neo-European countries in the nineteenth century.

The great French historian, Alexis de Tocqueville, drew attention to the resemblance between the United States of America and the then wholly feudal Russia. His great work, the first reasoned book about American democracy, came out in 1835. Neither he, nor his readers, gave enough weight to the physical problems of Russia. These physical problems still dominate the country. Most people today believe that man controls the environment in which he lives. People who can be half-way around the world tomorrow in person, or see it all on simultaneous television, or eat food from anywhere, any place, any time, are impatient about physical geography. In Russia, facts about climate, geology, botany, are paramount. The environment represents a serious challenge to settlement. Russian response to this challenge cannot be ascribed to political or doctrinal lapses in the recent past. Russian leaders are changed, with normal, human frequency, according to power-ratings and operational effectiveness. The ecology remains, and changes, if it does at all, very slowly.

Russian answers to the challenges of climate are very different to the responses of Americans to the challenge of living in North America. It is essential to try to distinguish between cause and effect. European Russia extends from the Arctic to the Black Sea, in a north-south line and from the Urals westward as far as Muscovite power has been able to extend. The Russians are Eastern Slavs, and have been living in the Moscow area only since just before the Norman Conquest of England. The tribes settled in this now sacred heartland about the same time that Christianity was accepted in Kiev, in about AD 988.

The climatic zones are very important, because they break the rules of the rest of the world. In the extreme north, there is tundra, which can only support lichens and mosses. Upon these unpromising materials the reindeer are supported, and with the reindeer there are Lapps living an existence originally nomadic. The tundra gives way to the forest, irregularly, but a timber line is clearly visible from the air. The northern timber is almost exclusively spruce and pine; further south, and in the milder pockets, needle-leaved trees give way to mixed woodlands, broad leaves predominating in areas of better soil or climate. South of the forest, which is the largest wooded area in the world, lies the steppes, a sort of savannah. The steppes runs from Hungary to Mongolia, south of the Urals. It was the pathway for all the Eastern invaders, and the commercial route in the Middle Ages, before the Black Death, and the parade ground for the Mongol Golden Horde itself. The steppes also have a more agricultural function.

The largest proportion of the steppes are composed of Black Earth. The soil contains up to 15 per cent humus, the age-old product of decayed grass, bushes, scrub trees. In Russia, the Black Earth is in a layer up to 2 metres deep. Handled properly, the Black Earth of the Ukraine, as of Iowa, is one of the most valuable agricultural soils in the world. North of the Black Earth is the podzol of Russia proper. In the podzol grows the forest: mixed round Moscow, boreal or 'taiga' further north. This runs from between 45° and 50°N to the tundra at the Arctic Circle. The forest is a zone of sand and clay, in patches with no pattern. There are many bogs and marshes. Streams and rivers run slowly, without much fall, since no part of European Russia is more than 400 metres (1,313 feet) above the sea. Rivers start in swamps and lakes, and run mostly in a north–south direction. The main rivers in European Russia are the Volga and the Dnieper. Together with their many tributaries, they formed a network, with easy portages, for trade at an early date. Frozen far longer than rivers in North America, they were perhaps an even more convenient passage in winter.

The secondary fact of life in Russia was, is and will remain, the climate. Leningrad, formerly Petrograd, and once St Petersburg, lies on about 60°N, the same latitude at Stockholm or Bergen, the southernmost tip of Greenland, or the northern border of the Canadian provinces – Manitoba, Saskatchewan, Alberta and British Columbia. The far north of the Canadian provinces is more unsuitable for agriculture even than the area round Leningrad, and no Canadian would today think of growing grain in those latitudes.[36] The southern tip of Greenland, with its Atlantic climate, and Bergen, washed by the Gulf Stream, were sites for Viking farming which lasted in Greenland for nearly five hundred years, and has survived in Bergen. No one, in modern times, could grow wheat or rye economically in either location. Stockholm is more moderate in climate than Leningrad. Though the Baltic exercises an influence smaller than the Gulf Stream, Stockholm is warmer in winter, cooler in summer than Leningrad.

The peculiarity of the Russian climate is that lines of constant temperature, isotherms, lie not east and west as in the American landmass, but north and south. The winter gets colder the further away from the warm air of the Gulf Stream; this warms Western Europe, losing heat as it moves east, and is no longer much of a moderating influence by the longitude of Minsk, let alone Moscow. These are important and interesting considerations. From these derive the short Russian summer.

In the north, on the podzol, in the taiga, round Novgorod or Leningrad, the frost-free farming season is less than 120 days; round Moscow it is less than 150 days; in the Black Earth it is 180 days. In Sweden, round Stockholm, the season is longer than it is in the Ukraine; in Bergen or the Shetlands, it is longer again.

The winter breaks suddenly in Russia. The thick snow which has lain on the ground for up to 180 days melts. The ice in the rivers breaks up. There is a sudden flush, a sharp rise in temperature, and spring is soon over. For the peasant, spring and summer was and is a back-breaking period of toil. The short, hot, summer involved another risk, rainfall.

The warm westerly winds which encompass the earth bring much rain to the north-west of Russia, to the Baltic Provinces, and to the taiga around Leningrad. Inland, the rain falls at the wrong time of year. In Moscow, the precipitation, snow, sleet and rain, is about 550 mm (22 in) a year. This is a little less than London or San Francisco, but good crops are still possible. Unfortunately, July and August are the wettest months of the year, with 23 per cent of rain falling in those two months. A drought in May and June can prejudice both winter and spring grain crops. Too much rain in the next two months makes harvesting very difficult. But another structural problem remains. The rain in Russia falls mainly on the poorer soils. In Leningrad, precipitation is a quarter more than in Moscow. In the Black Earth region, it is often below 400 mm (16 in) per year, too little for a good crop of grain. This would not matter if there were any tradition of good husbandry.[37]

If there is too little rain in any one year to grow a decent grain crop, there is an answer. Since the Greeks were farming in the same area of Southern Russia more than 2,500 years ago, it is to fallow one year in two or three, and 'use' the 'saved' moisture to grow a good grain crop in the other year or years. This is especially apt in the Black Earth which is so high in humus that it retains moisture from one year to another. But there was never any tradition of good farming in Russia. Husbandry was unknown to any class. No one was interested. There were good historic reasons why this was so, and why it has affected the whole history of Russia, up to and including the present.

The Slavs were originally a pastoral people, and nomadic. They took over the area round Moscow about a thousand years ago, and had no means of cultivating the soil properly. If they had proper harness from China (see page 56) they certainly did not have a proper plough. The usual medieval Russian plough was a scratch-plough, without a mould-board, called a *sokha*. (This was in use on Tolstoy's lands as late as 1870.) In the Russian heartland, the usual crop was rye. When the productivity of Russian grain fell below a minimum of say, 3–1, the peasant broke in new land. The slash and burn technique – applied to the forest – yielded a decent series of crops for a short period, and the peasant passed on. This was fine, if the population did not increase too fast.

When measured, the Russian peasant birthrate in the nineteenth century was running at a rate of more than 5 per cent per annum. This meant, allowing for life patterns of a century ago, that one in ten of every adult couple was producing a child; one woman in five of childbearing age was either pregnant or suckling an infant. If the death-rate of under-fives was more than 50 per cent, population growth did not follow birth-rate; in the absence of disease then there was grave danger of starvation or famine or worse. Russia was saved from this fate by two forces.

One was low density of population. Using the boundaries of today, yet excluding land in what used to be Poland, Romania, Czechoslovakia, Finland, Estonia, Latvia, Lithuania and East Prussia, gives European Russia an area of Black Earth greater than the whole of France, at least 270,000 square miles, as big as the whole of Texas, and nearly twice the size of Iowa. This gives European Russia about 270,000 sq. miles of the best grain-growing soil in the world. This is quite separate to the podzol further north. Russians moved, always, south and east to the Black Earth, which was easier to cultivate, and produced a better return in a shorter period than any forest soil.[38]

There was a struggle which went on for several hundred years between the Russians and the Turkic pastoral nomads who occupied the Black Earth steppes. When the Russians won a battle or a campaign, they took over an area. When the Turks from the khanates of Kazan or Astrakhan won a battle or a campaign, they destroyed the Russian settlements and made the Russians prisoners and sold them into slavery. Further west, there was another solution to Russian progenitive capacity. For a thousand years, roaming bands of Cossacks and Tartars made the hinterland of the Black Sea a recruiting ground for fair-skinned slaves for sale in Constantinople or Cairo. It was the huge Russian birth-rate which made this possible. Russian slaves were a feature of Muslim life for 1,000 years. Slavery ultimately ended, the surplus remained. The problem of population growth would not be solved except in the most brutal modern fashion.[39]

Towns certainly never offered a solution. Peasants could not emigrate into towns, nor grow grain for urban consumption. Surplus grain was never worth growing. There was no growth of towns to encourage any kind of trade. Most European towns were established in the four centuries before 1600. In the same sort of timescale, three Russian efforts had been destroyed. Between 800 and 1200, there was a string of Viking settlements between the Baltic and the Black Sea, which followed the rivers, and formed a useful 'back door' to Constantinople. This was cut in the south when Asian nomads severed the route to Constantinople.

Before and after the Black Death, Novgorod had been a member of the Hanseatic League, and Western European merchants traded furs and metalwork in that town. Jealous, inward-looking Moscow destroyed first the trade, then the city itself. Finally, Ivan the Terrible sacked the city in 1570, killing, it is said, 60,000 people, and enslaving 10,000. If so, he was less terrible than the Black Death, the true cause of the earlier decline. In 1467, 1508 and 1533, more than 100,000 are said to have died of pestilence.

There was one final post-Renaissance effort at Russian urbanization. The Renaissance was not, of course, Russian, but Dutch and English adventurers set up trading posts on the river line from the Baltic to Moscow. This lasted from about 1540 till 1580, when the Russian government bowed to its own merchants who were jealous of Western success. After that, there were no towns in Russia other than military or government centres. Even in 1846, the urban population of this huge country of 65 million people did not exceed 6 per cent. By the beginning of World War I, the total population had increased to 170 million. Only 17 per cent were dwellers in towns and cities. Urban population had increased from about 4 million to less than 30 million. They would be hungry very often.

The Russian population increase of over 160 per cent between 1846 and 1914 was not matched by technological answers. Emigration was of minor importance. In 1783, the Russians had annexed the Crimea, and tamed the Tartars as well as the Cossacks. Three million are reckoned to have migrated into the Black Earth region before 1846; nearly 10 million between 1846 and 1914. In the same period, 4 million went to Southern (Black Earth) Siberia, and 2 million to the less favoured Central Asian steppes.[40] Only 4 million went to the New World.

After Emancipation in 1861, the peasants who moved were free serfs.

They were deliberately assisted by the government, and the Russians established new Europes in the same way that Western Europeans also unconsciously established neo-Europes.[41] The colonial expansion of Russia, which had begun in the time of Ivan the Terrible, the Tsar, in 1552, was initially of unfree serfs, attached to their migrant masters. Siberian immigration also included political exiles, entrepreneurs amongst the aristocracy, foreign concessionaires interested in mining or timber.

There were two reasons why the Russian peasant was a poor farmer. Both derived from the availability of ample land. Like the American, the Russian could always bring virgin land into cultivation. This was worth much more than trying to farm better at home. When the time came that all the virgin land had been cultivated within the technological abilities of the time, then trouble ensued. But that time would not come until the nineteenth century. Yet the influences which made the Russian serf such a rotten farmer were in place long before.

There was no winter occupation, and no outlet for surplus grain. So three consequences ensued. Much surplus grain was turned into vodka, and there was a serious peasant drink problem after every successful harvest. During the long, long winters when no work could be done, drinking became a relaxation, a solace. But it also made a grain shortage worse. The Russian weather made work possible for only half the year. The rest of the year had to be endured, in a very cold climate. Being huddled on top of a communal stove may have been one way to spend the winter. Vodka could have helped. Livestock enterprise was never, apparently, considered. The number of farm animals in relation to the population fell throughout the nineteenth century. Between 1867 and 1913, the number of horses, cows and pigs increased by 50 per cent, the people by more than 100 per cent. Sheep numbers actually fell, absolutely.

The second point is the communal nature of the peasants' work. When was this kind of communality established? It was long before any idea of socialism. It probably derived from the very earliest pioneer days under Ivan the Terrible. This organization of the extended family, so character-istic of historic Russia, probably descended from the primeval Slav tribal organization, of a group of about 50–100 related people. This broke down into the communal organization. In turn, the commune was the legal tenant in many settled places. This did not mean that the Tsarist *mir* bore any relation to the Soviet collective.[42]

Miserably low returns in Russian agriculture are nothing new. They are, today, between 30 and 40 per cent of what a Western farmer would get in the same conditions. They always were. When in 1846, a good English or Dutch farmer would get a yield per hectare of over one tonne, average Russian yields were 350 kg (772 lb). In Russia, in 1913, the average yield for wheat over the previous five years was 0.7 tonnes per hectare; this was twice the 1846 yield per hectare, but still only one-third of the English yield. No attempt was made to solve the problem. Russians walked away from the difficulties. They still do.[43]

Virgin land, as has been seen, was one answer. Another was to find other employment. Instead of sitting on the stove all winter, drinking vodka, one option was to trap furs. The forests were very rich in animals in early times, and Russians became great exporters of furs. Another winter possibility was to cut timber in the forest zone. The Baltic became the great source of timber for the West. Russia is still a great supplier. Another answer was mining. Russia, like India, became a country noted for precious jewels and metals, even if it was also very poor. Another choice was home manufacture on a village basis of craft products. These activities were communally carried out, requiring neither great brains nor much capital.

Russia was unique in the world in that she had no shortage of land or people. If neither the problem of productivity per hectare nor of productivity per man exists, how do you manage? By solving neither. In the absence of challenge and the profit-motive, can there be efficiency?

Before any competent practical farmer answers the question, it would be as well to remember that nineteenth-century Russia was the only country in the world in which this problem was posed. If they had been short of land, Russians would have learnt how to manage husbandry properly; if they had been short of humans, they would have learnt how to grow food with early attention to labour-saving devices. As it was, Russians neither learnt to be good farmers in the English sense, nor learnt to be efficient ranchers or monoculturists, like contemporary Americans. Any visitor, from almost anywhere, was appalled by what he saw.

A structural problem was the nature of the emancipation of the serfs in 1861. It had had left them so badly indebted that the debt tended to grow rather than be paid off. In 1907, forty-six years after emancipation, more than 85 per cent of the peasants were still in debt, most of them for a sum twice that of the original computation. In 1907, Stolypin abolished the debts of the ex-serfs. But in the ensuing six harvests of peace, grain yields per hectare did not decrease or increase significantly. Apologists have always deplored the Russian climate, with its uncertain rainfall. But hardly any irrigation or drainage was practised, even in areas close to rivers which would have obviously benefited. The introduction of new crops was an intellectual burden comparable to the labours of Sisyphus.[44]

Potatoes were introduced in 1833, and coincided with an outbreak of cholera. By 1913, potato production was still less than that of Germany, which had half the population. Sugar beet took twenty-five years to reach half a million hectares (over 1 million acres). In 1913, sugar production was less than that of France, with one-quarter the population. Maize was not really grown, however well suited to the Black Earth, till the four hundredth anniversary of Columbus's voyage in 1892. In 1913, Russian maize production had not reached that of Italy, whose population was less than one-quarter that of Russia.

In 1920, an expatriate Russian put the available grain per head in exporting countries in 1910–14 in the following terms: Canada 1,696 kg (3,740 lb), USA 1,151 kg (2,536 lb), Argentine 1,322 kg (2,915 lb), Romania 875 kg (1,929 lb), Russia 445 kg (980 lb). Contemporary importing countries had the following available: UK 680 kg (1,500 lb), Germany 497 kg (1,100 lb), France 480 kg (1,060 lb), Italy 442 kg (974 lb). Russia, with 445 kg (980 lb) available, exported 60–70 kg (132–154 lb) per head, leaving the Russian people with the lowest amount of grain per head in Europe – 381 kg (840 lb). This was one kg (2 lb) less of grain per head than available in Spain, a much warmer country.[45]

The Russian Revolutions of 1905 and 1917 were ascribed by contemporaries to political injustice, a marked distaste for the autocracy, and an overwhelming desire for liberty, equality and fraternity and so forth. Has enough been said to suggest that a much simpler cause existed? Faced with no imperative, in very early days, to farm efficiently by any yardstick anyone would today use, the Russian peasant, leaderless, was left to look after himself. When help was forthcoming, it took a political form. The commune gave way to the collective. Soviet dictators after 1917 bent all their efforts on improving the armed forces, industry and communications. The same has been true of subsequent Russian rulers.

In fact, did not population pressure, plus masses of virgin land, operate in such a way so as to stultify all the responses with which contemporaries in other countries were answering the challenge? In the United States, a relatively small population increased production and food supply per head to heights never before achieved. In the other neo-Europes, the same sort of pattern also emerged. New Zealand, Australia, Canada, South Africa, the Argentine, all became increasingly able to produce at such a low cost that they could export all over the world and leave their own populations far better fed than the same sort of people in Europe.

In Europe itself, production per hectare became of increasing importance as land rents rose. Even after they fell after the crucial year, 1879, the profitable way to farm was still to select a product which the farm or the farmer produced with efficiency, and then optimize output per unit area of land.

Russians never addressed themselves to these problems either in the form of government action, intellectual discussion, or university, college or even landlord tabletalk. As a result, Russians were often hungry. In some years, they were hungrier than anyone in Europe, Spain included, which suffered two real famines in the 1870s. There is no better recipe for revolution than insufficient food. It was, in all probability, the true cause of the French Revolution, idealistic talk notwithstanding. But the statistics do not exist to prove or disprove the thesis in relation to 1789.

In relation to both 1905 and 1917, the figures are available. Do they prove, beyond all reasonable doubt, that the reason for the revolutions was hunger? Population growth was pushing, not against the supply of land, which is not yet a limitation in Russia, but against the supply of capital, technique, applied intelligence, curiosity, the rules of good husbandry, and a real love of the land which is an essential ingredient in good farming.

These qualities are still absent in Russian agriculture. Every intelligent young person wishes to leave agriculture, and parents encourage children to abandon collective drudgery, and to become desk workers. Truth is never told, *glasnost* notwithstanding. Practices which any good Western farmer would call wrong, bad husbandry, even immoral, are common. There is no honest criterion for success; only reports to and from corrupt bureaucracy.

European Russia, allowing for the use of fertilizers, pest control, and machinery, produces less today than in the five years 1909–13. During that period, Russians were the worst fed in Europe. They still are. But for the secret police, there would have been several revolutions since 1917. There still might be. Well-wishers in 1913 waited for improvement. They still do.[46]

Far more devastated than Russia, with far fewer resources than any European state, without much indigenous fuel, or arable land in quantity, or animals or machinery to cultivate the soil, or merchant marine for essential imports, or much help from former enemies, and with a worse image than most defeated foes in history, the Japanese in 1945 would have been considered a candidate for long-term convalescence, not triumph. Nor could Japan have been anyone's contender for great wealth, greater wealth than every other country in the world within forty years. Nor would anyone have believed that in just over a generation Japan would produce 50 per cent of the world's ships, 25 per cent of its cars, 90 per cent of its videos, and 40 per cent of its integrated circuits.

Any study of Japan, instead of being directed at the aberration from the 1920s to the 1940s would have led wiser, more farsighted Westerners to perceive the possibility of a Japanese miracle. The omens were there. With the wisdom of hindsight, it is possible to explain how it happened.

The name Japan derives, via 'Cipangu', from an East Indian corruption of the Japanese word 'Nippon' or 'Nihon' which is what they call their own country. 'Cipangu' was what the Mediterranean world called Japan in 1492. It would be many years before any European reached even the main southernly island, Kyushu, and then trade and intercourse between various foreigners and the Japanese would only last for a century. It would not be until the late nineteenth century that the full extent of the Japanese islands was known to Europeans.

There are over 4,000 islands. The number is always increasing, since the geology of the archipelago is volcanic, and new islands appear from time to time. More land area is added because of the efforts of the Japanese themselves. They have reclaimed more land than all the Europeans put together – they have 'created' nearly half their coastline; the whole of the centre of modern Tokyo, for example, was reclaimed in the seventeenth century. Land is in permanent shortage in the Japanese psyche. There are nearly 143,000 square miles in the islands, which extend from the subarctic of Hokkaido, frozen for 150 days in the year, to the subtropical paradise of Okinawa. The stretch is as great as most of the mainland United States in a north–south direction, 20° latitude.

The oranges, sugar cane, pineapples and bananas of Okinawa have to be contrasted with Hokkaido in the far north, home, according to legend, of primeval, 'treeliving' *Ainu*. Hokkaido all lies south of the forty-sixth parallel, about the level of Lyons, France or Portland, Maine. Hokkaido, and the west coast of the main island, Honshu, have cold, wet winters. By contrast, the twenty-sixth parallel which runs just south of Okinawa, is far south of anything in Europe, on the same parallel as the Sargasso Sea, the Bahamas and much of Florida. Okinawa is cooler than the Bahamas in winter; the west coast is cooler than the east since the winter weather comes from the north-west from Siberia, with bitterly cold wet winds, full of snow. Tokyo Bay, in the middle of the archipelago and on the east coast, is more moderate from a January average of 5°C (40°F) to 25°C (78°F) in July. There is a current analogous to the Gulf Stream, from the south.

The seasons are much more regular than those in the British Isles, with which Japan tended to be compared a hundred years ago. There is an especial regularity about the renewal of spring. Cherries blossom in a regular pattern, the front advancing one degree of latitude in each couple of days, and taking forty days to travel from south to north. The climate is regular; the weather is not.

The Japanese islands are subject to the vagaries of two major seismic fault lines. The islands are volcanic in origin; the consequential effects are not only appearances of islands at intervals of about ten years, but there are forty still-active volcanoes. There are at least twenty minor earthquakes a year – 10 per cent of all those recorded in the whole world. This seismic activity also gives rise to avalanches, tidal waves, inland floods. The last great earthquake, far more destructive than that of San Francisco in 1906, was in 1923. The death toll was then over 100,000, and the loss of perhaps 70 per cent of the flats and houses in the Tokyo conurbation. It is said that there is a sixty-nine- or seventy-year cycle in the matter of these earthquakes. So the next is due in 1992 or 1993. Today, twenty-five times as many people live in the area as in 1923.

This figure illustrates Japan's problem. The population as a whole has only increased by about two-and-one half times since 1923. But they are crowded into flat land, of which there is a grave shortage. The density of population of the main island, Honshu, which has 75 per cent of the population, is slightly more than that of England, which has rather higher a percentage of the population of the UK. But, while there are 380 people per sq. mile in Honshu, and 360 in England, there is far less flat land per head in Honshu. There is, in fact, only about a fifth of the land fit to cultivate as arable or pasture, against more than three-quarters in England. So the density of the Japanese population becomes an obsession. Four-fifths of their country is fit only for forest, if that. The slopes of most of the extinct volcanoes, with Fuji-yama the most famous, are bare, sulphurous, sterile.

The *Lebensraum* problem of the Japanese is central to the history of the last five hundred years. So it is worth stating the problem another way. Each Englishman has a potential 0.28 hectares (0.68 acres) for all purposes; each inhabitant of Honshu 0.25 (0.63). But each Englishman has more than half-an-acre fit to carry building. Each inhabitant of Honshu has only one-sixteenth of an acre fit for buildings. Put in sq. metres, each Honshu-san has 300 sq. metres (250 sq. yards) for all building purposes; each Englishman more than nine times as much, 3,000 sq. metres (2,500 sq. yards). No wonder that real estate has entered the Japanese soul. Even 150 years ago, when they grew all their own food, each inhabitant of Honshu had only three times as much land as today, for all purposes. Or, in Japan as a whole, before the annexation of Formosa or Korea, in the original islands, there was only just about half-an-acre per head for all purposes except forest. That was to grow the essential rice, to produce the fruits, the vegetables, tea, silk, chicken and eggs, the oxen, the squat brown ponies, and everything else demanded by a pre-industrial country in 1860. It was thus that the Japanese had lived for four previous centuries.

Values for Japanese real estate have always been ridiculous. Today, the gross value of all the land in Japan, plus the infrastructure, is valued at twice that of the value of the whole landmass, on the same basis, as the forty-eight mainland United States. The continental United States, without Alaska or Hawaii, is more than twenty times the size of Japan. On a per capita basis, the land, buildings, infrastructure of Japan is valued at 35 times as much as Americans value the same assets in the 48 states. This is ridiculous. So is the fact that two tennis courts in the centre of Tokyo made five hundred million dollars, or four hundred thousand dollars per sq. metre, when sold for building purposes in 1987. People who regard London or Manhattan real estate as inflated should recognize that similar land and buildings in Tokyo cost at least one hundred times as much. If a million pounds or dollars outside the City of London or Wall Street will buy a respectably sized office or a very luxurious house or flat, the same kind of difference does not exist as between central Tokyo and the rest of the conurbation. Japanese real estate is even more expensive than that of Hong Kong or Singapore, whose island-states have, respectively, 5,000 and 4,000 people per sq. km against 3,800 per 'safe' sq. km in Honshu. Allowing for land unfit to build upon, Singapore and Hong Kong have more than double the density of population of Honshu. Yet land values in Honshu are about five times those of Singapore, three times those of Hong Kong. Not surprising since the Japanese, alone of all people, refuse to build except on flat land.

Five hundred years ago, probably no European had ever been to Japan.[47] It is true that Columbus's first voyage was known to be aiming for 'Cipangu', but Columbus never defined the products of this fabled country. Nor was the position of the islands very accurately charted. They were felt to be in the same latitude as the Bahamas. The distance was seriously underestimated. The earth was known to be a sphere, the longitude of, say, the Canary Islands known to be about one hour, 15°W of Barcelona; more elegantly, the nearest point of the Azores was also about 15°W, one hour from Lisbon. Yet Cipangu was placed in quite the wrong position and the earth thereby made smaller by nearly 40 per cent. This logic was never pursued, so that the longitude from Barcelona to the mouths of the Ganges, was known to be about 90° or six hours eastwards. But Cipangu was held to be only about five hours west. So what had happened to the rest of the twenty-four hours? According to this calculation, there were thirteen hours, 195° between the mouths of the Ganges and Japan. In fact, there is only about three hours, or 45°. One of the major causes of the 'loss' of nearly 10,000 miles or 195° at the latitude of Japan was the fatal dictum, widely believed five hundred years ago, that five-sixths of the world was terrestrial, only one-sixth water. In fact, of course, the surface of the earth is less than one-third land, more than two-thirds water. Even so, the extent of the knowledge and the ignorance of the position of the places to which Columbus was sailing remains one of the great mysteries of the year 1492. Whatever else happened, no one reached Japan in that year.[48]

The first categorically known European arrivals in Japan were three Portuguese passengers on a junk, travelling from Macao to Thailand, which was blown off course by some 1,500 miles and made landfall on Tangeshima Island, one of the string connecting Kyushu island with Okinawa. This was in 1542 or 1543. The Japanese were reported to be curious and hospitable. The Portuguese, eager to trade, gave them many Western artefacts. The Portuguese were most impressed by the quality of the Japanese steel swords – then, as now, the finest in the world – and exported in large numbers to China and Korea. The Japanese were more impressed by the Portuguese possession of the three personal firearms, crude arquebuses. These were characteristically copied within a month of the Portuguese arrival. Equally typically, the Portuguese weapons, having been stripped of their secrets and laid bare, were returned to their owners. The Portuguese trio, nameless pioneers, were followed by many more.

In the next few years, Portuguese merchants arrived in force. They traded between Japan and Goa, and between Japan, Macao, the Philippines and other East Indian islands. All would have been well except for the confusion between trade and dominion. The dominion sought by the Portuguese was not temporal, but the King of Portugal in 1547 deliberately encouraged Francis Xavier, the Jesuit friend of Loyola and fellow founder of the Society of Jesus. King John III had sent Xavier to Goa in 1542 as the 'Apostle of the Indies'. Xavier made thousands of converts in Goa, and went on to Malacca, the Banda Islands, Amboyna, the Moluccas and Ceylon. Concentrating in feudal societies upon converting rulers and nobles, Xavier found that this policy multiplied his effective work many times.[49] The feudal rulers' followers were converted by the native nobles without any further intervention by Xavier. Whether the simple peasants understood Christianity in the many separate languages of the Indies is another matter. Francis Xavier started his work in Japan in 1548. It was to lead directly to the success of modern Japan, which is not noted for its Christian ethic. Xavier's efforts would be almost wholly counterproductive.

Francis Xavier himself visited Kagoshima, Hirado, Kioto, the last a huge city, with 96,000 houses, according to a Portuguese estimate of the time, and thus bigger than Lisbon. Xavier stayed twenty-seven months in Japan, and during that time, he had made several hundred converts. He left in 1552 for Goa, and died on the voyage. He never attempted a mission in China.

No language is more difficult for Europeans to learn than Japanese, the construction of the language does not lend itself to alien philosophical concepts; nor was Xavier a good linguist. In fact, he was a very bad one. But the Portuguese traders linked quite clearly the possibility of trade with the degree of toleration shown by the Japanese to the Christian religion. The Japanese, who imported small foreign consumables to make their lives more pleasant, plus the oriental spices controlled by the Portuguese, plus occidental weapons, were usually willing to swallow their philosophic doubt and pride and accept Christianity as the price of trade. There was also at that date, and to the great detriment of Japanese national unity, massive and expensive feudal wars between various sections of the country.

Two examples of this process suffice. On the island of Amakusa, the chieftain became a Christian, and forcibly converted his followers. This was in 1555 or thereabouts. The chieftain quite clearly associated conversion with trade. But no Portuguese ship appeared, so the chieftain smartly converted himself and his followers back to Buddhism, and expelled the European Christian missionaries. In Nagasaki, then a little fishing village, a more positive development took place. In 1567, a church was built; Sumitada, the feudatory, encouraged the development of the port. In 1572, five years later, the inhabitants numbered 30,000 and there was an annual visit of at least half a dozen Portuguese ships. By the 1580s, most of the island of Kyushu had some kind of Christian presence, balanced by the annual visit of at least one Portuguese ship. In 1581, there were said to be over 125,000 converts in Kyushu, out of a Japanese total of 150,000. At this point, Christianity was not only confused with the positive virtues of trade with the Portuguese, but also with the negative virtues of not being Buddhist. Many of the Buddhist monasteries were hives of feudal industry; they were often defended camps, supporting local feudal lords against the centralizing influence of the great trio of Shogun overlords: Oda Nobunga, Toyotomi Hideyoshi, and Tokugawa Iyeyasu. Hideyoshi, in particular, used Christians as a counterweight to the Buddhists. He allowed a church to be built in Osaka, then the capital. A year later, he changed his mind. The pretext was that Christians ate useful animals like oxen and ponies then no part of the Japanese diet.

The reversal of Hideyoshi's mood was perhaps due to the intolerance of the Christians when they found themselves in a majority, as was the case in parts of Kyushu, where converts had been compulsorily turned to destroy Buddhist temples and other holy places. In 1587, the Christians were expelled. The next year, this order was rescinded. The Portuguese once more made clear that without a tolerance of Christianity, there could be no foreign trade. The Japanese judged the foreign trade too important to be able to dispense with Christianity.

This tolerance lasted for ten years, and was broken by rivalry between

Spain and Portugal. Though the Iberian countries were united in the joint crown from 1580 to 1640, there had been a demarcation agreement between the two countries, and a Papal bull which gave Portugal a monopoly of trade with Japan. The Spanish Dominicans and Franciscans in Manila, having largely converted the (not very many) natives of the Philippines at the point of the sword, sought fresh fields to conquer, and landed in Japan in 1593.[50] There was also the singular incident of the *San Felipe*, a galleon, loaded with wealth from the Spanish Indies, on track for Acapulco in Mexico, blown off course by a hurricane, landed in Tosa. Shown all the wealth onboard, worth $50 million in today's money, and a map of the Spanish and Portuguese kings' dominions in the world, after 1580 most of the earth, the pilot of the ship told the Japanese: 'Our kings begins by sending into the countries he wishes to conquer, missionaries who induce the people to embrace our religion, and when they have made considerable progress, troops are sent who combine with the new Christians, and then our kings have not much trouble in accomplishing the rest.'[51]

On learning of this speech, Hideyoshi reacted with fury; the Franciscans were to be mutilated alive, then crucified, at Nagasaki, the Christian epicentre in Japan. One hundred and thirty-seven churches were demolished in Kyushu, the Jesuits were to be sent back to Goa. The Japanese penalties of the period were merciful. Only the lobe of one ear was cut off, and crucifixion consisted of tying the victim to a cross, and driving a spear through the heart. Death was instantaneous, as with the Christian Samurai who were deemed to have to commit suicide. Hideyoshi died the following year. Though his policy was initially reversed, his successor, Tokugawa Iyeyasu, ultimately arrived at the same philosophic position.

Japanese statesmen were wedded to toleration; they also believed in a national consensus. Both aims were challenged in feudal Japan. Philosophy was confused with party interest; consensus was sacrificed to the internecine feudal warfare. The foreigners brought in more dissent. Spanish friars quarrelled with the Portuguese dependent Jesuits; Portuguese traders fought with the Spanish who followed the priests from Manila. Spanish government emissaries demanded the expulsion of the Dutch (arrived in 1602) and the Dutch, though they traded without the imposition of missionary Christianity, sought to fight the English, who arrived in 1613. The Japanese sought to separate the European enemies by allocating a different port to each nationality. But there was also the problem of the Japanese Christian converts. These took up positions in the feudal battles then going on in Japan, ultimately in the nearly successful Shimabarra rebellion in 1638. The Spanish had been expelled in 1624, the Portuguese in 1638, because the latter were thought to be conspiring with the rebels. These were not the first anti–European edicts, just the most effective. Between 1600 and 1640, there were many anti-Christian incidents encouraged often by one faction or another. There was also the question of firearms. Perhaps, in the end, gunpowder was more important than alien religion.

Japan in the seventeenth century was far ahead, in iron and steel technique. Japanese pig-iron, smelted by cottage-industry methods, was far cheaper than European. Japanese steel was acknowledged to be the best in the world. Japanese swords had a unique quality. The blades were so formed, beaten and hammered for weeks on end to have a characteristic which few sword-makers have ever been able to achieve since. The blade can sheer a fairly thick nail, without damage to the sword. One sweep of the samurai's two-handed sword, correctly used, can remove a man's head, clean, at one blow. A sixteenth-century Japanese sword can cut through any sword made in Europe of that or any other date. A supremely difficult art had been mastered, of making the edge of the blade a series of thin laminates, each forged until the edge was sharper than anything made anywhere in the world, as sharp as a modern razor blade. But the body of the sword, in order to avoid being brittle, had to be soft, to avoid shattering. The edge was high-tensile and unbelievably sharp, and the body low-tempered so that it might accept shock without damage. The Japanese sword of quality was far superior to the best Damascene products of the Muslim world, until then the swords which Western nations most admired.[52]

The sword also had a personality, a life of its own. A great sword was passed down from one feudal warlord to another, from one swordsman to another, from one soldier to another. It was no disadvantage that the sword had been used by a samurai to commit suicide. The sword was not buried with the corpse, as in some Western funerals. The sword went on and on. Indeed, since a great sword might take several years of a great steelmaster's life to make, it was just as well. In all probability, steelmasters were less common than samurai.[53]

There was a ritual about fighting with swords. It was icily polite, had important gracious preliminaries to bloodshed, sincerely courteous in its formality. No such ritual could exist with large numbers of men drawn up with muskets or arquebuses. In this case they just fired the guns.[54] And then there was the class problem. Gunpowder had destroyed the validity of the feudal European castle, and then brought to an end the host of mercenary soldiers who rampaged through late medieval Europe. Anyone could shoot with a gun; only a nobleman could use a sword. The knight was no longer a match for an infantryman. Technology democratized warfare. No one would express such a sentiment until the 1800s; but it was true. These fears were mouthed by Japanese noblemen, as well as by Frenchmen after poor yeoman archers at Agincourt had unhorsed the flower of chivalry, even if they did not speak in class-conscious terminology. So the gun threatened the Japanese way of life. The gun could only be banned from Japan if the foreigners were also banned. Perhaps too much has been made of the disruptive nature of Western Christianity in the Japanese reaction to Europeans. Perhaps the vile nature of the gun was more important. Perhaps there was a third reason.

The extraordinary and very advanced nature of Japanese society in the time of first European contact was not properly recognized, then or now. This was a highly educated people, with a far greater degree of literacy than in any European country, higher, even, than in Florence, in 1598.[55] Tokyo, a city of half a million in 1610, built largely on reclaimed land, had an aqueduct opened in that year which brought pure water to a city centre for the first time since the Romans in the first century in the Mediterranean. The nature of Japanese diet was not understood by the carnivorous Europeans, and before 1870, the Japanese did not eat meat, nor kill domestic animals for flesh.[56] Their consumption of fish, then as now, was at least ten times the European level; perhaps this helped with the intelligence of the race as a whole.

Above all, Japan in 1600 had a very large population. Its 22 million people compared with about 10 million Iberians (then under one Crown), about 16 million Frenchmen, and just over half as many Germans or Italians. The great trading people, the Dutch, numbered only 1.5 million, and the English a mere 4 million. The Japanese were in 1600, as in 1900 or in 1990, the best educated in the world. No Japanese knew of these facts or figures, but they knew that there were 22 million of their own countrymen long before any European country had done an accurate census. The Japanese also knew of the size and power of their two neighbours.

China was immense, disorganized, self-contained, with a great reluctance, since 1521, to engage in any kind of foreign intercourse. The only material in which there was a serious deficiency was copper, and this the Japanese supplied. The Koreans, with whom the Japanese had conducted a war in 1592, successful until the Chinese intervened, as in 1950,[57] had a much smaller population than Japan, probably known to them as about one-sixth of the Japanese. Neither China nor Korea represented a threat. Even without gunfire, the Japanese argued, they were inviolate. Japan was too difficult a country to invade, too tricky to move in, almost impossible to occupy. The warlike temper of her people made a foreign adventurer an unlikely arrival. The Japanese too, had a great sense of superiority, equal to their sense of harmony, the importance given, then as now, to consensus.

This contradiction arose because of the peculiar circumstance of the Japanese triumph over adversity.

What had a hundred years of foreign intercourse produced? A new philosophy, or religion, Christianity, which preached an alien and sub-versive creed, that the loyalty offered to God was greater, far more important than loyalty to one's feudal master. This directly threatened the status quo. Christianity should be banned. It was. The Europeans had also brought in various vegetables, some of which proved useful or beautiful. Tobacco was banned, as were other drugs, such as opium. But legumes of various sorts were welcomed by thrifty Japanese gardeners and farmers. New sorts of rice may have also been introduced in that century, and maize for use in the drylands, and different millets, or sorghums, and barley, and capsicums, or sweet peppers from South America via Manila, and some of the other Columbian plants, such as yams and sweet potatoes, which failed to challenge the native giant radish. The white potato did not appeal either. It is possible that pyrethrum reached Japan from the Arab world in the same time, but not derris root. The Japanese gained a great deal from the hundred years intercourse with Europeans, including a belief that they were better off isolated. It was this conviction which saved the Japanese from any kind of sub-European colonial status, such as that which every other country in the world (Thailand excepted) has suffered.

Since 1950 the yen has appreciated by nearly eleven times against the pound sterling and by nearly three times against the United States dollar. Yet in none of the years since 1950 has Japan had a trading surplus of more than 1 per cent of gross domestic product. In seven years, there has been a deficit, supported by the United States. In most years, there has been a surplus of about 0.55 per cent of GDP. The economic virtues of Japan are less obvious than the consumerism of others. Against the Swiss franc, for example, the yen has maintained a parity limited to a movement of about 5 per cent. At the moment of writing, it is within 1 per cent of its 1950 rate. This may merely mean that the Swiss and Japanese economies are success-ful, those of the United States and the United Kingdom, less successful.[58] Even the currency of the most successful EEC economy, that of West Germany, has declined by over 20 per cent against the yen since 1950. Against almost every other currency, the Deutschmark has appreciated. For the West Germans, this has been a challenge. Possessing the hardest currency in the Common Market, they have had to export their hardware with the handicap of an automatic and rising Deutschmark in relation to the devaluation or depreciation of the currency of their competitors and customers. This the Germans have succeeded in doing; but the Germans have only been 80 per cent as successful as the Japanese, who now export more cars than the next three exporters combined. In the 1960s, it started with ships. Today, the Japanese cannot compete with the South Koreans in either shipbuilding or steelmaking. By the time that Korea, or Taiwan, or Brazil is able to undercut Japanese cars, other products will have been invented which other people will take a long while to copy or surpass. For this nation of one-time 'imitators' now originates a great many products.[59]

This was a people nurtured in an earthquake zone; yet they prospered. There were so many people living in paper houses that tobacco had to be banned, not on health grounds, but because of the fire danger. This was a people of 22 million, with a density of settlement unknown in Europe. Today, the Japanese have people/flat land ratio eight times as dense as the English. In 1660, the same ratio was four times as unfavourable. Today, flat land has to include buildings, roads, factories, railways, airports and so forth. In 1600, flat land had to produce enough food to keep five times as many Japanese as there were Englishmen. To do this, there was only one-quarter as much land as in England, per head of population. (Hokkaido, with more than one-fifth of the land area, was not occupied until the nineteenth century.) Japan, more so even than China, had a marvellously developed pre-industrial economy, with perhaps the most efficient agriculture in the then world. No one, of course, knew the facts. England, in the seventeenth century the best fed in Europe, had four times the land per head of the Japanese; Japan was the best fed country in Asia. She still is. The extraordinarily efficient agriculture of Japan made possible the splendid isolation of the two centuries from 1640 until the white man came again. In turn, the splendid isolation made continuous and essential the efficient agriculture. The magnificence of the Edo period which lasted until the Meiji restoration in 1868 depended, in the end, on sufficient food, upon an end to feudal warfare, upon an absence of foreign intercourse, and upon consensus being allowed to play its part. This period of isolation was an essential precursor to the extraordinary story of modern Japan.[60]

Notes

1 Review of *Seeds of Change* in Smithsonian Magazine, 1986.
2 It should not be forgotten that the United States, acknowledged by the world in 1783, was followed into nationhood by Iberian America within forty years. This time, the British encouraged those who believed in Independence.
3 This was almost a deliberate policy, that overseers and managers should be half-breeds. There was a feeling that they could act as intermediaries between the black slaves (or Amerindians) and the white owners.
4 Many consider the potato arrived indirectly from Spain, but the plant was important in Ireland by 1620.

5   There was a very early comparison with the climatic difficulties for European manual labour in Virginia compared with the same sort of work on the same sort of farms in New England. In fact, summer temperatures are often very similar. The slave trade to Virginia can be seen as a cultural matter. It was a very different problem when cotton came along in the nineteenth century, in an important way.

6   George Vancouver was a Royal Navy officer who accompanied Captain James Cook on the second and third voyages, from 1772–80. After the Treaty of Versailles of 1783, which gave the United States true independence, Vancouver was sent as commander of an expedition to the north-west coast of America, north of the Spanish settlements in California, and south of the Russian settlements in Alaska. The impulse was as much anti-Spanish and anti-Russian as anti-American. *A Voyage of Discovery to the North Pacific and Round the World in 1790–95*, London, 1798.

7   This perception was of great importance in building Puritan morale.

8   'The Indians', wrote William Bradford, of Plymouth, 'fell down so generally of this disease as they were in the end not able to help one another, no, not to make a fire, nor fetch a little water to drink, nor any to bury the dead.' *Of Plymouth Plantations*, ed. S. E. Morison, New York, 1952.

9   There was an interesting selection process at work. Settled Indians were hit harder than hunter-gatherers. Did smallpox over, say, two centuries, induce Indians to cease being settled, as did the horse? By extension, have diseases, deep in history, inhibited or retarded early settlement of land, the establishment of agriculture? Have diseases dependent upon density been responsible for mankind's rather short period as a farmer? Ten thousand years of farming, a generous figure, is a short period compared to half-a-million years of *homo sapiens* with most of the time spent in small groups, and less susceptible to disease.

10   The Common Law is shared with every English neo-Europe, except South Africa, which has its own complicated system. The ex-colonies, starting with the United States, have produced judicial decisions which have then become part of the laws of England. Seven once-Spanish Western states in the USA also have specific, non-English laws, such as communal property.

11   The chief long-term permanent effect of the now-forgotten Swedish colony was to make fashionable throughout the American colonies, Nordic construction for houses, now known as log-cabins, unknown in England. 'Clapboard' was the English timber method of the time.

12   The 'fall line' was the point on rivers on the Eastern Seaboard where ships met the first serious waterfall or set of rapids. This was further inland on the Hudson than on the Connecticut River, but the fall line existed on every river as far south as South Carolina. The extent of navigation possible below the fall line often dictated the rapidity of development of the colony; the Chesapeake Bay area was outstandingly well placed.

13   This problem of 'poor' land, impoverished by settlers, in fact, was an issue within a generation of arrival in every colony, especially where the exhausting crop tobacco was grown.

14   Average size of ship, as measured in those days, under 100 tons. This was smaller than all but the smallest individual ship crossing the Atlantic other than Spanish, whose minimum in 1587, was raised to 300 tons. It was not a question of safety so much as the relationship between crew and cargo which was much more favourable in large ships than small. But English and American sailors were free men, did not favour over-manning, and were often largely employed on 'shares' like ancient and modern fishermen. Small ships also gained favour after 1650, because developments in guns made the small ship much closer to the large in a fair fight.

15   The great Mississippi valley offered a southbound waterway from a few miles eastwards of the Appalachians in Western Pennsylvania and Virginia, and the Great Lakes were connected to the Hudson by the Erie Canal in 1825. A network followed, connecting Lake Erie with the Ohio and Wabash rivers, Lake Michigan at Chicago with the Illinois River at La Salle, and two others which crossed the Appalachians. These were mostly in place before the slump years 1837–44. The Chicago–La Salle canal was not finished until 1845, and was exceptional in carrying sewage, and in falling from Lake Michigan to the Mississippi River. Most of the canals were state funded. Eight Western and Southern states defaulted by 1840, thus confirming the view that risk was best taken by private investors.

16   Chicago was made by the railroads. Before 1830, it took three weeks to reach New York; in 1860, two days; in 1890, one day; in 1910, 16 hours. Before 1840, wagons would stream across the surrounding plain to deliver grain for the waterborne trade at Chicago. By 1870, there were 12 railroads meeting at Chicago, by 1900, more than 20, after which date there was some amalgamation and rationalization. The population has followed the railroad into the great city: in 1830, less than 100 people; in 1840, 4,479, after which the city grew at 8.6 per cent compound per year until 1900, when its population was over 1.6 million. The great fire of 1871 caused hardly a dent in this material progress, which was celebrated at the World's Columbian Exposition in 1892–3.

17   The rate of growth of the white American population before 1846 reached annual increases of 3 per cent – not so many died in childhood as in Europe. Black slave increases were sometimes at a higher rate. Both impressed Malthus with the extraordinary reproductive capacity of human beings in a favourable situation. Ireland, of course, proved Malthus's gloomy predictions right, not America, but the Irish surplus turned up in America in any case. Or the more fortunate did.

18   No one should be impressed by the anachronistic sentiments which are current about the early white settlers in Australia, mostly convicts. They were extremely lucky, most of them, as many realized when they looked back, in prosperous old age, at their progress since being reprieved from the gallows. To claim, as some have done, that they should not have been transported, is to use today's attitudes to criticize actions two hundred years old.

19   In the Finnish famine of 1697, 35 per cent of the population died. In the most recent famine, that of 1867, 8 per cent still died, but huge numbers went to the United States.

20   Average for Iowa in 1900–5.

21   Clarence Darrow, the great liberal lawyer, after the Pullman strike, 1894.

22   The critical problem is not frost, but snow. Frosted land can be ploughed; to plough snow into the ground is very difficult, and creates trouble for future cultivation.

23   The gold-equivalent cost today would be $12.50 which would buy a good deal of simple food, steak, potatoes, bread, vegetables, coffee, eggs, bacon, cornflour.

24   Australia was at times a great source of supply of horses, often as army 'remounts' exported to British possessions in the East, in South Africa, even to Egypt. There were great stories about Australians and horses, cf. *Breaker Moran*, 1902.

25   American wagons, unlike those in Europe, carried grain in bulk, not sacks, from at least as early as 1840, during the canal era, and before railroads were widely spread. These wagons were 'tippers' long before those in Europe. All this to save labour.

26   Yield tended to fall, on average, after the first few seasons.

27   One searcher after artefacts found a hundred-year-old plough, in a creek, near Waterloo, Iowa, in 1976, just in time for the Bi-centennial.

28   The continuous cheapening of the 'factory' chicken has proved to be both virtuous and vicious. Ostensibly, poultry meat is now available for far less, in real terms, than in 1910. But the means to this end are unpleasant for the birds and the process offensive to many consumers. Dietary value is also suspect.

29   Mendel never affected plant breeders or geneticists consciously until the years around World War I, and Mendel was not wholly accepted until 1930 at the earliest. There was a contemporary saying that a cross between black and white would produce: one white, one black, and two khaki. This was the extent of understanding of Mendel in about 1910. It was on a par with Disraeli who, when asked in the 1870s, with reference to Darwin, whether he thought mankind was descended from apes or angels, replied, 'On the whole, I am on the side of the angels.' This saying has since been misunderstood.

30   Successful farmers ceased to be primary producers and became converters of (often imported) feeding stuffs, tailoring the product – milk, eggs, meat – to the demands of the market. Business acumen became more important than husbandry, even more important than technical skills. Survivors amongst farmers became people who could survive at any job.

31   Chemical expertise in Germany was essential to their expansion before 1914, and their wartime efforts afterwards. This was in every area of life, as well as farming, but agriculture benefited, then, as now. Western Germany is now home to three of the world's largest agrichemical companies.

32   See *The Great Wine Blight*, George Ordish, Sidgwick and Jackson, London, 1987.

33   To *empolder* land, the first step is to surround the area with high, raised 'quays' of soil, to keep out the external water, and to control that within. The next stage is to pump out the water within the polder. This may take two years by windmill, and is a continuous process, since the new polder must needs be drained for all time. Water-pumping by windmill became cost-effective about 1560, and after about 1850, steam was substituted. Much of the Netherlands is now below sea-level, and is provided with drainage pumps which need 12 hp (now electrical) for every 1,000 hectares (2,471 acres) which is 1 metre (3 feet) below sea-level. In most of the Zuider Zee, empoldered in this century, this means about 1 hp per 100 hectares (247 acres). The drainage channels, which are higher than the new polder, are used as navigation and irrigation canals. The reclaimed soil may take 10 years to become fully desalinated.

34   Mussolini's Fascist regime was not a great economic success, leaving aside the incompetence and cruelty associated with bully-boys and castor oil. He was praised in some Conservative circles in the 1920s and 1930s because 'he made the trains run on time'. Despite this, and cleaning up the drains of Venice, and removing malaria from the Pontine Marshes and some of the Po Valley, there was nothing consistent or competent about Fascist 'planning'. The weakness of Fascism was the same as that of Nazism or Communism. No economy can operate efficiently in a climate which does not permit plural political or economic opinion, i.e. choice. In the end, this is what has saved democracy throughout the world. Current examples (1988) may include Russia, Poland, Burma.

35 Since Roman times, white bread has been a status symbol. Until 1870, modern white bread was impossible to make. White bread flour needs steel-rollers, which are easy to adjust and maintain, and use one-fifth the power of stone rollers. Steel-ground flour is far easier to sieve, since the particle-size is far more uniform. Steel-rollers, which came from Austria–Hungary, about that Empire's only contribution to technology, and fine sieves had, by 1890, rendered the bread of the poor little more than energy, of little greater value than white sugar.

White bread of a hundred years ago contained no vitamin A or D and little vitamin B_1. Iron and Niacin (vitamin B_4) were nearly halved by the exclusion of the fibrous portion of the flour. The lack of fibre, plus the low level of value in the white bread, led to malnutrition amongst the poor, who might eat little else, in London, in 1890–1900, besides tea, margarine, and condensed milk. At that date, none of these products were fortified by vitamins. (See *The Englishman's Food*, London, 1957.)

Army officers were horrified by the low physical state of recruits during the South African War of 1899–1902. Compared to soldiers from the neo-Europes, the British had 5 cm (2 in) less height; thinner bones, less muscle, and far less chest expansion; their teeth were also of low quality. This military horror seeped through into the national consciousness and conscience; but it would be forty years before action was taken to protect the poor by the reinforcement of bread and margarine, by raising the extraction rate of flour to 85 per cent, by encouraging consumption of fresh vegetables and milk and by increasing the awareness of food values. During 1940–53, food became a weapon of the Welfare State fairly distributed to all, largely rationed. After the War itself, 'Fair Shares' became a social and political policy, which proved to breed unwanted and uncovenanted side-effects.

36 A great deal of grain is grown in Sweden, even north of Stockholm, and small quantities in Iceland and Eastern Siberia, for strategic reasons.

37 Any serious student should consult an atlas with good climatic charts.

38 Ratio of people/soil remains considerably more favourable than the same ratio in the United States, less favourable than in Canada.

39 The fierce Russian reaction to Muslim nomads from the days of Ivan the Terrible (d. 1584) was supported by peasants and nobles alike; presumably this was a folk-memory of the slaving sweeps from the south and east. The capture and sale of Christian boys to become the Mamelukes of Egypt did not stop until 1798, but this largely affected the hinterland of the Crimea.

40 It is worth noting, perhaps, that the plague still raged in Central Asia. Russian railways were built to avoid ancient cities and plague itself.

41 Russian peasants moving south and east took with them their own micro-organisms. These diseases acted like white man's diseases in the Americas, and the biological experience of the natives in the new settlements in Siberia were similar to that of the Amerindian.

42 'The *mir* was not a collective; farming in it was carried out privately, by households.' *Russia under the Old Regime*, Richard Pipes, London 1974.

43 A primitive man, achieving a small increase of seed garnered over seed sown, and in 1900, this might be only of the order of 6 or 7/1 against an increase in England of 20/1, might well decide to try a different piece of land, or a different farm. In the absence of soil analysis, cultural expertise, fertilizers, proper implements, what better alternative was there? Today, the Soviet Union ought to have solved the problem.

44 Sisyphus, father of Odysseus, cheated death for a time, was punished by being forced to roll a stone up a hill; each time the stone nears the top, it rolls down again. This was considered a just punishment for a crafty, deceitful politician, which Sisyphus was. The labours of Sisyphus are commonly experienced in the development of ideas before their time, or if beyond the audience, or in any good idea badly managed.

45 Professor Nordman: *Peace Problems*, London 1920.

46 Statistic used derived from *European Historical Statistics, 1750–1970*, B. R. Mitchell, London 1975. Caution should be exercised in this area. There are Stalinized statistics still at large.

47 Trade had been carried on by Japan, Korea and China, from about AD 700, and Chinese navigators knew of the extent of the Japanese political empire. Some of this information may have reached Europe upon Marco Polo's return to Venice in 1295. For the next two hundred years, scanty information about Japan was blown up into mythological wonderland territory.

48 It also remains a mystery as to how long Columbus went on thinking that those few islands in the Caribbean which he *did* discover in 1492–3 were part of Asia.

49 Jesuits then, and ever since, have found it economical of manpower to convert Top People, and let example, authority or fashion operate upon Top People's followers.

50 The pre-Spanish population of the Philippines was of the order of half-a-million, against today's 50 million. The total land area is almost exactly the same as that of the whole of the British Isles. The native Filipinos were ignored by their neighbours until in 1570 they found themselves the bone of contention between Spanish from Mexico and Muslim *Moros* from Borneo. The Spanish won, without a great deal of difficulty.

It was no accident that the Philippines were colonized from Mexico. They thus became the most westward of the Spanish Dominions, though they should, under the Treaty of Saragossa, 1529, have been the most eastward of the Portuguese. The Spanish, of course, cheated, and to make their deceit legitimate, they continued to approach the Philippines from Acapulco.

This had two results. The first was that the Philippines became the Asian port of entry for all American cultivars: tobacco, cocoa, pineapple, capsicum, tomatoes, maize, the potato, and so forth. Maize reached China before it reached India; tobacco reached Japan before it reached Persia; capsicum reached Hungary from the Philippines and became paprika. Secondly, antagonism between Spanish and Portuguese Far Eastern traders informed their behaviour in Japan, even after the nominal unity between Portugal and Spain, under the Spanish Crown from 1580–1640. The Japanese always distinguished between the two nations as far as traders were concerned.

51 Translated by Captain Frank Brinkley, RN, *The Times* correspondent in Japan, and historian, 1906.

52 Connoisseurs of Sir Walter Scott will not forget the Muslim sword, given by Saladin to Richard the Lionheart which would cleave a cushion, a feat impossible for any Western sword. Japanese swords were even better, able to cleave the traditional human hair. *The Talisman*, Sir Walter Scott, 1825.

53 There were from 5–7 per cent of noble samurai and their families in the population. It is difficult to believe that there were more than half of one per cent of skilled swordmakers.

54 There was, of course, the fabled meeting of the French and English Royal Guards at the battle of Fontenoy in 1745. The two lines met, face to face, and an English officer ran forward and asked the French to fire first. The French refused, whereupon the English fired, and nearly 1,000 French Guards officers and men fell at the volley. Such niceties of conduct were uncommon in Europe, nor did this case help the English, who, with their German and Dutch allies, lost the battle.

55 In 1980, 99 per cent of Japanese were 'functionally literate' against 80 per cent of Americans, and this with a much more difficult language than English. Japanese IQ is the highest in the world, 7 points above that of Japan in 1938, and 10 points above the US or Western Europe. Two per cent of Western Europeans' and Americans' IQs are above 130, 10 per cent of Japanese. Yet Japan spends a lower proportion of GNP on teaching than any other advanced country. Classes of 70 are common; but there are no drop-outs, no streaming, no underachievers. There is a national consensus that education is an absolute necessity for nation and individual alike, not a battleground, nor a privilege, nor a pressure-group. Nor is there much abstract love of knowledge. The whole Japanese success in the last forty years is due to the relationship of the intelligence of the nation to conceptual skills. It is a function of attitude, not money.

56 Buddhist attitudes to fish and game are not the same as feelings for other animals, otherwise Japanese intelligence would not be as high as it is.

57 Chinese intervention in 1950 prevented the United Nations defeating the Communist North Koreans, after the latter had invaded the South.

58 This is a comparative term. Constructing a 'basket' of the world's 10 least successful economies reveals that such an index against the yen has declined by over 300 times since 1950. Burma, which is poorer than it was in 1922, has declined in relative prosperity since the Greater Asian Co-Prosperity Sphere came to an end in Japan's defeat in 1945, by 1,000 times, compared to Japan forty years on.

59 Watchman, Walkman, RAM, world's newest rail system, magnetic levitation, low-temperature physics, compact CDs, etc.

60 The magnificence of the Edo period, of almost complete isolation, was made plain to the West in *The Great Japan Exhibition*, London, 1981–2. What was not obvious was that the unique nature of the civilization was due to the response of the Japanese to the Forces of Change. No other people responded in exactly the same way to its own space challenge.

CHAPTER FIVE

Malthus Defeated?

In the last century, world population has multiplied by four times. In other words, it has doubled twice. This simple arithmetical truth is a causative factor stronger than any other action of mankind. Procreation has become more important than politics; increases than economics; population pressure than popular belief.

The taming of disease has been a prime reason for this increase. Perinatal mortality at one end is matched throughout childhood and adolescence, while at the other, lives are extended far beyond their natural span. This may prove to be admirable in rich countries able to feed themselves, or to buy food from others. Not so happy for the poor.

Yet food supply has advanced in this century to meet and match population increases in Western Europe and in the neo-Europes. Shortages of food are limited to second and third world countries. Inappropriate management policies are the main problem. In Soviet Eastern Europe, a 25 per cent increase in fertilizer usage between the 1970s and 1980s only produced 2 per cent more grain. In North America, 11 per cent more fertilizer produced 23 per cent more grain. In Africa, state control does even less well. In some countries, not only in Africa, 'planning' has been directly responsible for starvation.

Poor countries do not have the money or distribution systems to use first world surpluses properly. Technology transfer may be the best policy. In some countries, peasants have even forgotten how to use basic manual tools, bemused as they are by pretentious agricultural policies propagated by ill-educated urban civil servants. In other countries, the Green Revolution – sensibly organized – meets human need without difficulty. In India, and Mexico, and China, and Indonesia, productivity increases have been important. The world as a whole has every reason to believe itself capable of feeding its people – at a price.

The price is that no demographer can seriously see a future in which the world population stabilizes at less than double today's number. With natural control measures defeated, the world stares at several 'options' – war, new sorts of incurable disease, famine on a wide scale, or the world drowning in its own ordure, wrecking the fragile ecosystem of One Earth. The only alternative is to work for some improvement in every process to prevent the kind of breakdown which will otherwise assuredly happen before populations level off.

In the second half of this century, the rate of change in every kind of human activity has speeded up and continues to do so. In some areas, the acceleration has become a mental health problem. In others, the process threatens the environment. In yet others, the whole moral base of human life, the sacred nature of creation, is jeopardized. We live in an age when anything appears to be possible. Anything goes, as the song says.

These truths are self-evident, however much they may baffle priests, elude the philosophers, and render anxious ordinary men and women. What is not obviously clear is the cause of these changes. It is the purpose of this chapter to examine the driving forces in our own times. Not surprisingly, these turn out to be the same three which have formed a triangle throughout history. Population growth is the engine of change. Population growth in turn is much modified by disease and food supplies.

In this century, world population is poised to double nearly twice. The 1900 figure was 1,625 million. The first doubling occurred at some time in 1964. The second doubling will probably take place before 2005. The first doubling in the twentieth century took sixty-four years: the second will take, perhaps, forty-one years; logically, the third doubling should take place in about 2033. This is logical, but unlikely. The one certitude about population projections is that they are nearly always wrong.[1]

This is both a comfort and a cause for anxiety. The comfort is that such uncertainties create jobs for many professional people: actuaries, economists, demographers. The cause for anxiety is that what they have to say in terms of the future is often worthless. There is one absolute certainty. That is that population growth is a profound cause of our present condition. Things would be very different but for sustained population growth. Without the pressure of population, the world would not be as it is. With the same population as in 1945, about 2.2 billion, the rate of change would be slowed down; there would be an almost continual first world agricultural slump, not surpluses; inflation would not have to be resisted; pressure on resources such as oil would be so much reduced as to render the Arabs impotent; the third world would be a backwater – charming, quaint, visited for its ethnic qualities – and not a cockpit for the first and second worlds. Few land animal species would be endangered. The sea would not be an area of deep anxiety; polluted by man's activities, short of fish and devoid of whales. There would be no acid rain; no greenhouse effect; no threat from aerosols; no hydrocarbon related smog, not even in Los Angeles, which, incidentally, would probably have a population one-third what it is now. This fantasy has only to be stated to be denied.

Population growth is a fact of life. It has been much accelerated by mankind's activities in the last half-century. It has been much modified by the retreat of disease in the recent past. The twentieth century is also notable for personal cleanliness.

Cleanliness declined after 1492, for at least 350 years. First of all, bathing became suspect, because of syphilis. The daily, weekly, monthly public bath taken by both genders in Renaissance cities in Europe disappeared from the ritual of life. To the fear of syphilis, and to the connection between the bath-house ('bagnio') and prostitution was added the high cost of heating water as wood became unobtainable and coal had to be imported.

Cleanliness implies drains, which were one of the great pathways for disease. There were no main sewerage drains as we know them today until the nineteenth century, on any kind of city-wide scale. Londoners, proud occupants of the then largest city in the West, used so-called 'cesspools', which were, literally, pools of polluted effluent, soaking away into the surrounding earth. From the local earth, these cesspools drained into the local wells, which supplied the local population with water and their own (and other people's) enteric organisms. It was the connection between wells and cesspools which killed people as eminent as Prince Albert (he died in 1861 from typhoid fever) and many, many more and humbler inhabitants of large English cities. In very hot, unfavourable years, it is probable that 10 per cent of the population of all ages in poor districts would die of some sort of enteric disorder in the mid-Victorian period. In London, in 1862, there were nearly 400,000 cesspools, draining into 100,000 drinking-water wells. The bacterial connection was not made for another generation.

There was, however, a view, identified in particular with North-West Europe and the United States, that cleanliness was connected to Godliness. This implied that there was a connection between dirt and disease. From this partial truth emerged the great clean water movement.

New York City was the first in the modern West to divide water and sewage: this was done by reaching further and further out for fresh water. By 1900, water was piped from the Catskills to Manhattan, from Wales to Liverpool and Birmingham, from the Pennines to Manchester, Leeds, Bradford and Sheffield. The inhabitants of the Thames Valley, from Oxford to Greenwich, had to rely on the river which acted as both water supply and sewer, and still does. In between these two functions are a number of purification plants, much chemical activity, and more than 20 million people. This treatment removed a fundamental restraint upon population growth, probably reducing mortality more than much medical effort.

After pure water, the second important contribution to health from the United States was anaesthesia. The Chinese have used acupuncture for at least a thousand years. Hypnotism was employed in India and Persia, and by some Arabs. Ether was suggested by the English polymath Michael Faraday, who also experimented at length with nitrous oxide (laughing gas). The heroes of early operations were, however, American dentists, not doctors. Dr Horace Wells of Hartford, Connecticut, removed his own tooth while under nitrous oxide sedation in 1844. Dr Morton of Boston used ether as a general anaesthetic (on others) for tooth extraction and general surgery. Mr Robinson of London worked with Liston, the great surgeon, on several operations before the end of 1846. Sir James Simpson applied ether to midwifery the next year. By the time of the Crimean War, 1854–7, and, even more, by the time of the war between the States, 1861–5, anaesthesia was in general use. Antisepsis was another matter.

So little was survival from surgery originally considered likely or possible, and so unknown were the actions of micro-organisms, that surgeons never even changed their bloody clothes, or washed their hands before the work of Lister, Pasteur and Koch. Lister, a surgeon son of an inventor and developer of microscopes, was intellectually well placed to combine the two disciplines and use antiseptics to increase survival rates after surgery. Previously, the operations had been successful, but more than three-quarters of the patients died. They died from shock, loss of blood, and, more usually, septicemia. Anaesthesia overcame shock. Lister's work on ligatures stopped internal bleeding. His use of carbolic acid stopped sepsis.[2]

Pasteur was the son of a tanner, and trained as a chemist; he worked on ferments, and set out the rules for preventing putrefaction in processes such as winemaking, milk-handling, brewing. The word 'pasteurization' derives from his discoveries. Though milk can be made safe by pasteurization, humans do not survive such treatment. So antiseptics, which kill germs but not human flesh and bone, were substituted. Robert Koch, the third hero, was an early Nobel prizewinner who specialized in bacteriology, and worked on tuberculosis, cholera, rinderpest and other diseases.[3]

Surgery a hundred years ago was still daring, if no longer as painful for the patient. Before World War I, the appendicectomy was the fashionable new operation, being first performed in 1886, and on Edward VII in 1902. Operations on diseased kidneys, lungs, ulcers were all performed before 1900. Surgery was improved just in time for the carnage of World War I and the annual increase in road accidents in every country in the world in the twentieth century. Outside Europe and the neo–Europes, surgery was insignificant in affecting population growth.

Drugs, pharmaceuticals and more sensible habits were of greater importance than surgery in most countries. In the middle of the nineteenth century, both morphine and cocaine were in use by the time that proper needles were widely available for injection. This was in the 1870s. As a local anaesthetic, cocaine was compounded with various other substances, and even used, at one time, in medicated chewing gum, as a dental painkiller. The great drug of all the malarial areas was quinine, which became freely available in the 1880s, and cheap enough, at one-farthing a day, for general use. Quinine probably had more effect upon population growth than all the efforts of all the doctors ever born. Later, it was preventive measures, like drainage, which did much more than quinine in combating malaria.[4]

Preventive medicine, vaccines and drugs have made light of what had once been killer-diseases. Scarlet fever, measles, diphtheria, whooping cough, German measles and tuberculosis have all been rendered relatively harmless in the first world. The common cold defies defeat. Influenza, with its ability to change its very nature, a characteristic it shares with AIDS, is always a possible pandemic. The outbreak in 1918–20 killed more people in Western Europe than did the battles of World War I. Antibiotics and the sulfa drugs have cleared up all sorts of local and generalized infections, often undiagnosed and treated before they were identified; this happened before 1970 in most advanced countries. A new generation of doctors is less certain about the merits of the blanket use of antibiotics. The habit of the 1960s: 'Here are some pills; come back if you're not cured', is no longer regarded as good medicine. Careless medical men have bred all sorts of new, antibiotic-resistant organisms. Some hospital walls are covered with drug-resistant organisms of great power. So far, the drug companies have kept ahead of the germs. If this position should ever be reversed, a serious pandemic would ensue.

Simple, cheap drugs are now widely used on a daily basis by millions of people at home. Aspirin (1898) was often compounded with phenacetin (1887), and both are widely used today. Chloral hydrate, the first (stinking) hypnotic, was followed by others, less smelly, paraldehyde (1868), sulphonal (1880) and barbiton (1898).[5] From these came a long sequence of barbiturates, all synthetic, which held sway before librium (1945) and valium (1947). Iodine, which occurs naturally in seaweed, was synthesized in 1885, and became a household antiseptic, until superseded after World War II.

Two massive developments required no hardware, no technology, no modern industrial base. They both required a change of attitude. This has often proved harder in history.

The first was the general view of mental illness. Graeco–Roman attitudes were more humane than those of the Middle Ages. In extreme cases, the mad were regarded by Christians as being possessed of the Devil. In an age of Conformity, it was comfortable for the Establishment to consider dissent disorder. In London, lunatics were housed in institutions like the Bethlehem Hospital (1247), hence Bedlam. There were similar institutions in other cities. In villages, the local idiot was more tolerantly treated.

Renaissance attitudes were more easy-going, less dogmatic. The first inkling of a modern approach was to split the 'mad' into what remains a modern starting-point: neuroses are natural disorders; psychoses are unnatural fantasies; the latter may or may not be accompanied by organic changes in the body, the former never. Gradually, people recognized that mental health was a problem associated with the environment. 'Madness is a disease of civilization' became a common comment, and the observation that the talented were not far removed from the demented was often made.

By 1900, some sort of organized 'science' had supplemented philosophy. There was a physical school, which sought to treat the insane with aural or electric shocks, or by drugs. The school, founded by Sigmund Freud, passed from hypnosis to 'free association' to the interpretation of dreams. The oedipus complex was the overwhelming desire of the infant to have exclusive possession of the parent of the opposite gender; this was suppressed by the ego, the awareness of self. The id, the unconscious, was the home of repressions, and is responsible for the content of dreams. The libido, the third element in the mind, was responsible for the emotional energy applied to work, sexual activity or creative living. The super-ego was the conscience, which developed later, and controlled the ego.

Freud's disciples and followers have accepted most of his postulates, as have most workers in the field ever since. Two famous disciples were Adler, who invented the 'inferiority complex' and thought that desire for triumph was a most important driving force, and Jung, who believed that the key was the motive driving the libido. Was it psychic energy, or religion, myths, the collective unconscious, perhaps?[6]

Of all three, Freud, Adler and Jung, and of all modern practitioners, it would be fair to say that they are men of their time. Nearly everything they postulated was known to the Greeks, and to artist-genius figures ever since, in literature, painting, music.

To a post-Christian society, nominally liberal, this whole industry can often be a prop, an alternative to personal morality, brutally misused in Stalinist Russia and Hitler's Germany; its impact has been greatly increased by the use of drugs, in every sort of society. The profession, divided into psychologists, psychoanalysts and psychiatrists, is thickest on the ground where the lifestyle is furthest removed from the natural: Los Angeles and Manhattan. To be without a shrink amongst the smarter classes is equivalent to the humbler sort of person being without a car.

In the Counter-Reformation, Freud, Adler and Jung would have been burnt at the stake. Their crime would have been to relieve mankind from the consequences of belief. What would the Inquisition have made of modern nurses?

The answer is that nursing was an old gentle activity, performed by patrician Roman ladies from the fourth century onwards. Throughout the Middle Ages, nursing was associated with nuns and the order with the largest number of graduates is that of St Vincent de Paul, founded in 1633. It was in Northern countries, after the Reformation, that the connection between nursing and domestic duties was first made.

Gradually, the patrician, almost professional competence of the nursing sister gave way to the deplorable old soak, the gin-sodden Sarah Gamp of Charles Dickens's imagination.[7] It was, in turn, Florence Nightingale who rescued the profession and made of nursing a modern skill. She grasped the principles of hygiene long before most doctors, the essential nature of the educated girl, properly trained to be a sick-nurse, and the subsequent lifelong status of the professional woman. Florence Nightingale did more for women than to reform and rebuild an ancient semi-charitable sisterhood fallen into decay. She gave girls from good families an opportunity outside marriage for a worthwhile career, better in many ways than the archetypical governess of the period. Florence Nightingale stamped upon the whole of hospital life the type of inspired common sense which she called 'scientific cleanliness'. No longer was the old-style muddle and dirt permitted to survive. She also believed in the virtues of Christian love and fresh air.

From this mid-Victorian beginning has grown what is the largest economic sector in every advanced country. In the first world, the health industry is huge. The British National Health Service, an unmanageable monolith, is the largest employer in Europe, after the Red Army. More is spent on health care in the United States than on any other sector of human activity except eating. These two items are not unconnected. Most health care expenditure in the first world puts right what results from expenditure on unsuitable food, alcohol, tobacco or other follies.

Hospitals have developed a momentum of their own. The young are nearly all born in them. The old nearly all die in them. They are a natural dockyard to repair all the casualties of modern life: victims of street violence, bodies dead on arrival, the wounded from car accidents, even people who need a stitch or two because of a hand that went through a pane of glass. But should the hospital dominate society as it does? No baby has been born in a northern English or Scottish city at a holiday weekend for the past ten years because births are induced for the convenience of the staff. The chronically old and sick are kept alive, sometimes beyond their natural term.[8]

The very nature of those born is altered by the absence of perinatal failure. High-tech operations of every kind, to brain, to heart, to kidney, are regarded as professional challenges, without thought of whether or not they should ever happen. The health industry, so magnificently served by so many, and occupying more than one in ten people in every first world country, contributes much to the survival of so many at both ends of life. Does it know where it is going?

There are two basic problems about modern health care. They appear to be social, political, economic. But they go to the root of public morality. Needless to say, the problems are rarely articulated. If touched upon, the questions are fudged.

The first point is that high-tech medicine costs serious money. An acute heart attack, brought into an emergency ward, attracts, in England, expenditure on drugs and intensive care of not less than £10,000 and an average of £17,000. Organ transplant operations, with 'new' organs taken from a dying, but not dead, person, involve several fudges. The cost may be as high as £100,000. The chances of success may be as low as 15–20 per cent. 'Successful' operations may prolong life for a few years only. The survivor can rarely live more than an invalid's existence. Questions are never asked: should organs be taken from biologically live people? Should such huge resources be employed on high-tech operations in order to keep medical men happy? Are the lucky patients the right people to operate upon, or are they just guinea-pigs? Who is to decide who the beneficiaries of all this high-tech attention should be? In some countries, it is the market. In the Soviet bloc, it is the rule that only favoured party members get all the care and attention available. Ordinary people over fifty are not carried by ambulance in some second world countries, and no person in Poland of over sixty, unless an *apparatchik*, is allowed into hospital. Like the market, this system is logical. In Western Europe, there is an uneasy feeling that any method of selection is wrong, that everyone should be able to benefit. This is obviously impossible. A service free at the point of delivery can never work.

The effect of such contradiction at one end of life is matched at the other. Old people are sometimes kept alive as cabbages; young people are born who have no chance of a normal life. Before every birth took place in hospital, general practitioners, or midwives, especially in rural areas, did not strive officiously to keep alive. If a child was the product of incest, or spastic, or malformed, or was born blind or diseased, then it did not survive. Today, such conduct, performed in public, amounts to murder. A hundred years ago, perinatal mortality took between 20 and 50 per cent of all births in the slums of London or in rural Russia respectively. So no one noticed the unnatural selection process which favoured the fit. Today, in Western Europe, perinatal mortality is down to such a low figure as would make many ask why those who die should. In some hospitals in Scandinavia, perinatal mortality is felt to be a disgrace to the institution. Those who are kept alive are often a burden on the state for the rest of their lives. The care of the unfit, which literally took a fraction of 1 per cent of the gross national product a century ago, because there were not many wholly unfit, will increase every year in the first world. It could well be as much as half of all 'health' care before the end of the century, as much as 5 per cent of national income in some countries. These matters make people feel uncomfortable. The decision not to keep a child alive· at birth, so simple a hundred years ago, when there was no one present at the birth except a faithful colleague and the mother, is today so complex. Who makes the decisions? Who has the right to do so? It is not surprising that these matters should be fudged. Who, in all conscience should wish to rule in such cases? Who would dare to judge the matter?

There is, of course, a sea change involved in the population of so-called 'caring' countries. An increasing proportion of the population can be categorized as 'disabled'. There are said to be 18–20 per cent in every Western European country. In the sense of not being able to run a four-minute mile, *and* understand the difference between the baroque and the rococo, *and* between fission and fusion, *and* to articulate the theory of relativity, everyone is virtually disabled. That is, only a tiny minority can perform in every department as a dedicated, discrete specialist. The 'disabled', however, all have some strength which makes them outstanding. But if they are labelled 'disabled', and if society sees itself as responsible for them, two dependencies are created. One is that of the 'disabled'. The second is that of the 'caring professions' which have a vested interest in the existence of the 'disabled'. This is another burden which has been imposed upon society without conscious thought.[9]

The problem is accentuated, perhaps created in its present acute form, by another sea change in the world. Christianity has abandoned the primacy of the hereafter. Conduct in this world importantly obscures belief in the next. Few sophisticated Muslims are strong enough in their faith to put heaven before the mundane. Even in Israel, Jews are probably just as secular. Most countries in the world follow the example of the United States and profess a constitutional laicism. This makes death officially a difficult business. It must be avoided at all cost. Health care is devoted to prolonging life; proponents even talk about 'saving life' as if such an action were possible. For those who do not understand the immense effects of not believing in the hereafter, a visit to a hospice might convince. To be in an institution whose purpose is dignified (even cheerful) death, is far removed from the ultimately hopeless task of prolonging life. If people accept the hereafter, the whole health care business becomes much easier to manage.

Obviously, ample provision for the young and unproductive and the old and unproductive implies an unequal burden on different economies. The 'compassionate society' cannot harm a country where each farmer feeds a hundred other people, and enough houses, factories, cars, washing machines, electronic goods are made by modern means to meet maximum demand at a low price. But to establish lavish standards as 'normal' and 'civilized' is grotesque when they are transferred to the third world. To replace family responsibilities for the old by institutions is a luxury that the third world cannot afford. Time may tell whether or not the first world has been wise so to do.

To remove from parents ultimate responsibility for the care of their young, which is what the first world has also done, may save a minority of children from discomfort, even danger. But a society in which nearly half of all marriages end in divorce is more likely to neglect its children than one which has no provision alternative to the family. Indeed, the existence of an alternative may make unsatisfactory parents easier with their conscience, and neighbours less critical. It is possible that easy divorce combines naturally with the removal of parental responsibility for children.

As to the young, African experience is valid. Sub-Saharan Africa increased its population by 25 per cent in the first quarter of this century; by 45 per cent in the second; by 100 per cent in the third; in the fourth, the out-turn looks like being at least 125 per cent. Nearly all this increase was by reason of survival of children who would previously have died. Some of this medical success was because of vaccination and inoculation; some was by the apparent, and local, elimination of malaria, bilharzia and sleeping sickness; some was much simpler, obvious, known to every non-medical person in the West: use only clean water, wash the hands before a meal, encourage clean clothes, wash vegetables, avoid parasites. By such simple means were the survival rates of infants increased many times.

All very admirable. But there is no food for the increased African population – 300 million of them under 15. There is plenty of land.[10] There is enough water – at a cost. But to grow food requires capital – simple capital, tools, seeds, animals. This might cost no more, no less than $500 per head. The capital does not exist in Africa, and it is unlikely that the first world will provide $150 billion for this purpose. Put another way, each sub-Saharan born requires a matching $500 of investment in order that the child becomes an adult. This is far more difficult than keeping the child alive. Unfortunately, none of the aid agencies can ever think in a long enough time-scale to address the problem with logic. Far easier to be compassionate today, lay up trouble for the future. This is a respectable form of improvidence. It is practised by a veritable army of the good.

Nor is this a problem which will go away. Rural 'congestion' or extreme density of population has existed in Europe, almost within living memory in southern Italy, parts of Ireland, and in the Balkans. Such local overpopulation was solved by emigration or by industrialization.[11] The emigration of poor, unskilled, illiterate people is no longer a possibility. The industrialization of most of Africa is a capital intensive exercise which only has to be mentioned to be dismissed. The African case will therefore continue to haunt those who think of it.

African overpopulation is not solved by pop concerts. A single concert may raise funds to keep alive a proportion of the population for a year. What then? Another concert? Each year, nearly 30 million sub-Saharan babies are born. This means that each year, someone, somewhere, in Africa, should invest $15 billion, or more than the surplus product of half the United Nations. To state the figure is to realize that it will not happen. Yet, to keep each of those babies alive, over and beyond the efforts of the mother may only cost $10. Three hundred million dollars to keep alive one year's crop of African babies is much easier. It may well be within the abilities of the aid agencies, if not a pop concert. The problem, never faced, is what happens next year, and the year after, and so on.

We live in a squeamish age. To state the African problem of population is to invite the use of birth-control. But disease and hunger, perinatal mortality and the loss of two-thirds of the children born before they reach the age of ten used to be the means of population control in Africa. No African, educated at the London School of Economics, is impressed when told that these were once the methods of population control in Europe, too. If Africa can be visited by jet, then all the latest, high-tech methods of birth-control should be also available.

Overpopulation cannot be gainsaid. If it is not solved in one way, it has always been solved in another. There is no avoiding this truth. In Africa, population control will have to be famine, or disease, or interfering with reproduction. There are other, even less acceptable alternatives.[12]

Famine is a comparative term. It is entirely possible that tropical and sub-tropical Africans could survive for years on a diet half that of Europeans, say 1,500 calories.[13] Disease could return as the great controller of infant numbers, especially if there were any kind of social breakdown.[14] The problem with physical birth control methods are the same as they were in India, and likely to be much worse.[15]

Most countries in Africa, South Africa included, are probably beyond any comfortable ability to feed their increase. Even in South Africa, the task is daunting. In the Republic, there are nearly 30 million Bantu. The Bantu birth-rate is over 1 million a year. No one, of course, invests $500 per head, $500 million in all, each year, in Bantu agriculture. This is far more important than an absence of apartheid.

Bantu, like perhaps half of all Africans, use maize as a staple source of starch. This Amerindian plant has been raised to its high current potential by Anglo-American methods. The British ambition has been transferred all over the world: output per acre within a renewable system, a 'rotation of crops'. The American aim, originally with the target of output per man, was transmuted by the vastly increased use of machinery, fertilizers and plant breeding techniques into a much wider philosophy. When the two ambitions, of output per unit area and output per manhour coalesced, as in the more successful neo-Europes, the results are dramatic. This has been true of Canada, Australia, New Zealand, parts of South America and Southern Africa. These neo-Europes all derived their systems from both Britain and the United States. The English legacy was that of rotation of crops, and the essential involvement of livestock to make best use of the necessary grassland within the rotation. This spread wherever the British settled in the neo-Europes.

The same kind of philosophy, modified to circumstance, came to dominate advanced Western European countries. Scandinavia and Holland joined English husbandry methods with good transport and supplies of electricity to turn from butter, cheese and beef production to the provision of liquid milk. By World War II, liquid milk production had become the most important agricultural activity in Scandinavia, Holland, Switzerland and the United Kingdom, in that order. Milk not drunk 'fresh' was converted into the traditional butter and cheese, and into the new condensed and dried product; milk was put into chocolate, into canned soup, into prepared foods of every kind, into bread even. Great play was made of milk in 'health' terms.

In the United States, milk became healthy in direct proportion to the number of dairy farmers, and their influence on state legislatures. Thus, milk was healthier in New York State or Wisconsin than in South Dakota or Louisiana. In Europe, milk was much healthier in Switzerland than in any of the Latin countries. In France, milk was healthier in Normandy than in the Midi. Electricity and good transport made liquid milk a possibility all through the Alpine regions, and farmers in Austria, Bavaria and Northern Italy were offered the same opportunities as in Switzerland. In Switzerland in the 1930s milk became so profitable as to be taxed to subsidize the Federal Railways.

Liquid milk became identified with the care of children, nursing mothers, and the frail of all ages. Milk ultimately became a symbolic product of the Welfare State, a prop to agriculture in times of depression, wholesome, non-carnal, almost. The drinking of milk became a 'good thing'. After World War II, welfare milk in England became much more than a symbol, a shibboleth. When Mrs Thatcher, as Minister of Education, removed the subsidy from schoolchildren's milk in 1971–2, she was labelled 'Thatcher the milk-snatcher' by interested parties. In other countries, milk was already suspect. It was accused of making children fat, liable to adult cholesterol problems, prone to acne, even. Milk peaked, as a fashionable commodity, sometime in the 1970s.[16]

In the United States, the same process of Depression, plus refrigeration and good transport drove northern and eastern dairy states into milk. The opening of the 'bonanza' states to the growth of wheat because of railroads connecting with the Atlantic and the Great Lakes meant that millions of acres in the east went out of cultivation. In Kansas, Nebraska, the Dakotas, there was a restless search for inherent fertility, a 'mining' of the soil, and a tendency to move on. There were dry seasons; big blows, when crops had too little root-growth; plagues of insect pests; no fertilizers, neither rotations nor good husbandry were involved; bare fallow was the only alternative to grain cropping. This unsympathetic treatment of the soil ruined not only millions of acres west of the Mississippi, but millions of acres unable to compete in the east, or in Europe. Between 1879 and 1939, enough land went out of arable cultivation in Europe and the old United States to give an annual bread ration to 500 million people. By the time the need for such huge increases of supply became obvious, other crops used the 'old lands' of Europe and neo-Europe more profitably. Only in the 1960s would grain production widen to cover almost any flat field in temperate climates, if such use was economically appropriate.

The wide prairie was also to be found north of the 49th Parallel. Between 49°N, and some point in the middle 50s, Canada west of the Great Lakes was another strip of bonanza wheatland, either side of the railroads, stretching for mile after mile. From 1879 onwards, there were three sorts of wheat crop. There was the virgin prairie, ploughed twice and sown first, in August. Then the portion which had been summer-fallowed. Then that which had been ploughed in the previous winter and harvested in the current year. Harvest in the following year was therefore prolonged, made easier to carry out before being motorized.[17]

The internal combustion engine arrived on the scene just in time for World War I. Ex London and Paris buses gave troops what was often their last ride into the trenches; trucks of all kinds hauled food and ammunition and specially built tractors hauled guns; combat aircraft and tanks became possible. But the long-term effect of the internal combustion engine was greatest in transport and in agriculture. The tractor solved both the British and the American problem. Cultivation became more professional, more timely, more efficient; rotation of crops, and the proper exploitation of grassland other than by grazing or haymaking became much easier; so proper husbandry of the soil was more capable of achievement. By using bred strains of both cereals and herbage crops, fertilizers and pest control, output per acre potentially increased between 1920, when tractors first became 'serious' and available, and, say, 1970, by at least four times in cereals and by six to eight times in grassland. Output per man rose to such a level that it was possible in 1970 to grow a crop of wheat in England with one man-day per acre to grow four tons. In America, half the input of labour would have been applied to each acre, but the acre would not produce four tons of wheat. On the other hand, state of the art techniques would produce more maize-corn per man-hour in Iowa than anywhere else on earth, if that were wanted, even if Americans, New Zealanders, Australians and Englishmen were all using the same machinery.[18]

Canadian cereals were important from the 1870s. They still are. If world markets were open, Canadian barley, at one-third the cost of production in Europe, would be as important as Canadian bread-wheat or American maize. As it is, Western Europe, the biggest market before World War II, importing one-third of all grain requirements in an average year, is now a net exporter. Canadian farming has had to adapt to the same sort of crops as Old and New England; fruit production, vegetables, grain turned into meat, eggs, milk, butter and cheese, much more concern for the herbage crops than existed a hundred years ago.

Australia and New Zealand were countries whose formative years were made possible by technology, which in turn made them both part of the English farm in the period before 1939. Australia, now settled for more than two centuries, originally starved when the convicts tried to feed themselves. Indeed, it would be twenty years before the raw colony of the land around Sydney would even feed itself, let alone have a surplus for visiting ships or new arrivals. The state of the Aboriginal inhabitants is worthy of note. They were hunter-gatherers, and would remain so, without the white invasion, because there are no native plants, no native animals which can be domesticated. The Aboriginal people of the south-east corner of Australia may or may not have known the other Aborigines.

The individual Abo tribes may or may not have been similar people; they may or may not have had the same sort of habits. It is unlikely that indigenous people in lush New South Wales would have the same patterns of behaviour as people who survived round Alice Springs. The likely answer is that each group of Aborigines, perhaps an extended family or a small tribe, had a huge area of land to support them. There were berries, roots, meat from marsupials (two-thirds of all native Australian mammals) and fish and birds. But there were no ruminants of any kind; no apes, monkeys or baboons. There were few animals resembling any European species, the most obvious being the wild dog, the dingo. There were two interesting great birds: a black swan, and a white eagle. There are few carrion birds, no vultures, but sixty sorts of parrot. There were many edible birds, pigeon, duck, geese, plovers, quails, all unique to Australia. There was the emu, equivalent to the ostrich of Africa and the rhea of South America. The finest freshwater fish is the Murray cod, sometimes as much as 45 kg (100 lb) in weight. There are many salt-water fish and at least two turtles which humans can find useful as food. There are also crocodiles in the north, some swimming across the Tasman Sea from the East Indies. There are two other peculiarities. There are koala bears who live on eucalyptus leaves so tainted as to make koala flesh unattractive to predators, including humans. Secondly, there is no native method of recycling dung from ruminants; the dung beetle (scarab) had to be imported from Africa to deal with mountains of ancient, unrotted, fibrous dung from imported ruminant animals.[19]

The native, indigenous, ancient Aborigine had a thin life. But it was his own. He developed, as is known, especially spiritual qualities to deal with the feast-famine syndrome; an especial response to the challenge of a tummy first full, then empty, and an especial enzyme so that long periods of low intake did not produce so much pain as the same conditions in a white man. The Aboriginal attitudes to birth control and the survival of the old were severely practical. There were few unfit in an indigenous tribe. But they suffered from the white invasion. The first agents of destruction were not, as ever, men, but white men's parasites.[20]

There was an outbreak of a severe disease within months of the arrival of the First Fleet. Was it smallpox? If so, it produced the same kind of result as in Mexico or Peru. There was little further competition from the Aborigines in the area of Sydney. The next invaders, which moved more visibly than microbes, were pigs. They were released near Sydney in 1789, and ranged over the whole eastern third of Australia, and much of South Australia besides. Regardless of breed, feral pigs are selected by nature to survive if they are thin, long-legged, with snouts adapted to burrowing, with huge tusks in the male. This process of selection takes about ten generations, and is quicker than the reverse, which can produce a good bacon pig out of a modern wild boar. Wild pigs in both America and Australia have the same nick-name, razorback.[21] They were fierce, successful as a species, capable of killing a cow, a horse or a man with their sabre tusks. Despite all the modern efforts at killing swine with gun and lance and poison, wild boar still figures in the Australian landscape, as a semi-parasite, semi-independent animal, like the rate. Unlike the rat, they make for good eating.

Cattle became feral even earlier than pigs. The first Australian cattle were loosed from those brought over on board HMS *Sirius*. They were not English, but South African. What their bloodlines were, no one now knows. But they were great survivors. In 1789 eight animals strayed off. By 1804, fifteen years later, the herds ('mobs' in convict Australian) numbered nearly 10,000. They were untameable, a resource of wild food for anyone in the bush, and for any escaped convict or 'bush-ranger'. By 1830, despite an effort to kill African feral cattle, and substitute European alternatives, there were nearly 400,000. By 1850, there were said to be millions. Who counted? The introduction of the rabbit and its destruction of Australian sheep grazing is well known. Less well known, less damaging, but bad enough, was the import of the European rat.[22]

Sheep made Australia. Wool was the first crop to be a commercial success. There are many native grazing plants in Australia, grasses, sedges, but no legumes. These were introduced, and largely spread by sheep. The merino, introduced in the early days, produced an average of less than 1.5 kg (3 lb) per fleece in 1850. By 1900, this figure had doubled, by careful selection and adaptation of Merino-type sheep and by introducing European herbage seeds. Wool remain the largest single export by value until the 1960s. In the Bi-centennial year, 1988, appropriately enough, wool overtook coal as the greatest single Australian export. Its position in future depends on the merino wool price, which has ranged between A$2 and A$15 per kilogram in the last twenty-five years; on the strength of other currencies, on international prosperity, and to a lesser extent, upon fashion. Initially, merino wool from Australia was only of great value because of English technology in spinning and weaving and finishing. Today, every advanced country buys and uses Australian wool.

Wheat production in Australia followed the curve of the Australian (white) population. It was initially only the surplus which was exported. In the ferocious drought year of 1902, wheat was actually imported. Modern Australians would find this hard to believe.

Breaking land in the absence of modern tractors was more difficult in Australia than in America, Canada or New Zealand. Soil often lay in pits and troughs, and tree stumps proved impossible to handle economically before the native invention of the stump-jump plough. Arable land might take ten years to become fertile. In Australia, more even than in America, man-shortage was always more serious than land-shortage, which has virtually never existed. Yields before the introduction of superphosphate in the 1880s were lower than in medieval England, as low as 10–12 bushels per acre, less than one ton per hectare. To be fair to Australia, this was about the same as contemporary yields in Southern Russia, on much better soils. Together with superphosphate, better management of the soil helped defeat drought, and yields rose in those areas with more than 20 in (500 mm) of annual rainfall. But wheat was pushed out of the higher rainfall areas.

Cattle, largely feral until 1900, began to be important as a source of hides, tallow and salted meat before 1880. Refrigeration made the export of butter, cheese and frozen or chilled beef, mutton and lamb possible. Great efforts were made to round up the wild cattle, or make better use of them with imported beef or dairy bulls. By 1914, there was an important refrigerated trade, with at least one ship a week leaving each of the six main ports. Successful as was this development, Australian beef did not compete in quality or price with the Argentine trade. This was 7,000 miles nearer Europe, and the grazing was better. There may have been significant differences in the feral cattle stock: Longhorn Spanish of the sixteenth century, Anglo-African of the nineteenth. Did this factor make for higher quality beef from the River Plate?

Dairying in Australia started in Victoria, then spread to New South Wales and Tasmania. Rye-grass, cocksfoot and clovers were sown on partly-cleared land. Pastures took as long as arable land to come into full production. Sometimes, it seems that European grasses had to turn into something uniquely Antipodean in order to thrive. This is true of clovers and of rye-grass in both Australia and New Zealand, and even of agrostis in Western Australia.

New Zealand has a much more favourable climate than Australia for the successful invasion of European flora and fauna. The European human was less favoured. The Maoris were more numerous, more advanced, more warlike than any Australian Aborigine. They were also more crowded by a factor of over 100–1 on the North Island in 1850. There were no other land mammals before the white man, except for the two brought by the Maoris, the edible dog, and a black rat. Both are now extinct, or very rare. The early Europeans imported ferrets, cats, stoats and weasels, which did so much damage so quickly that three islands had to be established as sanctuaries for native fauna. Acclimatization has been the name of the game of settlement in New Zealand.

Pheasants, deer of five kinds, ducks, and brown and rainbow trout all colonized with ease. So did grain of every kind, rich grasses, fruit trees, vines, and long before any of these, white man's diseases. The one great failure was the salmon. More than a hundred efforts all failed, regardless of whether the salmon was Atlantic or Pacific.

The Maoris were debilitated by syphilis, acquired from white sailors off whalers, off sealing ships, and spread by the Maori practice of polygamy and sexual hospitality. Within a generation of Captain Cook's first arrival in 1769–70, venereal disease had joined Maori infanticide as a population control measure. The Maori population plummeted. Within another generation, Maoris were also dying of 'consumption'. By 1830, there were thousands of muskets on the islands, acquired by Maoris in exchange for European crops grown under European direction, for visiting Europeans in European ships. In 1830–1, there were fewer than 800 whites in all New Zealand. Inside fourteen months, Australia alone exported 8,000 muskets to New Zealand, and three times that number came from Europe. In 1835, Charles Darwin arrived on a visit, and found hundreds of acres of white man's crops, and pigs, horses, cattle, wild and in profusion, as well as rats everywhere.

There does not seem to have been an outbreak of smallpox in New Zealand comparable to those in the Americas or Australia, but measles acted as powerfully as smallpox in Australia. Missionaries were very active in the 1830s and 1840s, and they tried to introduce Maoris to examples of white culture other than alcohol, tobacco, gunpowder, muskets and barley, wheat, potatoes, clover, apples, pears, apricots and peaches. By 1840, when the resident white population in New Zealand was less than 2,000, Maoris had been reduced by disease to 60,000. By 1860, when the Maori Wars started, the Maori race had been halved compared with only fifty years previously. By the end of the wars, the Maori population was only about 40,000, that of the whites over 250,000. The wars did not make much difference to population, as always. Disease killed more Maoris than did muskets. It was the gold rush that brought the whites into New Zealand. That was in the 1860s. As in California and Australia, the chief long-term effect of the gold rush was to increase permanently the local population. Gold rushes a generation later leave so many people per million ounces extracted. This is an important and very interesting ratio yet to be established.

No one thinks of gold in terms of New Zealand today, unless gold be butter. It is the pastoral products of the country that matter. Lamb, butter, cheese and, to a lesser extent, beef, are the products of this most efficient grazing country. Almost no nitrogen is used in fertilizer form. Almost every grazing field is supported by an abundance of clover, which draws nitrogen from the air and enriches the soil, the companion grasses and the clover itself. The clover seed originally came from England. Kent, Suffolk, Devon, the Midland counties are represented in the genes of New Zealand clover. New Zealand White is a definite type, more prolific than its ancestors, and encouraged by the magnificent climate, the most suitable for clover in the world. For twenty years, clover did not thrive in New Zealand. There was an absence of bees to work their fertility-giving magic upon the flowers. Bees were imported in 1839. Since that date, clover and bees have been part of the essential fabric of New Zealand life. Clover makes New Zealand pasture the most efficient in the world. Bees made the conqueror of Everest.[23]

Clover, in an Atlantic context, will produce its own herbage, and 'subscribe' up to the equivalent of over 100 'units' of nitrogen.[24] In some parts of Europe, nitrogen gain from clover is so small as to make its culture uneconomic. In Holland, West Germany, Scandinavia, some parts of Eastern England, on specialist dairy farms devoted to silage-making all over Western Europe, grassland may contain no clover at all. For nitrogen, the farmer depends upon the chemical company. In some systems, 300 'units' of bag nitrogen are used, three to five times what clover could provide. There is a straight line pay-off between nitrogen usage on suitable grassland and yield, and this line does not change on suitable soil, species of grass and climate until the 500 'units' level is reached. In New Zealand, no one has ever made any money using bag nitrogen.

Phosphates are another matter. The use of superphosphate manures only came in to fashion after their success in Australia.[25] They were not in general use on New Zealand pastures until after World War I. Together with tractors, milking machines and herd-testing to improve butterfat, the pastures of New Zealand started to support a considerable secondary industry. Milk was turned into butter and packed for shipment in co-operatives; lambs were slaughtered and frozen or chilled for transport over 13,000 miles to England; wool was sorted and graded and sold by a Wool Board. Beef, wheat and sisal, which had been important in the early part of the century, gave way almost entirely to the processing of clover. Modern New Zealand was formed by exploiting clover for fifty years, from 1920–70. It is fair to say that if the clover had not proved to be the boon it was, New Zealanders would have found something else to exploit as they have more recently – deer-farming, tourism, 'kiwi fruit'.[26] It is also fair to say that New Zealand might never have prospered without clover. It is a country built on clover. All over the islands, there is not a statue, amongst many other statues, to the humble Wild White Clover.

The Argentine and part of Uruguay became involved with European food for a shorter period. Beef was not important as an export from the Plate until after 1900. The beef came from the pampas, and they had been there since before 1580, when the first permanent successful Spanish settlements were made. Cattle, not native to any of the Americas, had presumably been left somewhere by former (failed) settlers. The pampas of the Plate were virtually free of any indigenous competition for the cattle; nor were there many predators. Indeed, the pampas were originally virtually empty. There was nothing for the jaguar and puma to eat on the plains until horses and cattle arrived. The predators came down from the mountains when the food appeared. So did the Amerindians. The long-horn cattle resembled those of Texas, having been descended from the same Iberian stock. Between, say, 1550 and 1850, they developed, over perhaps, more than 120 generations, into fierce tribal animals, roaming in great herds like the North American bison. Long of horn, speedy in reaction, sure of foot, they had been selected by their environment into two groups, the quick and the dead. Only the fit survived.

The multiplication process was sure, producing an estimated 50 million by 1750. (Who counted them?) Thousands were killed every year for the hides. There was not much tallow in them. They were mean, thin, rangy cattle, more dangerous, more difficult to tame than the accompanying wild horses. Living with them, off them, having changed their habits, were Plains Indians, having become carnivorous as a consequence of the feral Iberian animals.

When the Anglos arrived in Texas, the Argentine, or Uruguay, they sought to improve the wild cattle. Herefords (called 'hurfords' in Texas), Shorthorns, Devons, Aberdeen-Angus were all brought in to improve the native stock. In the Argentine, agriculture had been neglected in the Spanish way; this led to a wheat shortage in the 1870s in a country capable, even then, of exporting several million tons a year. In that same decade, the last of the Indian wars cleared the Plate pampas, and huge areas were sold, feral cattle and horses included, to largely English and American settlers for £80 per sq. 'league' of 6,669 acres. This amounted to less than 3d. per acre.

One second son of a Gloucestershire landlord bought £10,000 worth of this land in 1882. This amounted to over 323,760 hectares (800,000 acres), or over 1,250 sq. miles. On this land were an estimated 6,000 cattle, 10,000 horses, not a fence or hedge in sight. There were more than 400 Indian families living off the cattle and horses. The 'native' grasses, of course, were Iberian. The introduction of alfafa (lucerne), British grasses, European cereals, bred strains of maize brought in from the United States, transformed the situation. The Indians went to work as agricultural workers and cowboys. The cattle were thinned and improved; the horses transformed by careful choice of stallions, a railway built to a central wheat silo. Wheat, beef and live horses were exported. By 1910, the property contained five towns, roads, railways, electricity generation, hundreds of miles of road. It was sold to a meat-packing company on the death of the childless pioneer. In one of the towns was to be born the unrepeatable Eva Perón.

It was Eva's husband who brought the export trade of the Argentine to an end. In 1930, the country was the sixth richest in the world. A combination of low primary prices, war and, above all, bad government, made the Argentine twentieth in order in 1960. In 1985 the country was deep in debt. Perón had greatly assisted the process. Beef was eaten at home, rather than exported. Urbanization and secondary industries were much encouraged. Voters were bribed by competitive political parties. Brutal regimes stifled enterprise as well as inhibited freedom. The social stability which existed in Australia and New Zealand was absent in the Argentine. The English have no doubt as to why this should be. In the essential English Common Law, the Anzac countries follow the United States; they are themselves in other matters. Argentinos are over 95 per cent excitable, carnivorous, unEnglish. Peronista law was arbitrary, corrupt, commercially impossible.[27]

There is another non-racial reason. The population density of Australia is 2 people per sq. km, that of the Argentine is 10. The agricultural production of the Argentine is far less per unit area than the Australian. Australia, the lucky country, is far richer in natural resources, has minerals beyond the dreams of the Argentine. Argentine urbanization is expensive, unconvincing in economic terms. Though 'new Australians' come from every country in Southern Europe, the population is much more homogeneous than the Argentinos, and Australia does not have a majority of indigenous people resentful of a much richer Europe-oriented class. When the European dominance, especially English dominance, of Argentine agriculture was brought to an end in the late 1940s, progress ceased. There have been no advances since comparable to those in Europe, the United States, Australia and New Zealand. The agriculture of the Argentine is now backward. Concentration on the urban proletariat, and its perceived needs, is as damaging as the same policy in third world countries.

The failure of the Argentine, the most populous Southern Hemisphere neo-Europe,[28] should be compared with New Zealand, the most homogeneous neo-European country. The population of New Zealand is only 3.5 million, with a density of 12 per sq. km, compared with over 5,000 for Hong Kong, 30 for the continental United States, 360 for

England.[29] The prognosis for New Zealand is good. Low population density combines with unpolluted, fragrant, productive countryside, efficient industry. Even the restrictive practices of twenty years ago have been curbed. Racial problems are less onerous than those of Australia; much less onerous than those of the United States; few whites or Maoris really resent intermarriage, which is the key to racial harmony.

A secure agricultural base in a country once intellectually insecure made it, only a hundred years old in 1940, the then richest nation in the world. Since then, other countries have become richer as evaluated by the United Nations. The change in the world agricultural scene since 1960 has been a challenge. The challenge has been met and been turned into an opportunity.

The mild, equality-conscious, social security-minded New Zealanders have surprised themselves. Like other countries who have survived the Forces of Change, the New Zealanders have proved that when the going gets tough, the tough get going. Like that of Australia, the New Zealand Labour Party has abolished its belief in planning, embraced the free market, welcomed 'Thatcherite' reforms. Such a turnaround indicates at the very minimum, a vigorous political culture. It may also represent the renewal of the Left, conscious of the failure of socialism.

In one other neo-European Southern Hemisphere country, socialism has never entered the equation. South Africa, unlike Canada, the Argentine, Australia and New Zealand, has never produced any form of socialism in any kind of party. It has a long and complicated history, which in 1910 found the Union of South Africa in the British Empire. This lasted fifty years, until Harold Macmillan, in 1960, made his 'wind of change' speech in Cape Town. A few months later, South Africa left the Commonwealth.

For two centuries after its 'discovery' by the Portuguese in 1487, South Africa was little more than a barren shoreline, an inconvenient land to be rounded, with a few natural harbours. Cape Town slowly became a stop for water; and food and refreshment at a later stage, being occupied by forty-nine Dutchmen from 1654. By 1700, there were about 1,500 Dutch and French Huguenots in the Cape. At that time, there were only about 50,000 Bushmen and Hottentots west of what is now the Fish River. Eastwards, in modern Natal, the Orange Free State and Transvaal, there were as many as, perhaps, a million settled, cattle-raising Bantu, living on both slopes of the Drakensburg.

As is known, the Dutch were pushed north by the British, and then defeated by them. In 1902, when 'peace' arrived, there were probably 1.2 million whites, outnumbered by nearly 4 million Bantu, and half a million Cape Coloured and Indians.

South Africa is a country tormented, not only by hatred and apartheid, but by the force of population growth. If there is any wickedness in the tragedy, there is also the force of the importance of human population increase. In the middle of all the sharp political debate, it is worth noting that South Africa is at the limit of all but the best possible agricultural husbandry. Like its black-ruled neighbours, it only needs a little 'bad luck' to go hungry.

By the time of the Union in 1910, the white population was about 1,200,000. Today, it is rather less than four times the 1910 figure. In 1910, the non-white population was about 4.6 million; today it is about six times the 1910 figure. By 2000 it is likely that there will be 5.5 million whites; perhaps as many as 40 million non-whites, perhaps more. The absolute and relative increase is significant enough, and does much to explain the 'laager' mentality of the stubborn whites.

Political concentration upon the evils of apartheid has obscured the very real demographic problems. The white population increase is of the order of 1 per cent, that of the non-whites at least twice as great. Non-white birth-rates have fallen from a high of over 4.5 per cent in the 1950s to the present level of about 3.5 per cent. Non-white infant mortality is higher than that of the whites. But an increase of 2 per cent a year, unmatched by agricultural increase and investment, is likely to cause serious trouble by the end of the century.

Two per cent a year means a doubling every thirty-five years. It is unlikely that South Africa can double her agricultural production at present-day relative prices, or perform any comparable miracle. As to providing the capital for jobs for between 500,000 and 750,000 who come on to the job market each year, that is another challenge. South Africa's mineral wealth depends heavily on cheap coal, without which many gold mines would be unprofitable. In turn, all the minerals, coal, gold, copper, uranium and diamonds depend on cheap food. South African yields of maize and European cereals are up to world standards on white farms, using as they do tractors, modern implements, hybrid or pedigree seed, fertilizers, pest control, irrigation, and so forth. On the overcrowded little patches of land in the Bantu homelands, 'yield' is another matter altogether. Output is not properly measured, grain being grown for subsistence only. The homelands, of course, do not feed many 'workers', but only men, women and children not working in South Africa proper. The homelands have a population density many times greater than the white areas. It is this lesser known fact which is at least as important as the segregation of black workers in places like Soweto.

Even if apartheid were abolished overnight, and an earthly paradise established, the same danger would exist as it does in other third world countries: overconcentration on the town, promotion of uneconomic industries, low prices for farm products, agricultural under-production and lots of rural 'bad luck'. This has led to poor performance in every African country except South Africa itself. In each of the others, of course, there are special factors much cited by apologists. The truth remains that in any foreseeable political future, South Africa has to depend upon an industrial base founded on mineral wealth. Both are dependent in turn upon food supplies increasing faster than population. This is unlikely to happen.

One of the features of the colonial phase of many third world countries was that subsistence was left to the natives to work out for themselves while the expertise of Europeans was applied to export crops. This argument has been much deployed by anti-Imperialists in the United States of America. They are not always conscious, of course, that the same criteria exist in Latin America, operating for the benefit of American consumers. One great country, amongst all the developing nations, has probably done more than most to lift itself by its own bootstraps. That country is India.

There was, of course, a long way to go. India is less fortunate than most countries in its climate, in its huge area of land unsuitable for cultivation, in the high proportion of suitable land already in arable, in the tendency of the main human cultures to be fatalistic. India's density of population is the same as the whole of the United Kingdom, 250 per sq. km (97 sq. miles). Unlike the UK, Indian population, and therefore density, is increasing at more than 2 per cent per annum. Before Independence, population growth was only about 1.3 per cent, but food production was growing at less than this figure. Indian nationalists claim that this was because of concentration upon the export sector. As the chief exports of India in the first fifty years of this century were inedible: jute, cotton, raw and manufactured, tea, and until 1908, opium, this argument is unconvincing. The chief agricultural exports since Independence in 1947 have been, surprise, surprise, the same.[30]

Early Indian plans for the reinvigoration of the country after several centuries of European dominance were based on an industrial sector, especially a heavy industrial sector. This plan poured capital into capital-intensive plant at the expense of less capital intensive consumer goods and with a static farm sector. In years of bad luck or bad weather, 1958, 1967, 1973, India had to rely on foreign aid merely to maintain basic food levels in the villages which had failed to grow enough to subsist, as in the European Middle Ages. In good years, 1950, 1955, 1962, 1965, 1971, the situation looked much more optimistic; the talk both inside and outside

India was of surpluses (even exports) and the world food situation was viewed in a more favourable hue. This rosy perspective lasted until the next bad year. The swings between good and bad years were beyond the ability of storage to cope, being of the order of 25 per cent of average. Losses during storage and distribution, from India's host of rodent and insect pests was rather high, perhaps as much as 30 per cent. Not enough care, attention and imagination were being applied to agriculture. This was all characteristically socialist, and the same faults have occurred in this century in every 'planned' economy, of whatever type. The mistake has universally been a failure of recognition. A strategy which encourages the industrial sector is only valid if the agricultural area produces a sufficient surplus to feed the industrial worker. In the event of crop failure, or food shortage, the industrial sector may fare worse than the peasants. If this is reversed by the planners, the peasants object to food which they have grown being taken away from them and their families. This has happened all over the developing world. The behavioural forecasts of university economists are not always foolproof.

India's increase in food production has gone through several stages. The first, immediately after Independence, was to increase the traditional irrigation and apply more fertilizer. There was a huge programme of drilling wells all over India, to irrigate land to increase rice production. Rice increased in total yield by about a quarter in the first decade of independence, wheat by rather less. Much emphasis was placed upon a so-called 'Community Development Programme'. This produced far less yield increase than better irrigation, more fertilizer, more labour applied to more land in cultivation.

The only social or political change whose benefit could be measured was the abolition of the zamindari system of tax collection. The zamindar was a traditional, pre-British tax farmer, operating in Bengal. For reasons of administrative convenience, the British made these tax farmers virtually landlords. They were also turned into a hereditary class, and the zamindari system was imposed on other areas of India. To the British, who nominally always arranged the level of theoretical tax assessment, the system seemed just. To the Indian peasant, subjected to pressure from the zamindar, who might combine moneylending with tax collection, the whole system was corrupt, crudely unfair, and the zamindars had often become a privileged group of virtual landlords of large estates. The peasants, meanwhile, were in debt servitude.

More important than any political or economic 'planning' was the arrival of the so-called Green Revolution. This was based on new varieties of cereals capable of benefiting from more moisture, more fertilizer and making better use of both. This technology had been developed outside

Europe and the neo-Europes in some countries: Japan, for one. In the
1960s, it became a 'revolution' in many others. In India, the first harvest
after the drought of 1968 showed an increase of nearly 30 per cent in grain
production. Because rice is more difficult to hybridize than wheat, the
impact of new varieties has been much less in the irrigated portion of
Indian arable agriculture. Today, irrigation, always a strong point in
India, approaches one hectare for every three planted to food grains. This
usually means rice. The other grains are, in order of tonnage, sorghum,
millet and wheat. It is in wheat that the most impressive increases in
productivity have been made, as in the first world. Indian wheat yields per
hectare are now ahead of those in the Soviet Union, about a third of those
in Western Europe. There is in most years a wheat surplus in India,
available for export. Many opportunities exist to double-crop in India, the
limitations being fertilizer for each crop, and fuel for the irrigation pumps.
There is one time bomb ticking away as in all third world countries,
however well the economy appears to be managed.

Peasants can be satisfied with, say 220 kg (500 lb) of grain per head per
year. Of this, 80 per cent (176 kg/400 lb) would be eaten as cereal products.
The rest, a modest 20 per cent, would be eaten as the product of
domesticated animals, milk, butter, eggs, meat, etc. In India, as in every
other country, the rich eat as well as the same sort of people in the first
world. Such people eat more than a ton of grain a year – only 10 per cent as
cereals directly, pasta, bread and breakfast cereal, and 90 per cent as
converted by animals. The difference in food consumption between the
rich person in Bombay and the average European or neo-European is
minimal. The difference between the film director in Bombay and his
fellow countryman, the peasant on the Plains, is very great. The peasant
eats much less.

The modern history of eating has always been that the rich prefer
meat, eggs, milk and so forth, and as soon as they have more money, all
people have eaten more grain, not as grain, but converted by domestic
animals.

The trick is to prevent the majority of peasants in poor countries eating
like the majority of farmers in Europe or neo-Europes. This rationing by
price means that, of India's 750 million people, 700 million poor each
consume, say, about 0.25 ton per head per year. The 50 million richer
Indians consume, say, a ton per head per year. This means a total
requirement of 225 million tons a year. If even half the 'poor' consumed at
the rate of the 'rich', the requirement would rise from 225 million tons a
year to 487.5 million tons. If, more reasonably, only 1 per cent of the 'poor'
switched from being 'poor' at 0.25 ton per year to being 'rich' at 1 ton

per year, that would mean an extra 5.25 million tons a year. This is more than the extra grain, 4 million tons, needed each year to deal with the extra population. The extra population ratio is well understood. If, as in India, there are about 2.1 per cent extra people each year, and 2.8 per cent extra grain each year, happiness results. If the two figures are reversed, there is hunger, starvation, famine.

India, and a hundred other countries, including the USSR, depend upon the population not changing its habits too much. That means not allowing the peasant sector too much money to buy goodies like milk, meat and eggs. On the other hand, if the peasants are not given enough money, they don't produce, and deliveries fall. This has happened throughout the Eastern bloc, and in most of Africa. In China, the rulers have realized, since 1979, that the peasants have got to be energized by the market. Since that date, in the last ten years, the Chinese peasant has had the highest sustained increase in productivity in the world, 12 per cent per year; Chinese food increases per annum now comfortably exceed the Indian, having lagged for thirty years after 1948, because of civil war, revolution, and other political problems.

This time bomb apart, India seems well set to emulate Western Europe and the neo-Europes, where the 'Green Revolution' (so-called) has been going on for the last generation and a half, since the turnaround in the world food situation which started in the 1950s. It has been an evolution-ary process, not a revolution. The momentum of evolution may be maintained rather better than that of a revolution. There is no reason to believe that India should not be able to improve its position by a significant proportion each year. There remains plenty of room for improvement, especially in low-level control measures, village pest control, or interdic-tion against field ruminants, small birds, or insects. Pests still take more than 30 per cent of the potential crop, far more than in China. It has always been hard to persuade farmers that to control pests is an easier way to increase yields than any other. Indians are no exception.

America and Europe were agriculturally completely different a century ago; the inexorable forces of change have made the pattern of development such as to make the two continents much more similar.

A century ago, American agriculture was characterized by four virtues. First, inputs to farms were cheap, far cheaper than in Europe; land, of course, was far less expensive, but so were farm implements, animals, even taxes. Ultimately this arose from the very low density of population in the United States compared to Western Europe.

Secondly, output prices were necessarily much higher in relation to input prices than in Europe. Put another way, because of the low cost of inputs, value added (however measured) was much higher in America than in Europe.

Thirdly, land tenure, which was usually ownership-plus-mortgage allowed for technologically advanced methods to be adopted. In areas where there were sharecropping agreements, or British-style tenancies or other forms of long lease, innovation was much less likely to be pursued. In Europe, until recently, landlords determined farming methods in a way which Americans would generally have regarded as bizarre.

Finally, the American system of freedom of information was virtually unique in the agricultural world in 1876. 'Cow' colleges, financed by the land grants in the Morrill Act of 1862, widely advertised genuine research; there were also magicians and medicine men not much better than snake-oil salesmen. From this system grew the tradition, now universal in the first world, whereby farmers, alone of all producers, exchange information in a way unknown in mining or transport or manufacture. Most farmers today do not resent other farmers knowing the secret of their success.[31]

There were crises throughout the century. The cause of the crisis is always the same, whether it occurs in 1873, 1893, 1907 or in the 1920s. Agricultural production is elastic. Demand for food is not. This means that if food output increases by X per cent, food prices decline by more than X per cent. In order to offset a loss in total income, farmers who can afford to do so, increase total output. This has the effect of increasing total production of food, and the price inexorably declines further. During the 1920s, food prices declined in real terms by more than any farmer's ability to cope. By 1933, farmgate prices were only 20 per cent of what they had been in 1920. Whether the Great Depression was partially caused by the previous dozen years of low agricultural prices will be debated for years.

Before the 1920s and 1930s, in then less developed countries such as France, Italy or Germany, lower prices at the farmgate were not so devastating as in the neo-Europes. Peasants did not have to buy many inputs. Capital inputs such as machinery could be deferred. Animals were bred on the farm; food for the family could be grown at home; workers could be paid in kind or dismissed; fertilizer was generated in the course of the ordinary rotations, and by the preservation of animal residues. Cash was used by peasants for luxuries, not necessities. If there was no cash, retrenchment was in order. This happened in Europe whenever the growth in agricultural output exceeded the growth of population. After the railroads, the steamships and the refrigerated vessels, it was not only local agricultural output that affected prices in Europe; the output of every neo-Europe fed into the world-wide system. Whatever countries tried to do to insulate themselves against price changes in other places, in the end, economics could not be defeated. Nevertheless, European peasant communities were often much better able to sustain a slump than the industrial workers in the towns. At minimum, unless incompetent, they fed themselves. Many European peasant families went without coffee when times were hard, but they were better nourished than townspeople.

In the United States, in the 1930s, such an outcome was impossible. Every farm was part of a much wider network, which a generation later would be called 'agri-business'. This involved farm machinery, motor vehicles, electricity in all its forms, fertilizers and chemicals, petroleum, water, gas, textiles, metal, rubber, glass, wood and paper and plastic products. There was a huge and rising service element involved. There was the whole complex business of getting the food to the consumer's mouth. These trades, obviously, could not be allowed to go bankrupt. The farmer was saved in the United States because he was part of a much wider network. In much of Europe, and in most of the rest of the world, the self-sufficient peasant retrenched. Such an outcome was impossible in Western Europe, as well as the United States, which had to make the same kind of provisions for agricultural support.

Whatever it was called, the pattern was to set up compensatory devices. These devices gave the farmer more compensation for his product than he would have received from the market. Whether called 'guarantees' or 'subsidies' or 'controls', the devices worked in the same way, in the United States, Canada, Australia, New Zealand, South Africa, and in some other countries. In Britain, the devices were not properly in place until World War II. In Latin America, their absence did much to destroy the viability of the commercial agriculture of countries like the Argentine, Chile, Mexico or Brazil.

In the United States, farmers were paid to reduce the area planted to specific products. Storage facilities were built, and loan programmes instituted to regulate the rate at which products came on to the market. Sometimes the methods were bizarre: little pigs destroyed, grain burnt in industrial boilers, cotton piled up to rot. Meanwhile, other people, even in the United States, were hungry, or suffered from malnutrition, or could not clothe themselves properly. By the end of the 1930s, the United States agricultural support programmes had reached a generally acceptable level of activity. This raised compensation for the farmer, while controlling output at a level which neither forced up prices too much, nor meant that a great deal of surplus production had to be destroyed.[32]

World War II changed the agricultural scene throughout the world. A combination of shortages and of fragmented transport made discrete areas of Western Europe very hungry by VE Day; left to themselves, the inhabitants would have been even more hungry for the next five years. In

Eastern Europe, the combination of mindless Nazi brutality and calculated Communist social engineering made for starvation, famine even, rather than hunger. More people died from shortage of food, and the consequence diseases, in the East in the period 1941–8 than were killed in battle. Some, of course, were meant to die. These were Jews, or some of the middle classes, or any non-Communist who could not escape or make peace with the new rulers. No one will ever know the full tally. Nor will anyone ever know which of the two totalitarian regimes killed more people.

Outside Europe, disruption of transport and other infrastructures made for hunger and famine throughout Asia. India was badly affected, both because there was a shortage of shipping and a shortage of rail transport within India. China went into a long period of darkness resulting from the Japanese War, followed by the Civil War and later by the confusion of the Great Leap Forward (1937–72). None of these disruptions, nor the nationalization of farms, did a great deal for the hungry or starving. In Japan itself, rations for the natives in 1945–8 were down to about two-thirds of what they were in the 1930s. There were pockets of surplus due to poor transport. Australia and New Zealand could not export all they produced. In the Argentine, meat consumption was double that of 1938. Farms only a few score miles from big towns in France would be flush with food which could not be distributed. In Germany there was no civilian railway or road into Berlin passable in the summer of 1945; and deficit areas in the big towns in occupied Western Germany were as hungry as Holland had been a year before. Yet some farmers in Bavaria were living as well as ever, conducting barter deals with the occupying forces. There was some effort in democratic Europe to honour a relatively fair rationing system. Only in Communist countries was food used as an overt political weapon. The commissar fed well, as did the army and the secret police. Heavy workers and the 'productive' were reasonably well fed, if bored. Those the regime regarded as unnecessary were half-starved. In some countries, a thriving parallel, or 'free' or black market existed. There were strange currencies, preferred to the often worthless paper: cigarettes in Germany, petrol coupons in France, olive oil in Italy. The prudent neither smoked, nor used a car, nor cooked with oil. Very surprising fortunes were made by the abstemious.[33]

The political masters of the Western World at the end of World War II saw food shortage as one of the great failings. Such a belief was justified. There were great dislocations of normal channels of distribution and supply in almost every country in Europe, and in much of Africa and Asia. Perhaps the food supply of as many as half the humans alive in 1945 had been adversely affected by the War. There was a serious shortage of shipping, especially specialized ships such as refrigerated cargo–liners. Furthermore, areas of surplus had been prejudiced by the long slump in demand which had existed for twenty years before 1940. Even the United States, for the first time in history, had a marginal deficit between domestic food available and optimum food requirements. This was only between 1935 and 1940, and was primarily due to New Deal restrictions on farm output. As soon as the administration knew what was happening, the fault was corrected. The deficit was largely expressed by malnutrition amongst the poor and unemployed, rather than by any propensity to import food from other countries. None of the efforts of the politicians would have had any serious effect upon the world food shortage without advances in three areas of science and technology. All of these, in the end, derived from work done in other areas, often in pursuit of success in war. Almost literally, swords were beaten into ploughshares.

These advances derived directly from engineering, chemistry, and biology. In engineering, the very greatly improved metallurgy, machine-tool technology and batch production methods which had made possible tanks, aircraft and guns in huge numbers also produced cheap, effective and widely available tractors and implements. Internal combustion tractors had been used for nearly fifty years before 1950, but they were quite literally tractors. That is, they towed implements, mostly horse-type implements. Following the work of Harry Ferguson and others, the word 'tractor' became a misnomer. After 1950, 'tractors' more generally carried implements, not towed them. The design of the new implements was novel; so was the ability to control them by limiting draft, or depth of work, or wheel-slip, or horsepower applied, or by a combination. The power take-off made possible new implements driven directly from the tractor. These technical improvements were massive, far greater in effect than the substitution of the tractor-which-towed for the horse-which-towed. Such advances were only made possible because of cheap and effective hydraulics, derived from the wartime aircraft industry, new, cheaper and better steel mixtures originally brewed for war purposes, and the mass production of thousands of parts for tractors and implements. These were more precisely built than cars, and with the same advantages of meticulous assembly that had been needed for rifles, guns and armoured vehicles. Even simple nuts and bolts manufactured in 1955 were cheaper and far better than the same nuts and bolts manufactured in 1935.

The second great improvement was chemical and also derived from war. Fertilizer manufacture, in particular nitrogen manufacture, was a direct derivative from wartime explosives. Phosphate and potash became cheap and widely available because of mass handling techniques which derived, again, from the same elements as those which gave post-war tractors their competence: hydraulics, high grade machine parts, the use of special metals to deal with difficult materials. The end-user product was no longer a simple chemical, ground into a powder, with varying effects upon the long-term nature of the soil. Post-war fertilizers were often available as compounds of all three major chemicals, or with 'trace elements' added; straight nitrogen became available to fit particular needs. There were quick acting, or long-term, slow release forms of nitrogen; particular care was taken with the effect upon soil acidity, almost an unregarded after-effect in the 1930s. Fertilizers generally became notably easier to handle.

Derived directly from the war gases were the early 'miraculous' selective weedkillers. These attacked, for example, broad-leaved weeds and left alone the crop, which might be wheat, or barley, or grass, all of which were not susceptible to the weedkiller which liberated the European farmer from the red poppy or the yellow charlock. Once upon a time these had been inevitable in any field of winter or spring grain respectively. Other weedkillers quickly followed, for pests all over the world.[34]

Following weedkillers came fungicides to prevent the inevitable effects of excessive damp weather, or drought or too much nitrogen. Then came the even more controversial insecticides, which killed the beneficial ladybird as well as the aphid, or the beautiful, harmless butterfly as well as the bugs and beetles in the soil or on the plant.[35]

The combination of high nitrogen usage with the parallel advantages of pest control raised yields in the first world countries from a base in 1945–6 lower than pre-War to three to four times the output of the 1930s by 1970. Since the techniques have become widely known, an annual increase in yield has become possible; this is currently in the range of 2–3 per cent per annum, over rolling five year periods. None of this would have been possible without the further skills of plant breeding.

The integrated possibilities of new varieties capable of high growth rates had to await the presence of optimum water, plant food and pesticides. This has only been developed recently. Before the other elements were in place, the breeding of dwarf wheats or dense rice would not have met any of the local requirements. These were the same as they had been for centuries. A genotype, as in neolithic times, would be selected by local conditions, and less critically, by mankind, in each generation, and preserved for the next sowing. This process, carried out over 5,000 years or more, has produced, for example, about 30,000 kinds of rice. These have been collected by geneticists and used as a bank of source material for scientific analysis and propagation.

The rules of inheritance were first formulated by a yeoman farmer's son, then monk, then Abbott of Brunn, Gregor Mendel. Mendel, working with sweetpeas, had first arrived at the correct answers in the 1860s. The rules were rediscovered in the early 1900s. A shy, modest man, Mendel did not trumpet abroad what would one day be common currency. The work he did on the mode of inheritance of single pairs of alternative characteristics gave the world what is basically known about hybrids, dominant and recessive characteristics, and most of the science of genetics. If Mendel had not been an Austrian Augustinian monk, but a less humble man, he would have achieved in his lifetime the same kind of fame that was Darwin's. Their discoveries bind them together in a seamless robe.[36]

By 1945, the principles of hybridization and hybrid vigour were well known, and much work had been done in the United States on maize, and in various European countries on other grains. The hybrid methods of breeding require great resources, a huge data bank of original material and much time. The original material will have derived from the natural selection in a particular place which favours the development of certain characteristics. In most 'native' situations, nitrogen is in short supply, and in tropical soils, nitrogen is in more severe shortage than in temperate climates. In tropical heat nitrogen leaches, or vapourizes, and is used up more quckly than in cooler climates. So an increase in the rice or wheat crop in hot climates requires more nitrogen than the traditional ecotypes can use without the straw becoming weak and 'lodging'. So the solution to the third world food shortage was sought, in a large way, by hybridizing tropical rice and wheats. This work started in the 1950s.

Ultimately, this effort becomes a matter of numbers. The more lines hybridized, the more crosses made, the more chance there is of finding an outstanding answer to the problem. The first great result was in rice, and the result of eight years' work. This was a rice called, without fanfare, IR8. It was created by crossing Peta, a tall Indonesian rice with vigorous growth, with a Taiwanese dwarf variety. To achieve IR8, 10,000 other hybrids were rejected. Obviously, the numbers game is important. The International Rice Institute now has a gene-bank of 30,000 wild or cultivated, but unbred ecotypes. From these can be bred, in theory, new hybrids which can use water more efficiently, or take up nitrogen, or resist lodging, or contend successfully with disease or parasites. The yield, for example, of IR8, using 100 kg of nitrogen per hectare, is double that of one parent and three times that of the other. Some 'green revolution' hybrid grains can yield four times the original native ecotype. This is only because they can usefully use up to 150 kg per hectare of nitrogen. Such a fertility level would never occur in nature, and causes many problems in 'native' races of grain: lodging, excessive vegetative growth, huge leaf areas, fungus attack, other disease problems. What is true for rice is true for wheat, barley, oats, rye, maize and any other grain.

Obviously, the addition of 'artificial' nitrogen to the available plant food upsets the whole balance of soil nutrients; any additional nitrogen has to be accompanied by the necessary phosphate and potash and trace elements to balance the equation. Susceptibility to disease and parasites can be reduced by plant-breeding programmes. It may be cheaper to use fungicides and insecticides as a routine measure, and to concentrate plant-breeding effort on those genes which produce the highest yield. But the use of a given variety of wheat or barley in the first world will also be subject to another restraint; for more than two generations, Mendel's method of hybrid plant breeding has been used. In the United States, the maize programme begun in the 1920s was followed by cereal programmes in Europe in the next decade. The work of the Rockefeller Foundation in Mexico began in 1943, and proved that first world agricultural technology was transferable. In all these areas, it has been found that hybrids lose their vigour after a few years. With wheat in Europe, the time can be as short as two years, as long as six. In barley, lifespans in Europe have been longer, up to ten years, before a breakdown occurs. In maize, the time can be longer again, in grasses, longer still. There is opportunity for 'reselection' but the true hybrid cannot be guaranteed without recourse to a plant breeding institute. Left to a mere farmer, without the infrastructure provided by the men in white coats, most modern varieties would revert, relapse, or suffer from gene-decay. In fact, it was one of the most salutary lessons ever dealt out to plant breeders, when it was discovered that certain 'resistant' varieties became susceptible to 'new' races of fungoid disease. No one but a fungologist could tell whether the disease was really 'new' or just previously unrecognized.

The same general Mendellian rules, applied to cereals and grasses, are now used in animal breeding. Many animals are too slow, at a maximum of one generation a year, to produce results. But chicken and pigs have offered the same opportunities to the geneticist as do the plants. Commercial chickens and pigs in the advanced countries are now tailored hybrids and the original basic stocks from which the hybrids were derived are now 'endangered species'.[37] Sheep, to some extent, have been improved by establishing new, stabilized hybrids to act as dams or sires, comparable to long-term successes such as half-breeds.[38] In cattle, the generation span stretches out to at least 24–30 months. This is too long-term for the establishment of hybrids. The advance here has been limited to the use of semen instead of a live bull, and the upgrading of the whole national herd in most countries of Europe and neo-Europe. The use of artificial insemination has done more for milk and beef production in the United Kingdom, for example, than any effort other than the science of nutrition in relation to economic production. There are three dangers involved. All of them would have been unthinkable fifty years ago.

The first problem is that successful cultivars tend to come from a very few families: Western European wheats come from only a dozen families; sugar cane from four, coffee from three. A new cry has developed for 'biological diversity' as an antidote to excessive kinship. Genetic vulnerability was seen as a major threat to crops throughout the world. The experience of the kind of problem which might arise on a world scale was familiar to every 'progressive' modern Western farmer. He used, say, a 'new' variety of wheat in the 1960s. By 1970, this wheat was seen to be host to a 'new' race of the fungus *septoria*. Such a fungus made the use of fungicide obligatory. Such fungicides might have to be applied five or six times in the season. No matter that no one had ever heard of this particular race of *septoria* ten years previously. A generation before, few people outside the charmed circle of microbiology had even heard of *septoria* of any kind. By 1970, the particular wheat had become, in the plant–breeder's term, 'outclassed'. By 1975, elaborate patterns were recommended to plant wheats, and other cereals, in varietally mixed sowings. This was called 'Varietal diversification to reduce risk of fungus attack'. The irony that a mixture of one grain from each of six different varieties would produce a mongrel harvest was not lost upon plant breeders. At least, each of the six varieties was well bred in itself.

The second problem was that the 'new' varieties could only perform with the use of considerable nitrogen input. This meant, of course, that the drains were more or less full of unused raw nitrates. By 1980, this had become a clear health problem in parts of both Europe and the United States. Raw nitrates, ingested in the drinking water, are unpleasant for the population at large, dangerous for the young. It was a form of pollution of the very basis of modern life: clean water. More vital, in the long run, was perhaps the obvious fact that at some point in time, nitrogen, the cost of which was linked to the price of oil in the world market, would become both more expensive and more difficult to obtain. A green revolution which was sustainable as well as more productive would obviously have more value in the future than one which is wholly dependent upon infinite supplies of a commodity which most authorities expect to be in very short supply within fifty years. This shortage of nitrogen will also coincide with what looks, at the moment, like a further doubling of the world population.

The third problem is consequent upon development of bred strains of grain or grass which need both high levels of fertilizers as well as other

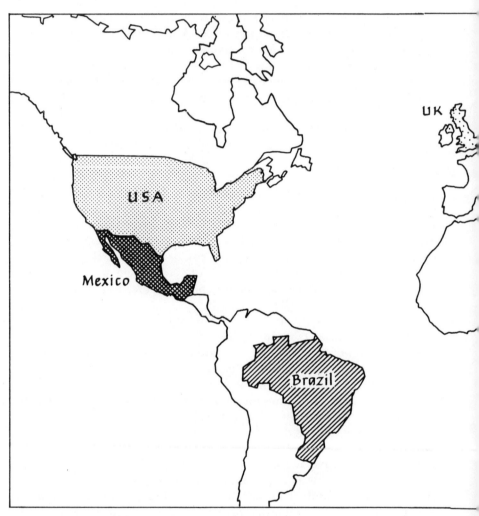

The World
Showing Slow and Rapid Growth Countries

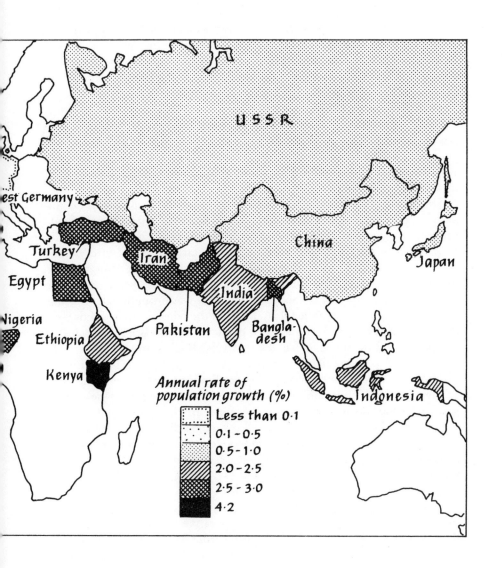

Annual rate of
population growth (%)

	Less than 0·1
	0·1 – 0·5
	0·5 – 1·0
	2·0 – 2·5
	2·5 – 3·0
	4·2

chemical inputs. More than half the cost of growing a crop may now be in seeds, fertilizers, other chemicals, as well as the cost of application. While the relationship between the cost of inputs and harvest value remains constant, no problem exists. But if commodity prices fall, as they tend to do if productivity increases, then the farmer or peasant is squeezed. The cost of inputs remains constant, or rises: the value of the harvest falls. The farmer, or peasant, may find that work is in vain. The crop makes a loss, and does not, in some cases, even cover the cost of the farmer's labour. All the farmer has done, in that immortal phrase, is 'to work for the bank'.

There are strong reasons why this state of affairs should not continue. The opportunities offered by genetic engineering are rather great. Working on the principles of Mendellian mathematics, and enlightened by the chemistry of the Double Helix, the biotechnicians can now see much to alter the whole nature of crop husbandry. By the end of the century, even more will be possible.[39]

The world is only about ten years away from the commercial exploitation of DNA transfer. This would mean 'designing' a plant which would provide its own nitrogen as do clovers. A wheat plant that had the ability to produce 4 tons per acre/10 tons per hectare of grain without any nitrogen would solve as many problems as it created. Supposing the men in white coats added the ability to resist fungi, so the plant needed no fungicide; while they were about it, a repellent was brought in from some other plant, and added to the DNA/RNA of the wheat so that aphids were discouraged. The farmer now has a plant which needs no nitrogen, no fungicide, no insecticide. What about weeds? Well, some plants have the capacity to discourage all but their own species near them. It is the method provided by nature for slow-growing seedlings to survive in the shadow of their parent. This could be provided so that nothing but wheat could grow near the wheat plant. What other pests are there? Rodents, for one. Could they be as deterred as are the insects? Probably. What about weather, which is as great an imponderable as exists anywhere? Suppose the biological engineers attacked the Russian weather problem, which is that there is too little rain in May and early June, too much in July and August. How about one of two courses?

A grain could be developed to be planted in May, and need fewer growing days than most wheat. If this putative wheat needed no more days than the average Western European spring barley, it could be bred to be ripe in 120 days, or sown on 10 May, and harvested on or after 10 September, after the worst of the summer rains. Alternatively, the plant could be designed not to need a great deal of moisture until it was 'fully-jointed' as the expression is, with the ear formed, and the grain ready to swell. This would be in July. This would be combined with an ability to stand a great deal of rain when the straw was at its full height, and at its weakest. Are these ideas fanciful, or 'impossible'? Not to anyone who realizes that the first wheat bred to the prescriptions laid down by Mendel was not commercially available much before 1913. The first European spring bread wheat to challenge winter wheats was not available before 1945. The first European winter barley to yield significantly more than spring barleys was not available before 1960. Within a generation, most of the advances described as 'possible' today will be commonplace. There will be a high cost.

The employment today in the industries which are going to be super-seded – the bulk petrochemicals, the fertilizer manufacture, transport and distribution, the pest control industry, the huge mechanical effort to spread fertilizer and chemicals on fields, and even the fuel needed to do this – all these resources will be unemployed, their workers having to find new jobs. It is hard to believe that all this effort will be contained in the genes of the seed which the farmer buys, and which he sows, properly, according to prescription, and then very largely neglects. Is this the type of husbandry by which farmers have been able to feed the world? Of course not. Nor are farmers unaware of the nature of this revolution. Apart from anything else, it will very greatly reduce the value of land as well as of chemical companies. More cost will be contained in the correct seed, correctly engineered, than in anything else. It is possible that seed might amount to more than half the cost of growing the crop. It is also possible that many crops will acquire the characteristic of today's soya bean husbandry. This does not permit much benefit from any effort which the farmer may put into the growing of the crop. There is little the farmer can do to influence soya bean yield. It may well be, in a generation, that this applies to nearly all crops. It is not a prospect which the average farmer welcomes. [40]

It is not necessary to discuss and deplore the genetic possibilities in the animal kingdom. It is the potential for creating horror which have attracted public attention to the future of genetic engineering. The nature of the positive potential is much easier to see amongst the flora than in the fauna. The great value of genetic engineering in crop husbandry is that the technology is absolutely transferable. At the moment, the Green Revolution depends upon first world seed, first world fertilizers, pest control and machines for their application. Farmers have to be trained to apply nitrogen and other fertilizers at the right time, to spray with fungicide and weedkillers at the right moment, to look after all the machinery involved, and to learn to care as much as a yeoman farmer in Western Europe, who has centuries of husbandry behind him. This is not easy to instil. [41]

But if the rice grower in Indonesia or the Philippines or Burma can be told to dispense with all that husbandry, and just plant the seed, at so many kg per hectare, then leave it? Is this not transferable technology at its finest? Is this not a gift from the first to the third world which will solve nearly all the possibilities of hunger, starvation, famine? Even the *teff* of the obstinate, attractive Ethiopians, could be engineered to survive the damage done by past generations.[42] The maize grown in Africa can now be tailored to the requirements of the individual microclimate, as can the wheat in India, the sorghum in Pakistan, the rice in Indo-China, the barley in Iraq. The potential ability of the world to feed itself does not appear to have been so bright at any time before the present. With famine avoided by technology, and most diseases under control, what is to prevent mankind doubling in population before 2035? The real killer, to which the world should now turn its urgent attention, is pollution.

For the cold-blooded demographer, writing at any time since the 1960s, there has always been a fairly simple proposition. At no time in history has population increase been known to survive beyond 'sustainable levels'. Always, in the past, war, with its disruptive potential, or disease, has solved the problem, or sheer numbers have exceeded food supplies. In other words, warfare, which directly and on its own has never killed very many, would be joined by its inevitable allies, disease and famine. These two could alternatively perform their role in peacetime once again as they have so often in the past. These associates, disease and famine, are much closer allies than war with either, and have been close friends for centuries, enjoying a special relationship.

The world now has a new condition. Warfare between major powers is so dangerous, because of nuclear capability, that war cannot be entertained as a solution to demographic problems. Disease is so much perceived as an 'enemy' that public opinion in those countries capable of medical technology would not countenance the slackening of the 'life-saving' effort. Global food supplies are no longer a problem, if mankind is sensible and applies effort in the right direction.[43] So what will happen? All previous population restraints have been swept away. The world will have to learn to live with these conditions.[44]

Twenty years ago, world population was 'only' about 3,500 million. Today, it is at least 50 per cent more. Twenty years ago, no one had ever heard of three globally important effects of overpopulation. These are the direct result of too many people consuming too many goods. Consumption makes it quite possible that pollution in peacetime will replace pollution by nuclear warfare as a real killer. These three effects of pollution are the greenhouse effect; acid rain; and ozone layer depletion. Twenty years ago, these phenomena did not even have names. Today, they are familiar problems to every concerned person.

Since the 1950s, world population has doubled. The per capita income of the people in the world has also doubled. The use of fossil fuels has more than quadrupled, intermittent crises notwithstanding. Though arable farm-land itself is not fully utilized in the world, except in Europe (88 per cent), Asia (83 per cent), it has proved to be cheaper to intensify than to bring virgin land suitable for arable into production.[45] This means the use of more fuel, in one form or another. The burning of fossil fuels has now reached between 12 and 14 billion tons of coal-equivalent per annum. This releases so much carbon dioxide (more than 5 billion tons a year) that it threatens to raise the temperature of the earth by the so-called 'greenhouse effect'.

The cost to agriculture of adapting to the new climates in which rainfall and temperature are unlike anything in the past could well exceed the profits being made from the overuse of fossile fuels. No one knows how much carbon the world can burn without danger. The figure is certainly below the present level. It could be as little as 6 billion tons a year of fossil fuel. This is about half the present 'burn'. Evidently, such a reduction could not be achieved without a massive increase in the use of nuclear energy. Yet the very people who now campaign most against nuclear energy are the same sort of people who ought to be concerned about the much greater dangers of fossil fuel. There is a great irony in the short-sighted 'ecology' of the anti-nuclear brigade. There is no merit of any kind in their intellectual blindness.[45]

Fossil fuels do not only create the greenhouse effect. They usually produce acid rain. Americans are very satisfied with the favourable results produced by checking automobile emissions. This effort, which costs several billion dollars a year, is as nothing compared with the costs involved in eliminating acid rain. The use of 'scrubbers' in power station chimneys needs, in some systems, a ton of limestone for every ton of coal or oil burnt, and another ton hauled away and dumped elsewhere. There are other systems, somewhat less demanding in the bulk involved. To check and reverse acid rainfall would probably require the reduction of the fossil burn to 6 billion tons and a clean exhaust campaign. This means that the world would have to plan to use an average of half of its present energy of all kinds. At the same time, it would be necessary to agree that the whole world would become a smokeless zone, in effect. The world would have to be more than smoke free; it would have to be acid-free as well.

Such an extreme programme would take a dozen years to put into effect, but time is running out. Acid rain is destroying far more forest in Europe than man is using. Lakes are being turned from a neutral base into acid water which will not support life. It is not impossible that some seas will follow the lakes. Once again, the chattering classes have not comprehended the problem. There is a great movement against the use of tropical hardwood in domestic situations in the first world. Wholly admirable. But far more important than window frames, panelled doors or loo seats in suburbia are acid rains in Europe which have already affected half West Germany's forest. Acid rain, however, is less of a giggle for the trendies. The cure is also more painful.[46]

Nor in the loo-seat class is the third evident new problem. It is the destruction of the ozone layer in the Arctic and Antarctic. Chlorofluorocarbons (CFCs) are released into the atmosphere all over the high-consuming world every time a refrigerator leaks, or an aerosol is used. At the time of its invention, CFC was seen as stable, not toxic, and not likely to decompose in the lower atmosphere and cause trouble where released. Instead, the compounds rise and reach the stratosphere. In most of the world, CFCs are dispersed by ultraviolet light over 22 km above the earth (above 14 miles up). The chemical compound breaks down into harmless chlorine which reacts with nitrogen oxides and water and becomes locked up as chlorine nitrate and hydrogen chloride, both harmless. Over the Poles, the chlorine reaction does not take place, and in turn, the CFC compounds are able to destroy the ozone layer. This appears only to affect the stratospheric layer at the two Poles. But a more worrying question is whether or not the total amount of ozone in the world is finite. If so, the use of aerosols, mostly for vain and wholly frivolous purposes, and the use of CFCs in refrigeration are likely to damage life on earth as badly as acid rain or the greenhouse effect. There is an even greater worry.

These three great threats to our environment were hardly in evidence ten years ago. As noted, they were unknown twenty years ago. Acid rain only appeared as an issue at the end of the 1970s. Hard evidence for the predicted warm-up due to the greenhouse effect did not convince any sceptic until the early 1980s. The ozone layer depletion at the South Pole is quite clearly dated at 1984 as far as firm statistical evidence is concerned. There are three great consequences of this timetable.

First there is the 'threshold' argument. Suddenly, this argument runs, something tips a problem overcentre and it becomes insoluble. The greenhouse effect took everyone by surprise; as did acid rain, noted by German foresters in the 1980s in areas which had been carefully managed for centuries. There was a more complete shock about the effect of CFCs upon the ozone layer[47]. These three problems have crept up upon scientists and tipped over into insolubility within a few years. What other horrors are likely to surprise the world, and will not reveal themselves until too late?

Secondly, since the evidence for the damage has only been forthcoming in the last few years, how old are the actions whose side-effects are now being witnessed? It is logical to assume that the effects of CFCs are now being felt, belatedly, in respect of what was used in the past. The same with 'greenhouse' CO_2 and acid rain. But how long in the past? Could these three problems be yet more legacies from the 1960s? If so, if all corrections were applied at once, when would the situation beneficially reverse itself? Not before the end of the century, obviously. 2010? Too soon. 2020? Too optimistic. 2030? Perhaps.

Two massive disasters took place inside a month in August 1988. Both could have been predicted; neither was unprecedented; both were aggravated by careless, selfish, unthinking management of land and water resources, over the medium term, and by political troubles over the short. They both occurred in areas of rather large increases in population.

Sudan is a country whose population has more than doubled since independence in 1956. But the nature of political tension between the Muslim north and the Christian (or Animist) south has meant near-civil war division in a country which is much poorer than under colonial rule. The plains around Khartoum are of impervious clay, nearly flat, and an excessive rainfall (as in 1946) has devastating results. Since 1946, the flood-plain around Khartoum itself has increased its population by five times, against a national average of rather more than twice. The drift to the city had been caused by the usual third world causes, under investment in agriculture, the best brains leaving the countryside, the government cheating rural workers of the fruits of their labour. Khartoum itself has become a largely shanty town, like many others, bloated in numbers, ruled by leaders long on promises, short on delivery. On this insecure, undrained, physically unstructured area fell two disasters. One was the effects of about 200 mm (8 in) of rain on sunbaked clay. The second was the flooding of the Blue Nile.

In both Sudan and Ethiopia, the search for fuel and animal food has meant more and more trees, shrubs, bushes cut down every year to cook human food and to keep alive domestic animals. It is not only mature forests which are destroyed in this manner, but almost every living plant is removed in some areas. If this de-afforestation and defoliation on tropical hillsides is followed by excessive rainfall, then run-off is accelerated, erosion is multiplied many times, the rivers raise the level of their beds, and break banks or flood low-lying land automatically. The results are far worse in the case of the Blue Nile, which rises in the highlands of Ethiopia. In the case of the White Nile, which also flows through Khartoum, any rise in flow is buffered by the huge swamp, bigger than Wales, called the Sudd, which lies between the highlands and Khartoum.

The second disaster was in Bangladesh. This country, once 'East Pakistan', was 'created' largely by India, not from any noble reasons, but to weaken West Pakistan. More than half Bangladesh is just above High Spring Tide Level, by a margin which rarely exceeds 10 metres (32 feet). Equally, half the country is only 3–12 metres (10–39 feet) above the bed of the rivers whose normal area forms more than a quarter of the country's total surface. A heavy monsoon used to be of great benefit. Water would be retained hundreds of miles upstream, in Nepal, Bhutan, Northern India, and even China. It would gradually seep out from wooded mountain valleys, and become the irrigation needed to grow three crops of rice a year in a country with the highest density of poor agricultural people on earth.

Every square metre of the surface of Bangladesh which it is possible to cultivate has been irrigated, and is needed. Bangladesh has more than 1000 people per square kilometer of arable land, more than 10 people per hectare, more than 4 people per acre. This is more serious than India's population problem, 500 people per hectare of arable land, rather more in China proper, and should be compared with 800 people per hectare of arable land in the Netherlands, the last in a country where only 10 per cent, at most, live by the land. In Bangladesh, the proportion is nearly reversed. Eighty per cent of the population is dependent upon the land and its products for their livelihood. Bangladesh has damaged herself in a classic third world way. Population was 29 million in 1900, 40 million in 1948, at the end of the Empire, nearly 100 million today.

The rest of the damage has been done by bad water management upstream on the Ganges and Bramaputra rivers; unmanaged run-off from monsoon rain can be guaranteed to cause disaster in a low-lying country. To make possible the kind of water-management enjoyed by the Netherlands would require the investment of between $50 and $100 billion over a 10-year period. It would also require proper forest management upstream, and alternative fuel for hill country peasants and food for hill country animals. None of this is likely to happen. The Netherlands has increased its population from 1.5 million in 1600 to 15 million today, and during those centuries there has been heavy and continuous investment in water-management in a country as low-lying as Bangladesh. The Netherlands is fortunate, too, that it is not liable to tropical rainfall. All its upstream neighbours, Germany, Switzerland, France, Luxemburg and Belgium, manage their forests properly, and do not contain large numbers of starving peasants who have to cut down trees to live. The moral is quite clear, implementation apparently impossible, solution beyond reason.[48]

Critically, there is the problem of what else is going to be discovered. Without becoming hysterical, can anyone properly quantify the effects of new potential problems? Some can be identified already. They have not yet reached the point at which the public is prepared to countenance their solution. These 'new' problems are also closely connected with old problems. The basic enigma is the combination of high population increase in the third world, plus the desire of all first world people for 'growth'. It is 'growth' which produces the greenhouse effect and acid rain and a depleted ozone layer. It is the relationship between personal consumption in the first world and the destruction of the rain forest which has to be adjusted. It is the ratio between 'development' and fossil fuel use in the first world which has to be reassessed.[49] It is the production of sludge and sewage in the first world which threatens the oceans. It is the nitrate use of the past 40 years which pollutes drinking water supplies.[50] It is the unthinking emission of all sorts of chemicals which threaten natural chemical cycles.[51]

In an ideal world, there would only be a sustainable agriculture. There would be 'growth' only supported by natural ecosystems. There would not be any waste extruded into the atmosphere unless the effects were known. A world-wide effort to replace dead and dying forests would become a major campaign. Urban waste would be recycled to benefit agriculture and reduce the amount of inorganic fertiliser manufactured and applied. New advances in biological engineering would produce grains and grasses, bred for today's conditions; and trees would be developed which could survive acidity. The monitoring of naturally developing mutations, such as the algae which suddenly appeared in the Baltic in 1988, should be considered a priority. Perhaps most important of all, the safety of nuclear power must be made so much more credible that the fossil fuel burn can be substantially reduced. Mankind does not live in an ideal world.

There are certain optimistic portents. The use of modern control systems makes possible elegant efforts of fuel efficiency in new industries. The breeding potential in genetic engineering leads to a belief in the possibility of a more sustainable agriculture. Energy efficiency can be significantly improved in cars, electrical appliances, process industry, sustainable agriculture. Opportunities exist to cycle more efficiently, less destructively, the six most important chemical elements: carbon, nitrogen, oxygen, hydrogen, phosphorus and sulphur – these six making up 95% of all living matter. Ultimately, the hope is that fusion replaces fission, and nuclear power becomes demonstrably safe and clean.[52]

What is much more difficult to establish is the attitude of mind necessary to produce a future less stark than appears likely. Profits, markets, freedom to speculate and fail are all necessary to commercial and industrial efficiency. For the third world, overburdened by excessive population, overcrowded medical and sanitary facilities, congested land, filthy cities, food derived from droughty, dusty fields, the problems of the first world appear to be a small price to pay for enough to eat, and a job, a house, some education for the future. The doctrinal problems of the Russian Soviet Empire are akin to those of sixteenth century Spain. Unlike Renaissance Spain, the Russian Empire is a prime pollutor of the environment. It is to be hoped for the sake of the world that these problems can be solved without decay or explosion.[53] The first world inhabitant prefers to see no connection between 'affluence' and the destruction of rain forests, which recycle carbon safely and surely.

Nor are first world consumers, greedy both for rising standards of 'life' and the immeasurable virtues of clean air, beautiful countryside, fresh water, and a decent environment, impressed by calls to reduce consumption. The future has to be with higher efficiencies, in generation and use of power, in recycling, in land use, in building sustainable agricultural systems, and in stabilizing chemical cycles. Technological management has to be used to increase efficiencies by more than any rise in population or in consumption patterns.[54] This has to continue for a very long time, at least until total world population levels off; after that point, all increases in consumption will have to come from increased efficiencies.

Policies advocated by the hair-shirt brigade will for many reasons fail. One is because the degree of guilt required for their implementation cannot be kept up long enough to provide sustained motivation. Nor will self-denial achieve acceptance amongst the influential. Nor is self-denial the best policy. There is so much room for improvement in almost every process in everyday life that no one need look further. Such a policy is essential to prevent the kind of breakdown which unbridled abuse of the environment will otherwise assuredly bring.[55]

During World War II, the political idea of One World was launched. Predictably, it failed. We now live on only one Earth, whose natural ecosystem is overstrained, beginning to revolt. 'One World' was a political idea, a kite of the 1940s which failed to fly. 'Only One Earth' has to be the paramount ecological idea of the present. Without it, there will be a future only to be destroyed by pollution.

It would be an absurd end for mankind if, having defeated the restraints of disease, having apparently solved the food supply problem, and having avoided nuclear war, the species should fall victim to pollution, to drown in its own ordure. Malthus, apparently defeated, would be laughing in his grave.

Postscript

The English edition was criticised for abjuring prophecy. Two years on, a forecast is more possible.

The spread of HIV and AIDS appears to be less dramatic than once appeared likely. This is not true of Africa, but there is no doubt that some sexual habits have changed in a way which cannot be measured, even by earnest sociologists. If anecdotal evidence is to be believed, AIDS has become (in some places) a needle disease, not a sexual one. On the other hand, no clear indication of a 'cure' is yet in sight.

There has been much greater success in five major problems associated with the future: demography, topsoil protection, reafforestation, energy wisdom, debtor forgiveness for the Third World. The Worldwatch Institute has estimated the total annual cost of additional expenditures necessary to solve these problems and thus achieve a sustainable, managed planet at less than $150 billion per year. This is a far lower figure than would have seemed possible a few years ago. It has to be seen against the world's military expenditures, which are reckoned to be over six times as much.

The politically miraculous autumn of 1989 has apparently freed the satellites of Eastern Europe. Economic problems and a cultural dearth of management leaves the most polluted area of the World a basket-case with much hard work ahead. Every more fortunate economy must now help Poland, Czechoslovakia, Hungary, Bulgaria and Romania. The West Germans are strong enough to look after their own and assume a key position in Slavic Europe by the end of the century. They and the Japanese will also benefit their own economies greatly.

There remain philosophic barriers. The first is the strong lobby, which uses 'ecology' to promote its own distaste for 'progress'. This lobby favours a return to the romantic: horses, steam, sail, and windmills. The opposite is the nihilist, short-term approach which says that in the long run we are all dead, so why not be selfish while we live? In between, there are many attitudes. Anxious always to promote the kind of conflict which makes for good TV, commentators promote the theory that 'growth' and future well-being of the planet are essentially incompatible. This is as nihilist as the views of the determinedly selfish.

One essential requirement must be that politicians and bureaucrats recognise what is true in the real world: that the environment and economics have become wholly inter-related. This resumes a shift from short-term to long-term management objectives — always difficult for elected governments, and most difficult for governments which seek popularity.

The problem is often also one of time. 'Experts' often have to be trusted in their opinions. But 'experts' can be found to support or oppose almost any product or process. In the ultimate stages of a democratic and public dispute the *status quo* may win, if only by exhaustion.

The pity is that the *status quo* is often unsustainable.

Notes

1 A simple progression – 64–41–26. Years, in each case, for population to double.

2 It is important to remember that medical improvements have to follow previous improvements in microscopes. Magnifications of about × 20 were possible in 1800, × 100 in 1900. No germs are visible with the naked eye; without microscopes, pathologists would be blind. At × 250, not only the flea, *Xenopsylla cheopsis*, which carries the Bubonic Plague, can be seen, but the flea's own parasite. Doubtless at × 2000 the parasite of the parasite of the flea can be seen. The electron microscope has increasingly superseded the optical instrument since about 1960.

3 Robert Koch (1843–1910) discovered the bacillus of TB in 1882, of cholera in 1883–4, and the phthisis bacillus in 1890. In 1891, he was Director of the new Berlin Institute for Infectious Diseases. In 1896 and 1906 he worked on rinderpest and other African cattle disease. Nobel Prize, 1905.

4 Quinine Chapter of *Seeds of Change*, by the author.

5 Barbitone was discovered by Nebelthau, and christened 'Veronal' by his friend von Mering, since the latter considered Verona to be the most restful city in the world.

6 Disciples of Jung have spent many lifetimes arguing about what drives the libido.

7 Sarah Gamp, a character in *Martin Chuzzlewit*, 1843–4, was unwashed, selfish, opinionated and in terms of the infectious whom she nursed, a killer; she was not deliberately evil, just ignorant and careless, knowing and suspecting nothing about microbes. For a time, her typically English umbrella became known as a 'Gamp'. She was apparently representative of the period before Florence Nightingale, despite Dickens' record as a propagandist in other matters.

8 What is 'the natural term' is a difficult question. It is obviously far beyond the ability to reproduce, which is the natural term of most other animals.

9 There are alternatives: witness the imaginative and productive use of the superior tactile sense of the blind in Japan; in some industries, the blind perform very high-tech tasks.

10 According to *Scientific American* in 1976, unused potential arable land was as follows in each of these areas: Europe, 12 per cent; Asia, 17 per cent; USSR, 36 per cent; North America, 49 per cent; Africa, 78 per cent; South America, 89 per cent; Oceania: 90 per cent. Shortage of suitable land is not, therefore, a problem in America, Africa or Australasia. Population changes since 1976 will have modified these figures, but not by very much.

11 The drift into the shanty towns in Africa is a function of rural underinvestment. Ironically, it may be less difficult to fund rural areas than towns.

12 Ethiopia, an area in a repeated war-famine-disease syndrome since 1979, has always had a surplus population problem. In 2000 BC, Ethiopian slaves were on offer in the markets of Egypt, some of them voluntarily. It is probable that slaves also reached what is now Iraq at the same sort of time.

13 Medieval rations for workers in Cairo were lower than 1,500 calories a day; at the time of the Christian slaves who built the Citadel, after Saladin's victories over the Crusaders, there was an especial ration for the 'Franks' who were large men, larger than most native Muslims. This was in 1187–90. Smaller rations are appropriate in warmer climates.

14 Disease has been very greatly reduced in East Africa. As a result, population since 1900 has increased by nearly five times, since 1950 by nearly three times.

Forests have been destroyed, erosion increased, agricultural potential reduced, and intertribal warfare and horrors beyond imagination have become commonplace outside Kenya, which, despite its near 4 per cent annual population increase, is relatively well-managed. Not so elsewhere, where deafforestation threatens more than East African livelihoods. In addition to massive tribal killings in both Uganda and Rwanda-Burundi, there has been serious deforestation, which has threatened to affect the Nile flow. In 1988, the region was made miserable not only by savage acts of mankind, but also by excessive rainfall in some places, serious drought in others.

Tanzania, of which country much was expected in 1960, has become a notorious socialist slum, not far behind Burma in human-induced misery. However, economic unsuccess has at least kept down the population increase; Tanzania increased its population by 94 per cent between 1950 and 1975; Kenya by 126 per cent; Uganda by 140 per cent; Rwanda-Burundi by 100 per cent. The misery induced by population increase is plain for all to see in East Africa; most of the increase is due to reduced disease, unmatched by agricultural husbandry.

15   The pill is relatively expensive and can cause thrombosis; the coil is dangerous; the rhythm method is often ineffective if desire overcomes arithmetic. A successful birth-control programme involves a degree of literacy and numeracy as well as effective medical infrastructure.

16   During the Nigerian Civil War, in the late 1960s, dried milk was sent as a relief measure for Biafran babies. Much to the surprise of the milk-providers, many Biafran babies died when given milk to drink. Milk, to be properly digested, requires an enzyme in the stomach, lactase. This enzyme is peculiar to the milk of each species. Most babies have the enzyme necessary to digest their own mother's milk, or the enzyme is present in the mother's milk. Most humans in the world, except Western Europeans and neo-Europeans, do not have the enzyme, or the ability to digest cow's milk, or sheep's milk, or horse's milk. In most of the world, domesticated animal's milk has to be turned into cheese or yoghurt to make it available to humans. Countries which have the highest level of lactase in human stomachs are those with a long tradition of raw milk drinking: Sweden, Switzerland, some states in the United States. None of this was discovered before 1970.

17   The number of Canadian farm horses impressed the young A. G. Street who spent a year or two in Canada before World War I. There were 2 million in Canada, as many as in the United Kingdom. What also impressed him was the practice, in the prairie provinces, of letting horses fend for themselves during the winter. They apparently returned to work in the spring, as fat as butter, despite sub-zero temperatures for more than 100 days.

18   With a similar level of input of machinery and hand labour, fertilizers, pest control, etc., maximum output *per acre* has often returned to the country of origin of many crops. But some countries have been able to increase levels of certain inputs. So New Zealand leads the world for maize production, Holland for potatoes, France for tobacco.

19   This direct import of the dung beetle was an example of lateral thinking of a high order. There were no major herb-eating species in Australia until the whites imported them in the late eighteenth century. By the time that the Bi-Centennial was within sight, the more productive pastures of Eastern Australia had 150 years of uncycled dung, impossible to manage without physical removal, or ploughing of the pasture. Ergo, introduce a dung-cycling insect. The best available was the African scarab, an almost holy creature, for the same reason, in Ancient Egypt.

20   Aborigines were killed in large numbers by the parasites carried by the First Fleet and by every succeeding immigrant-ship. *The History of Smallpox in Australia, 1788–1900*, Australian Quarantine Service, 1914. Some Aborigines thought that the British deliberately brought the disease with them, to kill the natives. The British, at the time, did not make the imaginative leap necessary to realize what they were doing.

21   Research at the Copenhagen Zoo in the 1950s, produced a good Landrace lookalike after twenty generations of selection from one pair of wild boar. The genetic bank in a pair of pigs is almost as rich as that in a pair of humans.

22   The European rat, unconsciously introduced by every ship landing in the New World or Australia, often threatened the very lives of the human immigrants with whom they had crossed the oceans. Rats grew in size, aggression and numbers in the neo-Europes, multiplying far faster than humans. In the early days of colonies in America and Australia, rats also multiplied faster than human food crops; it was the humans who suffered, not the rats.

23   Sir Edmund Hillary, born 1919. First man, with Sherpa Tenzing, to stand indubitably on the summit of Everest, 29 May 1953. First man to cross the South Pole overland, 1958–9. The 'Conquest of Everest' occurred just before the Coronation of Queen Elizabeth II, and for a time, encompassed the Coronation Year with rosy expectations of new Elizabethan glory, of adventure, exploration and success.

24   A 'unit' of nitrogen is 1 kg per hectare (1 lb per acre), and the problem with a grass-clover sward is that in cold springs, or drought, or in very wet summers, production may be so uneven as to be unmanageable. It is better potential management which makes the use of nitrogen much more attractive to the farmer. In New Zealand, on the other hand, clover is worth much more, probably 3–4 times what it is in Europe. This is by reason of climate. It is worth mentioning here, for the sake of those who protest at the use of N, because of its effects upon nitrate in drainage water, that there is no difference in the drains between organic and inorganic N. Clover nodules, broken down in the winter, produce as much nitrate as inorganic nitrogen from the chemical works. The latter, of course, has to be largely converted in the soil to organic N before it can do its work, in any case. See *Bulletin 48*, Commonwealth Agricultural Bureaux, Farnham, England, 1970.

25   Australia and New Zealand are in many respects geologically similar.

26   'Kiwi fruit' is the Chinese Gooseberry, not much thought of in China, grown wild, a creeper, never domesticated, 'discovered' by a British botanist in 1900, and named *Actinidia chinensis*. Naturalized in New Zealand, and first harvested in 1906, it became fashionable only with *nouvelle cuisine* in the 1960s. Planted in southern Europe, California, before 1970. To the delight of anyone who knows its history, it appears in wooden boxes in England, marked: 'Genuine Italian Kiwi Fruit'. Fruit rich in vitamin C, it keeps for several months in cold store, as do apples.

If anything threatens New Zealand's future, it is not the absence of enterprise on the part of its business community. But racial disharmony, fuelled by White guilt and Maori birth-rate, hazards a reinterpretation of the Treaty of Waitangi; this was drawn up by no lawyer, but a Captain R.N., and intended by both parties to be deliberately equivocal. Current troubles will require a degree of good luck to prevent them becoming rather serious. If this happens, most of the entrepreneurial talent of the country will emigrate. There are plenty of opportunities elsewhere. New Zealand will then decline while the rest of the Pacific rim prospers.

27   The importance of an independent judiciary has always been understood in terms of human rights. A similar and perhaps equal importance attaches to a fraud-free, fair, unbribable system of commercial justice. No successful economy has existed without such a benefice, at least over a period of time. In some Latin American countries, it has been impossible to enforce the law of contract without bribery for as many years as in certain Asian countries.

28 Brazil, with about 150 million people, is much the most populous Iberian country but it is hardly a neo-Europe, being largely in the tropics. Argentina, with more than 30 million, is undubitably 'the most populous Southern Hemisphere neo-Europe'.

29 Hong Kong, with a population of 10,000 when ceded to Britain in 1842, has now a population of over 5 million; nearly all the massive growth has been in this century. It is a one-off city which defies analysis.

30 Cash crops, by definition, have to yield better than subsistence crops in a free society. In some landholding systems, the occupier has been compelled to grow an unprofitable cash crop. Not so, in India, today.

31 The way that farmers exchange information over methodology is in contrast to their discretion about actual markets. There is as much pride in showing neighbours the production-process as there is discrete satisfaction about achieving a good price in the sale of produce.

32 There was apparently a time when steam-locomotives in Brazil were fuelled with unwanted coffee. The smell was said to be unforgettable.

33 Cigarettes, accumulated by non-smoking free-market dealers, were the basis of several quite respectable West German fortunes. After the currency reform of June 1948, the cigarette ceased to have monetary importance; the West German 'miracle' began.

34 By 1965, twenty years after World War II, there was probably not a crop of any significance anywhere in the world which could not be protected from its associated weeds.

35 DDT, dieldrin and aldrin, in many ways the most effective, have given way to less persistent insecticides. Insecticides, in any case, are more persistent than weedkillers, since, by definition, weedkillers have to metamorphose to do their work. In reverse of the intellectual chemistry of the late 1940s, any country with capacity to make pest control products could now turn to the making of chemical weapons. This is suspected in the case of Iraq. In the 1960s, both East Germany and Czechoslovakia made use of the same sort of capacity to make LSD to help Western youth destroy itself. This kind of potential is the worst side-effect of such a capability, now in the hands of perhaps 40–50 nation-states.

36 Gregor Mendel, 1822–84; Charles Darwin, 1809–82. As far as is known, they did not meet or correspond, though one of Darwin's later works came close to Mendelism: *The Effects of cross- and self-fertilisation in the Vegetable Kingdom* was published in 1876. No published work on Mendelism until W. Bateson, *Mendel's Principles of Heredity*, Cambridge, 1902, also Royal Society *Reports*, 1902–6.

37 Pigs known a generation ago are now forgotten: Large Black, Tamworth, Gloucester Old Spot. A human generation is, however, potentially 60 porcine pregnancies and births; in human terms, 1,500 years.

38 There are useful sheep crosses, half-breds, between Cheviot and the Border Leicester, which do not breed true, and have to be 'renewed' in each generation; hybridizing sheep is another matter altogether, and more recent.

39 Two scientists at Cambridge University, James Watson and Francis Crick, discovered that DNA was a double-helix, with two strands intertwined. Each strand had four different chemical bases, A, C, G, T. The bases might be arranged in any order, but links could only be made between successive pairs: A to T, G to C. In 1960–61, Crick and others postulated that DNA was mathematically organized so that 'codes' actually specified the selection and assembly of amino acids which make up DNA. By 1970, this was proved. The codes were found to be in groups of three, called 'codons'. A series of 'codons' formed the sequence of orders to make a protein; each series of codons was, in effect, a gene.

Genetic engineers, who have now come out of the closet and are often hypercommercial, can be found in all sorts of places, usually linked to universities. By AD 2000, many would claim that a good geneticist will be able to take a gene from almost any living tissue and insert it into almost any other living thing. There is the problem of rejection which, it is anticipated, will be overcome.

In terms of human food supplies, the most important factor is that, of the improvement in crop yields since World War II, about two-thirds is attributable to genetic improvements resulting from selective breeding. Since fertilizer usage and pest-control chemicals may have reached a limit, why not let genetics take the strain? It is entirely possible that geneticists could engineer a 1.5–2 per cent compound improvement in crop yields without chemical inputs increasing. That is the good news. The bad news is the possibility of deformed animals, horrors like a man with a pig's brain, or a pig with a tiger's motives, or a rat the size of an elephant. Fortunately, this kind of horror-breeding is more difficult than breeding new lettuces. See *The Double Helix*, Cambridge, 1968.

40 Soya is a crop which has had to wait for technology. It needs especial machinery for successful husbandry; harvesting is difficult; drying was an insurmountable problem on a field basis before this century; the seeds require sophisticated extraction techniques, or too much of the original oil (typically 20 per cent) is left in the meal or flour. Over 10,000 cultivars can be used in various latitudes, and the crop is grown from the Argentine to Ontario, and from Indonesia to Manchuria. Seed is not produced with any success in Europe or Africa. The protein is very digestible, even by infants. As a garden crop, soya was (and is) the raw material of both *soy sauce* and *tofu*; each was (and is) made with the aid of a different benign fungus. There is today a huge trade in beans, meal and oil, amounting to over 75 million tons in all; world production of the primary beans is about 90 million tons. The crop is also grown for forage, hay and silage; the beans remain the world's best hope for increased vegetable protein, and the crop as a whole is a soil improver and an excellent 'entry' for maize. Yet, in 1942, only one million tons of beans were harvested for the market.

41 Transferable technology does not include husbandry, which is an instinct, not an art, even, let alone a science.

42 But the Ethiopians have also reduced their forest area in this century from 50 per cent of the country to 8 per cent, with dire results. For all of the 90 years of this century, except 6, Ethiopia has been ruled by Ethiopians, so it is not easy to blame Imperialism. The real conflict is population increase.

43 Given goodwill, even transferable technique is not a problem. Provided the third world will accept the gifts, the first would be only too willing to give the poor nations transferable technology; so much cheaper than giving food, or tractors, or oil supplies, or whatever hardware is needed today.

44 There is no respectable demographer who can honestly produce a levelling-off at less than 10–12 billions, twice today's population, most of the increase in the third world.

45 In private, Friends of the Earth will admit that they campaign against nuclear energy because it is more emotive than the greenhouse effect.

46 To clean up acid emissions from Western economies should cost about one half per cent of GNP as a capital sum, spent once, and wisely. In some socialist countries, it would be cheaper to start again. See footnote 51.

47 The number of scientists at the Pole, monitoring the ozone layer, is limited.

48 Men of goodwill are gloomy about the long-term problems of the Third World. For example *Electrifying the Third World* is a possible, enormously beneficial, very practical aim, especially promoted by reasearch bodies such as the Worldwatch Institute. The total capital cost of such a project would not be impossible, between $1000 and $2000 per head. What are missing are the management skills necessary to provide electricity on a sustainable basis. The chief beneficiary of electrification in the rural Third World is the forest, no longer despoiled for fuel, and no longer burnt with known, dire results, the despoiled forest lands washed down into the sea. On the other hand, early Europeans arriving off the mouth of the Amazon nearly 500 years ago, reported the sea coloured brown miles from land. So erosion may have existed before the huge increase in populations.

49 Seventy-nine per cent of world forest area existing in 1900 has been destroyed.

50 Nitrate has only recently become a problem, 80 per cent of synthetically-made Nitrate having been applied since 1945.

51 Centrally-planned economies are the dirtiest as well as the least successful. In kg of sulphur emitted per $1000 of GNP, Japan is the lowest, at (1). Czechoslovakia at (40) is the highest. In between are Sweden (4), France and West Germany (5) and the UK and the US at (7), Eastern European Socialist countries at (20) to (40).

52 This aim is inhibitied by an alliance between Big Coal and the Anti-Nukes.

53 Much more difficult than political *glasnost* or economic *perestroika* is the parallel clean-up of the environment, plus (doubled?) production.

54 'Efficiency' must be seen in the round. Ninety-five per cent *plus* of all fuel burnt in history has been wasted, less than 5 per cent producing heat, light, power. Yet without use and *waste* of fuel, mankind would still be hunting and gathering.

55 Opportunities for good management should make redundant the hair-shirt answer. *Sustainable* forest-management, or agriculture, or waste-management yields spectacular economic advantages as well as answers environmental imperatives. Unfortunately, the advantages are long-term, and democratic electorates and consumers often reflect the sour words of John Maynard Keynes in another context: 'In the long run we are all dead.'

Bibliography

Many of the books cited here are in the author's possession, therefore the edition or the place of latest printing may not be that of the books as identified.

Acland, J. D., *East African Crops*, London, 1971

Albion, R. G., *Forests and Sea Power*, Cambridge, Mass., 1926

Alngren, B., *The Vikings*, London, 1968

Altschul, Siri von Reis, 'Exploring the Herbarium', *Scientific American*, May 1977

Alvord, C. W., *The Mississippi Valley in British Politics*, Cleveland, 1917

Anderson, A., *An Historical and Chronological Deduction of the Origin of Commerce*, rev. edn 4 vols, London, 1787–9

Anderson, Edgar, *Plants, Man and Life*, London, 1954

Anderson, R. C., *The Rigging of Ships in the Days of the Spritsail topmast, 1600–1720*, Salen, 1927

Anderson, S., *The Sailing Ship*, New York, 1947

Andrews, C. M., *The Colonial Period of American History*, 4 vols, New Haven, 1938

Anstey, Roger, *The Atlantic Slave Trade and British Abolition 1760–1810*, London, 1975

Arnold, Edward, *Rural Economy and Country life in the Medieval West*, London, 1965

Arnold, Sir Thomas, and Guillaume, Alfred, *The Legacy of Islam*, London, 1931

Atkinson, William C., *A History of Spain and Portugal*, London, 1960

Babcock, W. H., 'Legendary Islands of the Atlantic: A Study in Medieval Geography', in *American Geographical Research*, New York, 1922

Baker, J. N. L., *A History of Geographical Discovery and Exploration*, London, 1931

Barbour, Violet, *Capitalism in Amsterdam in the 17th Century*, Ann Arbor, 1963

Barrett, W., *The History and Antiquities of the City of Bristol*, Bristol, 1789

Bastin, J., *The British in West Sumatra 1685–1825*, Kuala Lumpur, 1965

Bearce, G. D., *British Attitudes towards India 1784–1858*, Oxford, 1961

Beazley, C. R., 'Prince Henry of Portugal and the African Crusade of the Fifteenth Century', in *American Historical Review*, New York, 1910

Berlin, Isaiah, *Four Essays on Liberty*, London, 1969

Berlin, Isaiah, *Historical Inevitability*, London, 1953

Biddulph, J., *The Pirates of Malabar*, London, 1907

Birmingham, D., 'The Regiment of Mina', in *Transactions of the Historical Society of Ghana*, Lagos, 1971

Blegen, T. C., *The Kensington Rune Stone: New Light on an Old Riddle*, Minnesota Historical Society, 1968

Bloch, Marc, *Feudal Society*, London, 1961

Boswell, James, ed. Augustine Birrell, *The Life of Samuel Johnson*, 6 vols, London, 1904

Bougainville, L. A. de, *Voyage Autour du Monde*, Paris, 1771

Bourguignon d'Anville, J. B., *Nouvel Atlas de la Chine*, Amsterdam, 1737

Boxer, C. R., *The Dutch Seaborne Empire*, London, 1965

Bradford, E., *Christopher Columbus*, New York, 1973

Braudel, F., *The Mediterranean and the Mediterranean World in the Age of Philip II*, 2 vols, London, 1972–3

Brebner, J. B., *The Explorers of North America*, London, 1933

Broglie, Duc de, *The King's Secret: Being the Secret Correspondence of Louis XV with his Diplomatic Agents*, 2 vols, London, 1879

Broughan, Henry Peter, *An Inquiry into the Colonial Policy of the European Powers*, Edinburgh, 1803; New York, 1969

Bruce, J., *Annals of the East India Company*, London, 1810

Burke, Edmund, *Works*, 12 vols, London, 1808–13

Butzer, Karl W., *Early Hydraulic Civilisation in Egypt*, Chicago, 1976

Cambridge Economic History

Cambridge History of England

Campbell, John, *The Spanish Empire in America, by an English Merchant*, London, 1747

Campbell, W., *Formosa under the Dutch*, London, 1903; New York, 1970

Caraci, G., 'La Vinland Map' in *Studi Medievali*, Spoleto, 1966

Carus Wilson, E. M., *The Merchant Adventurers of Bristol in the 15th Century*, Bristol, 1962

Carus Wilson, E. M., *Medieval Merchant Venturers*, London, 1954

Chambers, J. D., and Murgay, G. E., *The Agricultural Revolution*, London, 1966

Champion, Richard, *Considerations on the Present Situation of Great Britain and the United States*, London, 1784

Chang, Kwang-Chih, *The Archaeology of Ancient China*, New Haven, 1978

Childe, V. Gordon, *The Dawn of European Civilisation*, 6th edn, revised, London, 1973

Chittenden, F. J., *The Royal Horticultural Society Dictionary of Gardening*, 4 vols, Oxford, 1956

Cipolla, Carlo M., *Before the Industrial Revolution*, New York, 1976

Cipolla, Carlo M., *The Economic History of World Population*, London, 1976

Cipolla, Carlo M., *Public Health in the Medical Profession in the Renaissance*, Cambridge, 1976

Clapham, Sir John, *The Economic Development of France and Germany 1815–1914*, 4th edn, Cambridge, 1966

Clark, Colin, *Population Growth and Land Use*, London, 1967

Cohn, Norman, *The Pursuit of the Millennium*, Oxford, 1957

Cook, James, ed. J. C. Beaglehole, *Journals*, 3 vols, Cambridge, 1966

Cooke, Alistair, *America*, New York, 1973

Crane, Eva, *The Archaeology of Beekeeping*, London, 1983

Crosby, Alfred, *The Columbian Exchange*, Westport, 1972

Curtin, Philip D., *The Atlantic Slave Trade*, Madison, 1969

Dalrymple, A., *An Historical Collection of the Several Voyages and Discoveries in the South Pacific Ocean*, 2 vols, London, 1770–1; New York, 1967

Dampier, William, *A New Voyage Round the World*, 3 vols, London, 1697; New York, 1968

Dantzig, B., and Pridds, A. V., *A Short History of the Ports and Castles of Ghana*, 1971

Darlington, C. D. and Wylie, A. P., *Chromosome Atlas of Flowering Plants*, 2nd ed., London, 1955

Davis, David Brion, *The Problem of Slavery in Western Culture*, Ithaca, 1966

Davis, Ralph, *The Rise of the English Shipping Industry in the Seventeenth and Eighteenth Centuries*, London, 1962; New York, 1963

Deane, Phyllis, and Cole, W. A., *British Economic Growth 1688–1959*, Cambridge, 1967

Deerr, N., *The History of Sugar*, Oxford, 1950

Defoe, Daniel, *Two Great Questions Considered*, London, 1700

Dickey, I. M., *Christopher Columbus and his Monument Columbia, being a Concordance of Choice Tributes to the Great Genoese*, Chicago–New York, 1891

Dodge, Ernest S., *New England and the South Seas*, Cambridge, Mass., 1965

Dols, Michael, *The Black Death in the Middle East*, Princeton, 1977

Dow, A., *The History of Hindostan*, 3 vols, London, 1768–72

Drummond, J. C., *The Englishman's Food*, London, 1957

Duby, Georges, *The Age of the Cathedrals: Art and Society, 980–1420*, Chicago, 1980

Dufferin, Lord, *Letters from High Latitudes*, London, 1857

Dunn, William Edward, *Spanish and French Rivalry in the Gulf Region of the United States, 1678–1702*, Austin, Texas, 1917

Edwards, Bryan, *History of the West Indies*, 3 vols, London, 1794

Encyclopaedia Britannica (editions since the 3rd of 1797–1801), London

Enterline, J. R., *Viking America*, New York, 1972

Ephson, J. S., *Ancient Forts and Castles of the Gold Coast*, Accra, 1970

Ernle, Lord (Rowland Prothero), *English Farming, Past and Present*, 4th edn, London, 1927

Fanfani, A., *The Vinland Map and the New Controversy Over the Discovery of America*, New York, 1965

Fernandez Armesto, F., *Columbus and the Conquest of the Impossible*, London, 1974

Ferwerda, F. P., and Wit, F., eds, *Outlines of Perennial Crop Breeding in the Tropics*, Wageningen, 1969

Fisher, H. A. L., *A History of Europe*, London, 1936

Fontana Economic History of Europe, ed. Carlo M. Cipolla, London, 1978

Fortescue, J. W., *History of the British Army*, 13 vols, London, 1899–1930; New York, 1970

Frankel, O. H., and Hawkes, J. G., eds., *Crop Genetic Resources for Today and Tomorrow*, Cambridge, 1975

Franklin, Benjamin, ed. A. N. Smyth, *Writings*, 10 vols, New York, 1907

Free, J. B., *Insect Pollination of Crops*, London, 1970

Freyre, Gilberto, *The Masters and the Slaves*, New York, 1970

Freyre, Gilberto, *The Portuguese and the Tropics*, Lisbon, 1961

Furnivall, J. S., *An Introduction to the History of Netherlands India*, London, 1934

Furnivall, J. S., *Netherlands India, A Study of Plural Economy*, Cambridge, 1944

Galbraith, V. H., *Domesday Book – Its Place in Administrative History*, Oxford, 1974

Gibbon, Edward, *The History of the Decline and Fall of the Roman Empire*, London, 1969

Gierset, K., *History of Iceland*, New York, 1924

Gillespie, Leonard, *Observations on the Diseases which Prevailed on Board a part of His*

Majesty's Squadron on the Leeward Island Station between November 1794 and April 1796, London, 1800

Gipson, L. H., *The British Empire before the American Revolution*, vol. X, *The Triumphant Empire; Thunder-clouds Gather in the West, 1763–1768*, New York, 1961

Gipson, L. H., Vol. VII, *The Great War for the Empire; The Victorious Years, 1758–1780*, New York, 1949

Gipson, L. H., *The Coming of the Revolution, 1763–1775*, New York, 1954

Glamann, K., *Dutch Asiatic Trade 1620–1740*, Copenhagen, 1958

Glass, D. V., and Eversley, D. E. C., (eds.), *Population in History: Essays in Historical Demography*, London, 1965

Goodrich, A., *A History of the Character and Achievements of the so-called Christopher Columbus*, New York, 1874

Gottfried, Robert S., *The Black Death, Natural and Human Disaster in Medieval Europe*, London, 1983

Grant, Charles, *Observations on the State of Society among the Asiatic Subjects of Great Britain . . .* , London, 1797

Gray, L. C., *The History of Agriculture in the Southern States to 1860*, Washington, DC, 1933

Greenberg, M., *British Trade and the Opening of China*, Cambridge, 1951

Greene, L., *The Negro in Colonial New England 1620–1776*, New York, 1942

Hakluyt, R., *The English Voyages 1494–1600*, ed. London, 1964

Hall, D. G. E., *History of South-East Asia*, London, 1964

Hamilton, E. J., *American Treasure and Price Revolution in Spain*, Cambridge, Mass., 1934

Hamilton, E. J., *Money, Prices and Wages in Valencia, Aragon and Navarra 1351–1500*, Cambridge, Mass., 1936

Hardiman, J., *History of Galway*, Galway, 1926

Harlan, J. R., de Wet, J. M. J. and Stemler, A. B. L., eds., *Origins of African Plant Domestication*, The Hague, 1976

Harler, *The Culture and Marketing of Tea*, Oxford, 1955

Harlow, V. T., *The Founding of the Second British Empire*, 2 vols, London and New York, 1952 and 1964

Harper, L. A., *The English Navigation Laws*, New York, 1939

Harrison, Gordon, *Mosquitoes, Malaria and War: A History of the Hostilities since 1880*, New York, 1976

Harrisse, H., *The Discovery of North America*, Paris–London, 1882

Hartley, Dorothy, *Made in England*, London, 1987

Hartley, W., *A Checklist of Economic Plants in Australia*, Canberra, 1979

Harvard Bibliography of American History

Haskins, C. H., *The Normans in European History*, Boston–New York, 1915

Hawkesworth, J., *Voyages in the Southern Hemisphere*, 3 vols, London, 1773

Herklots, G. A. C., *Vegetables in South-East Asia*, Hong Kong, 1972

Hermannsson, H., *The Northmen in America*, New York, 1909

Hilton, R. H., *The Decline of Serfdom in Medieval England*, London, 1969

Historical Statistics of the US, Washington, DC, 1960

Hobsbawm, E. J., *Industry and Empire*, London and New York, 1968

Holand, H. R., *Explorations in America Before Columbus*, New York, 1956

Hollingsworth, T. H., *Historical Demography*, London, 1969

Holroyd, John Baker, 1st Earl of Sheffield, *Observations on the Commerce of the American States*, London, 1783

Hourani, G. F., *Arab Seafaring in the Indian Ocean in Ancient and Early Medieval Times*, Princeton, 1951

Howard, E., *Genoa, History and Art in an Old Seaport*, Genoa, 1971

Howard, Michael, 'Power at Sea', *Adelphi Papers*, no. 124, London, 1976

Howard, Michael, *War in European History*, Oxford, 1975

Huffnagel, H. P., *Agriculture in Ethiopia*, Rome, 1961

Huntington, Ellsworth, *Civilisation and Climate*, New Haven, 1924

Hutchinson, Sir Joseph, ed., *Evolutionary Studies in World Crops*, Cambridge, 1974

Irvine, F. R., *West African Agriculture*, vol. 2; *West African Crops*, 3rd ed., London, 1969

Irving, W., *A History of the Life and Voyages of Christopher Columbus*, London, 1828

Jackson, Melvin H., *Salt, Sugar and Slaves: The Dutch in the Caribbean*, James Ford Bell Lectures, no. 2, 1965

Jacob, A. and Von Uexkull, H., *Fertiliser Use: Nutrition and Manuring of Tropical Crops*, 3rd ed., Hanover, 1963

Jenks, Leland, *Our Cuban Colony: A Study in Sugar*, New York, 1928

Johnson, W., *Genoa the Superb: the City of Columbus*, London, 1892

Jones, G., *A History of the Vikings*, New York, 1968

Keary, C. F., *The Vikings in Western Christendom*, London, 1891

Kershaw, Ian, 'The Great Famine and Agrarian Crisis in England', in *Peasants, Knights and Heretics*, ed. R. H. Milton, Cambridge, 1976

Klerck, E. S. de, *History of the Netherlands East Indies*, 2 vols, Rotterdam, 1938

Knott, J. E. and Deanon, J. R., *Vegetable Production in South-East Asia*, Laguna, 1967

Labaree, L. W., *Royal Government in America: A Study of the British Colonial System before 1783*, New Haven, 1930

Lacour-Gayet, Robert, *A Concise History of Australia*, London, 1976

Lambert, S. M., *The Depopulation of the Pacific Races*, Honolulu, 1934

Las Casas Bartolomé, *Historia de las Indias*, Madrid, 1875

Lawrence, A. W., *Fortified Trade-posts*, London, 1969

Leakey, C. L. A. and Wills, J. B., eds., *Food Crops of the Lowland Tropics*, Oxford, 1977

Lee, J., *Colonial Government and Good Government: A Study of the Ideas Expressed by the British Official Classes in Planning Decolonisation, 1939–1964*, Oxford, 1967

Ligon, R., *A True and Exact History of the Island of Barbados*, London, 1657; New York, 1970

Lloyd, C., and Coulter, J. S. L., *Medicine and the Navy*, 4 vols, London, 1961

Lynch, John, *The Spanish American Revolutions*, London, 1973

Lynch, J., *Spanish Colonial Administration: the Intendant System in the Rio de la Plata*, London, 1958

MacNutt, W. S., *The Atlantic Provinces: The Emergence of Colonial Society*, Oxford, 1965

McEvedy, Colin and Jones, Richard, *Atlas of World Population History*, London, 1985

Madariaga, S. de, *Christopher Columbus*, London–New York, 1940

Maheshwari, P. and Singh, U., *Dictionary of Economic Plants in India*, New Delhi, 1965

Major, H. R., *The Life of Prince Henry of Portugal, Surnamed the Navigator, and its Results*, London, 1868

Markham, C. R., *Life of Columbus*, London, 1892

Marwick, Arthur, *Britain in the Century of Total War*, London, 1968

Masefield, John, ed., *Dampier's Voyages*, London, 1906

Massal, R., and Barrau, J., *Food Plants of the South Sea Islands, New Caledonia*; South Pacific Commission, 1956

Matheson, J. K., and Bovill, E. W., *East African Agriculture*, London, 1950

Medawar, P. B., *The Hope of Progress*, London, 1974

Merrill, E. D., *Plant Life in the Pacific World*, New York, 1945

Milburn, W., *Oriental Commerce: containing a geographical description of the principal places in the East Indies . . . with their Produce, Manufactures and Trade . . .* , 2 vols, London, 1813

Mitchell, B. R., *European Historical Statistics 1750–1970*, London, 1975

Mitchell, B. R., with Deane, Phyllis, *Abstract of British Historical Statistics*, Cambridge, 1962

Mitchell, B. R., *International Historical Statistics: Asia and Africa*, Cambridge, 1982

Morison, Samuel Eliot, *Christopher Columbus, Mariner*, London, 1956; Boston, 1955

Morison, Samuel Eliot, *The European Discovery of America: The Northern Voyages*, New York, 1971

Morison, Samuel Eliot, *Admiral of the Ocean Sea: A Life of Christopher Columbus*, Boston, 1949

Morse, H. B., *The Chronicles of the East India Company Trading in China, 1635–1834*, Oxford, 1926; New York, 1965

Musmano, M. A., *Columbus Was First*, New York, 1968

Namier, Sir Lewis, *Crossroads of Power*, London, 1962

Nicolson, Harold, *The Congress of Vienna*, London, 1946

Norwood, Richard, *The Seaman's Practice, containing a fundamental Problem in Navigation, experimentally verified, viz: touching the Compass of the Earth and Sea, and the Quantity of a Degree in our English Measure, also to keep a reckoning at Sea for all Sailing, etc. etc.*, London, 1637

Nunn, G. E., *The Geographical Conceptions of Columbus*, New York, 1834

Ochee, J. J., Soule, M. J., Dijkman, M. J. and Wehlburg, C., *Tropical and Subtropical Agriculture*, New York, 1961

Oleson, T. J., *Early Voyages and Northern Approaches*, Toronto, 1964

Oman, Sir C., *A History of the Art of War in the Middle Ages*, London, 1924

Origo, Iris, *The Merchant of Prato*, London, 1957

Orwin, C. S., *The Open Fields*, Oxford, 1967

Oxford History of Technology

Parry, J. H., *The Age of Reconnaissance*, London, 1963

Parry, J. H., *The Discovery of South America*, New York, 1979

Parry, J. H., *The Spanish Seaborne Empire*, London, 1966

Parry, J. H., *Trade and Dominion*, London, 1971

Parry, J. H., *Spices: Their Morphology, Histology and Chemistry*, New York, 1962

Pendle, George, *A History of Latin America*, London, 1983

Philips, C. H., *The East India Company 1784–1834*, Manchester, 1940

Plato, *The Republic*

Plumb, J. H., *Man versus Society in Eighteenth Century England*, London, 1969

Pohl, F. J., *Atlantic Crossing Before Columbus*, New York, 1979

Pole, J. R., *Political Representation in England and the Origins of the American Republic*, London, 1966

Postlethwayt, Malachy, *The Universal Dictionary of Trade*, London, 1751

Price, A. Grenfell, *The Western Invasion of the Pacific and Its Continents*, Oxford, 1963

Purseglove, J. W., Brown, E. G., Green, C. L., and Robbins, S. R. J., *Spices*, 2 vols, London, 1981

Purseglove, J. W., *Tropical Crops: Dicotyledons*, London, 1968

Purseglove, J. W., *Tropical Crops: Monocotyledons*, London, 1972

Read, Herbert, *Anarchy and Order: Essays in Politics*, London, 1954

Rostow, Walt, ed., *The Economics of 'Take Off' into Self-sustained Growth*, Washington, DC, 1963

Rousseau, Jean-Jaques, *A Discourse on the Origin of Inequality*, London, 1952

Russell, E. John, *The World of the Soil*, London, 1961

Sadler, D. H., intro., *Man Is Not Lost: A Record of 200 Years of Astronomical Navigation with the Nautical Almanac, 1767–1967*, London, 1968

Salaman, R., *The History and Social Influence of the Potato*, Cambridge, 1949

Sauer, C. O., *Agricultural Origins and Dispersals*, New York, 1952

Sauvy, Alfred, *General Theory of Population*, London, 1969

Sawyer, P. A., *The Age of Vikings*, London, 1962

Schery, R. W., *Plants and Man*, 2nd ed., Englewood Cliffs, 1972

Scientific American: Food and Agriculture, entire issue of September, 1976

Sherborne, J. W., *The Port of Bristol in the Middle Ages*, London, 1965

Shetelig, H., *The Vikings' Ships*, Oslo, 1951

Simpson, J., *Everyday Life in the Viking Age*, New York, 1967

Sinclair, Keith, *A History of New Zealand*, London, 1969

Smith, Adam, ed. E. Cannan, *Wealth of Nations*, London, 1904

Steel, David, *Elements and Practice of Rigging and Seamanship*, 2 vols, London, 1794

Steel, David, *Elements and Practice of Naval Architecture*, 2 vols, London, 1805

Stefansson, V., *Ultima Tule*, London–New York, 1940

Tacitus, *Histories*, trans. Kenneth Wellesley, London, 1964

Tawney, R. H., *Religion and the Rise of Capitalism*, London, 1969

Tench-Cox, *A View of the United States of America*, Philadelphia, 1794

Thacher, J. B., *Christopher Columbus, his Life, his Work, his Remains*, New York, 1903

Thomas, Hugh, *An Unfinished History of the World*, London, 1979

Thomas, Keith, *Man and the Natural World*, New York, 1983

Thompson, E. A., *The Early Germans*, Oxford, 1965

Thompson, E. P., *The Making of the English Working Class*, London, 1965

Thordarson, M., *The Vinland Voyages*, New York, 1930

Thorndike, L., *A History of Magic and Experimental Science*, New York, 1934

Thrupp, Sylvia L., *The Merchant Class of Medieval London*, Chicago, 1948

Tornoe, J. K., *Norsemen Before Columbus*, London, 1695

Trevelyan, G. M., *English Social History*, London, 1942

Tucker, Josiah, *The Case of Going to War for the Sake of Procuring, Enlarging or Securing of Trade*, London, 1763

Tucker, Josiah, *The True Interest of Britain, set forth in regard to the Colonies: and the only means of living in peace and harmony with them*, London, 1774

United Nations, Department of Economics and Social Affairs, Statistical Office, *Demographic Yearbook*, London, annually since 1949

Verger, Pierre, *Flux et Reflux de la Traite des Nègres entre le Golfe de Benin et Bahia de Todos os Santos*, Paris, 1968

Villiers, Alan, *Captain Cook, the Seaman's Seaman*, London, 1967; New York, 1970

Wadia, R. A., *The Bombay Dockyard and the Wadia Master-Builders*, Bombay, 1957

Walpole, Horace, *Memoirs of the Reign of King George the Third*, London, 1845

Walter, R., *A Voyage Round the World*, London, 1748

Washington, George, ed. John C. Fitzpatrick, *Writings*, 39 vols, Washington, DC, 1931–44

Weber, Max, *The Protestant Ethic and the Spirit of Capitalism*, London, 1930

Weckman, L., 'The Alexandrine Bulls of 1493: Pseudo-Asiatic Documents', in F. Chiappelli, *First Images of America*, Los Angeles, 1976

Westropp, T. J., 'Brazil and the Legendary Islands of the Atlantic', in *Proceedings of the Royal Irish Academy*, Dublin, 1912

White, Lynn, Jr., *Medieval Technology and Social Change*, Oxford, 1962

Williams, E. T., *A Short History of China*, New York, 1928

Williams, Glyndwr, *The British Search for the Northwest Passage in the Eighteenth Century*, London, 1962; New York, 1967

Woot-Tsuen, W. L., and Flores, M., 'Food Composition Table for Use in Latin America,' Bethseda: INCAP-INNND, 1961

World Bank (International Bank for Reconstruction and Development), *World Bank Atlas*, annually since 1966, London

Worldwatch Institute, *State of the World, 1984, 1985, 1986, 1987*, New York, London

Index